AF443491

Paediatric Cholestasis
Novel Approaches to Treatment

FALK SYMPOSIUM 63

Paediatric Cholestasis

Novel Approaches to Treatment

EDITED BY

M. Lentze
Zentrum für Kinderheilkunde
Kinderklinik und Poliklinik der
Universität Bonn
W-5300 Bonn
Germany

J. Reichen
Institüt Klinische Pharmakologie
Inselspital
CH-3010 Bern
Switzerland

*Proceedings of the 63rd Falk Symposium held in Titisee/Black Forest, Germany,
October 9–10, 1991*

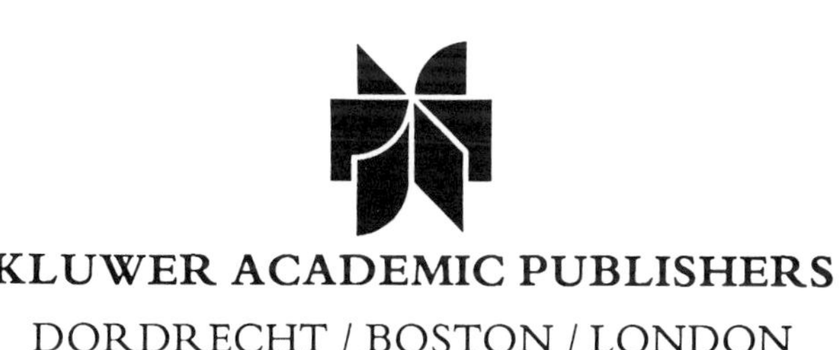

KLUWER ACADEMIC PUBLISHERS

DORDRECHT / BOSTON / LONDON

Distributors

for the United States and Canada: Kluwer Academic Publishers, PO Box 358, Accord Station, Hingham, MA 02018-0358, USA

for all other countries: Kluwer Academic Publishers Group, Distribution Center, PO Box 322, 3300 AH Dordrecht, The Netherlands

British Library Cataloguing in Publication Data

A catalogue record for this book is available from the British Library.

ISBN 0-7923-8977-8

Library of Congress Cataloging-in-Publication Data

Falk Symposium (63rd : 1992 : Titisee, Germany)
    Paediatric cholestasis : novel approaches to treatment : proceedings of the 63rd Falk
Symposium held in Titisee/Black Forest, Germany, October 9–10, 1991 / Falk Symposium
63 ; edited by M. Lentze, J. Reichen.
       p.   cm.
    Includes bibliographical references and index.
    ISBN 0-7923-8977-8 (cloth)
    1. Cholestasis in children—Congresses. I. Lentze, Michael J. II. Reichen, J. (Jurg)
III. Title.
    [DNLM: 1. Cholestasis—in infancy & childhood—congresses. 2. Cholestasis—physio-
pathology—congresses. 3. Cholestasis—therapy—congresses.   WI 703 F191p 1992]
    RJ456.C52F35 1992
    618.92′365—dc20
    DNLM/DLC
    for Library of Congress   92-15070
                                                     CIP

Contents

CONTENTS

SECTION 6: TREATMENT OF CHOLESTATIC DISORDERS 2: URSODEOXYCHOLATE

Preface

This book comprises the lectures and some of the posters presented at the 63rd Falk Symposium; this symposium, entitled 'Paediatric cholestasis: novel approaches to treatment', brought basic scientists interested in the physiology, ontogenesis and pathophysiology of bile formation, together with leading paediatricians taking care of uniquely large patient collectives of mundane and rare cholestatic diseases.

The organization of this symposium was stimulated by many exciting developments in basic and clinical sciences, many of them are already benefiting our small patients in a manner unanticipated a few years ago. Thus, for a long time paediatric cholestasis was of interest mainly to the pathologist, radiologist and surgeon who had to separate 'medical' from 'surgical' cholestasis; the 'medical forms' were ill-understood and only symptomatic treatment was available at best. This state of affairs has dramatically changed, thanks to our better understanding of the physiological basis of bile formation and its derangements leading to cholestasis. This has also permitted the design of rational forms of treatment, some of which are already incorporated into clinical practice, some of which are the subject of intensive clinical invstigations and others still are brilliant ideas which may or may not see the day as valuable novel treatments.

We hope that this volume can convey some of the excitement in the field. The contributions in the present volume contain many novel observations, reviews on accepted facts but also thoughtful and sometimes courageous speculations. Many new contacts were forged at this meeting; it will be interesting to see what will emerge from them in a few years time.

The editors wish to express their thanks to the contributors of this volume, to Dr Herbert Falk for his generous support and perfect organization, to all the workers behind the scenes of the Falk Foundation, to Ms Brigitta Oeschger for her help in the local organization and, last but not least, to Mr Phil Johnstone from Kluwer Academic Publishers for his help in editing this volume.

JÜRG REICHEN MD

List of Principal Contributors

W. F. BALISTRERI
Department of Pediatric
   Gastroenterology and Nutrition
Children's Hospital Medical Center
Elland and Bethesda Avenue
Cincinnati
OH 45229-2899
USA

M. BURDELSKI
Abteilung II im Zentrum für
   Kinderheilkunde
Medizinische Hochschule Hannover
Konstanty-Gutschow-Str. 8
W-3000 Hannover
GERMANY

J. C. COLLINS
Liver Research Center
Ullmann Building Room 517
Albert Einstein College of Medicine
1300 Morris Park Ave
New York, NY 10461
USA

J. COTTING
Service de Pédiatrie
CHUV
CH-1010 Lausanne
SWITZERLAND

J. B. DAS
Pediatric Surgical Research
   Children's Memorial Hospital
2300 Children's Plaza
Chicago, IL 60614
USA

V. J. DESMET
Universitair Ziekenhuisen Leuven
Sint Rafael
Patholog. Ontleedkunde B
Minderbroedersstraat 12
B-3000 Leuven
BELGIUM

S. ERLINGER
Service d'Hepatologie, INSERM U-24
Hopital Beaujon
100, Blvd. du Général Leclerc
F-92118 Clichy Cedex
FRANCE

W. GEROK
Medizinische Universitätsklinik
Hugstetter Str. 55
W-7800,Freiburg
GERMANY

A. F. HOFMANN
Department of Medicine, 0813
University of California San Diego
La Jolla
CA 92093-0813
USA

E. R. HOWARD
King's College Hospital
Denmark Hill
London
SE5 9RS
UK

E. JACQUEMIN
Division of Clinical Pharmacology
Department of Medicine
University Hospital
CH-8091 Zurich
SWITZERLAND

M. J. LENTZE
Zentrum für Kinderheilkunde
Kinderklinik und Poliklinik der
   Universität Bonn
Adenauerallee 119
W-5300 Bonn
GERMANY

A. P. MOWAT
Department of Paediatric Nephrology
King's College School of Medicine
   and Dentistry
University of London
Denmark Hill
London SE5 9RS
UK

J. M. NEUBERGER
The Liver Unit
Queen Elizabeth Hospital
Queen Elizabeth Medical Centre
Edgbaston
Birmingham B15 2TH
UK

M. ODIÈVRE
Service de Pédiatrie
Hopital Antoine Beclère
157 rue de la Porte de Trivaux
92141 Clamart Cedex
FRANCE

G. PAUMGARTNER
Medizinische Klinik II
Klinikum Grosshadern der Universität
   München
Marchioninistr. 15
W-8000 München
GERMANY

J. PAWLOWSKA
Department of Gastroenterology
Child Health Center
Al.Dzieci Polskich 20
04-736 Warszawa
POLAND

R. POUPON
Service d'Hépatologie et INSERM U21
Hopital Saint-Antoine
184 rue du Fbg Saint-Antoine
F-75012 Paris Cedex 12
FRANCE

J. REICHEN
Institut für Klinische Pharmakologie
Inselspital
Murtenstr. 35
CH-3010 Bern
SWITZERLAND

J. RUJNER
Department of Gastroenterology
Child Health Center
Al.Dzieci Polskich 20
04-736 Warszawa
POLAND

J. SCHÖLMERICH
Medizinische Universitätsklinik
Hugstetter Str. 55
W-7800 Freiburg
GERMANY

K. D. R. SETCHELL
Divisions of Clinical Mass
   Spectrometry and Gastroenterology
Department of Pediatrics
Children's Hospital Medical Center
Elland and Bethesda Avenue
Cincinnati
OH 45229-2899
USA

R. J. SOKOL
Section of Pediatric Gastroenterology
   and Nutrition
University of Colorado School of
   Medicine and the Children's
   Hospital
Box B 290
The Children's Hospital
1056 E. 19th Avenue
Denver
CO 80218
USA

R.-D. STENGER
Hospital for Paediatric and Juvenile
   Medicine
Ernst Moritz Arndt University
Soldtmannstrasse 15
O-2200 Greifswald
GERMANY

A. STIEHL
Medizinische Klinik der Universität
Bergheimer Str. 58
W-6900 Heidelberg
GERMANY

B. STRANDVIK
Department of Pediatrics II
University of Göteborg
S-41685 Göteborg
SWEDEN

F. J. SUCHY
Department of Pediatrics
Children's Hospital Medical Center
Elland and Bethesda Avenue
Cincinnati
OH 45229
USA

LIST OF PRINCIPAL CONTRIBUTORS

H. TSCHÄPPELER
Radiologie
Kinderklinik
Inselspital
CH-3010 Bern
SWITZERLAND

V. USONIS
Vilnius University Clinic of Children's
  Infectious Diseases
PO Box 2561
2015 Vilnius
LITHUANIA

J. de VILLE de GOYET
Université Catholique de Louvain
Cliniques Universitaires Saint-Luc
Département de Chirurgie Pédiatrique
Ave Hippocrate 10
B-1200 Bruxelles
BELGIUM

R. J. VONK
Department of Pediatrics
University Hospital
59 Oostersingel
NL-9713 EX Groningen
THE NETHERLANDS

P. F. WHITINGTON
University of Chicago Box 107
5825 South Maryland Avenue
Chicago
IL 60637
USA

B. M. WINKLHOFER-ROOB
Division of Gastroenterology and
  Nutrition
Department of Paediatrics
University of Zurich
Zurich
SWITZERLAND

Section 1
Physiology of Bile Formation

1
Physiology of bile formation

W. GEROK

Bile secretion is a unique and major function of the liver. Primary bile is secreted into the bile canaliculus, formed between two hepatocytes and sealed off from the intercellular space by the tight junctions. For the vectorial transport of various endogenous and exogenous substances from blood into bile hepatocytes, as secretory epithelial cells, localize distinct transport systems on their basolateral and canalicular surface domain; furthermore a vectorial intracellular transport is required. Therefore the normal process of bile secretion involves multiple transport and metabolic steps and is still incompletely understood. Nevertheless the following facts are well established (for reviews see refs 1–6):

1. Bile flow is driven by the formation of osmotic gradients between the blood, intercellular space and the hepatocytes on the one hand and the lumen of the bile canaliculus on the other. The pathway of fluid movement is transcellular and paracellular.
2. Conjugated bile acids are the most concentrated organic solutes in bile. The linear relationship between bile salt excretion rate and bile flow when bile acids exceed their critical micellar concentrations demonstrates that bile salt excretion is the major determinant of bile flow: bile salt-dependent fraction.
3. In the absence of bile acids a basal bile flow probably remains, defined by the extrapolation of the relationship between bile acid output and bile flow to zero bile acids. The size of this bile acid-independent fraction of bile flow has not been accurately measured and may be overestimated. Nevertheless, organic anions other than bile acids, e.g. glutathione and inorganic anions, e.g. HCO_3^-, are solutes responsible for this fraction of bile flow.
4. During passage through bile ductules and bile ducts the primary bile is modified by secretion and reabsorption of solutes and water.

In the following I will discuss some facts and open questions to four points:

1. Vectorial transport of bile salts as basis of bile salt-dependent fraction.

2. Vectorial transport of glutathione and inorganic anions for bile salt-independent fraction.
3. Modification of primary bile during passage through bile duct system.
4. Regulation of bile flow.

VECTORIAL TRANSPORT OF BILE ACIDS

The rate of synthesis of bile acids is very small in relation to their biliary excretion rate. Therefore vectorial transport of bile acids implicates three steps:

1. uptake across the sinusoidal membrane,
2. intracellular transport through the hepatocyte,
3. secretion across the canalicular membrane.

Sinusoidal uptake of bile salts

Bile acid uptake into the hepatocytes occurs against a high concentration gradient and therefore requires energy. At least two transport systems are involved: Na^+-dependent and a Na^+-independent transport system. Kinetic data demonstrate that under normal conditions the Na^+-dependent transport system is much more effective. Both systems transport conjugated as well as unconjugated bile acids, but the Na^+-dependent system has a clear preference for conjugated bile acids.

Na^+-dependent uptake of bile acids

This transport is carrier-mediated and uses the out-to-in sodium gradient as its energy source, which is maintained by the Na^+K^+-ATPase. So Na^+-dependent bile salt uptake is a secondary active transport process. Different bile salts show both saturation (Michaelis–Menten) kinetic and competition for uptake (for review see refs 1–6).

For understanding of the transport process on a molecular level it is necessary to characterize the carrier proteins. By photoaffinity labelling with photolabile analogues of bile salts[7–9,12] or chemically reactive derivatives[10,11] two bile-salt-binding membrane polypeptides of 48 and 54 kD were identified in the sinusoidal membrane (Fig. 1A).

The polypeptide with apparent molecular weight of 54 kD can easily be removed from the membrane by 2 mol/l NaCl solution, by sonication, and even by freezing and thawing. Thus, as a peripheral membrane protein, it may not be directly involved in membrane transport of bile salts, but may have an auxiliary function[13]. It is a glycoprotein with homologies of its amino sequence to the enzyme disulphidisomerase.

The 48 kD polypeptide may be involved directly in sinusoidal uptake of bile salts. It has recently been purified[14] and reconstituted into liposomes with preservation of Na^+-dependent taurocholate transport activity[15]. Binding studies with a monoclonal antibody which specifically recognizes this 48 kD

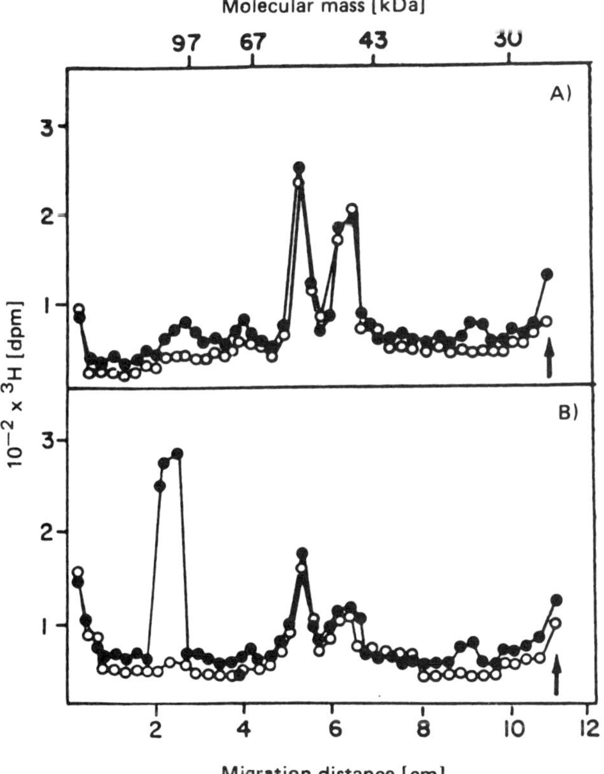

Fig. 1 Identification of bile salt binding polypeptides in (**A**) sinusoidal membrane, (**B**) canalicular membrane. Incorporation of radioactivity into polypeptides of membrane subfractions after photoaffinity labelling of liver snips with the sodium salt of the photolabile and ^{3}H-labelled analogue of taurocholate in the presence (●) and the absence (○) of Ca^{2+}. Separation of the polypeptides by polyacrylamide gel electrophoresis (from ref. 12)

polypeptide demonstrated influence on the bile acid transport system[16]. The expression of this Na^+-bile acid cotransporter in *Xenopus laevis* oocytes is a promising approach towards ultimately cloning the gene of this protein[17,52].

Although great progress in the understanding of uptake mechanisms for bile acids was achieved, several problems are unresolved.

1. Albumin effect: low concentrations of albumin stimulate Na^+-dependent taurocholate uptake and decrease the apparent K_m for taurocholate. The nature of this effect is not yet known; but does not involve an albumin receptor in the sinusoidal membrane[18–20].
2. Rheogenicity: evidence exists for both electroneutral (1 Na^+/1 TC) and electrogenic (2 Na^+/1 TC) cotransport[2,3] (TC = taurocholate). In isolated vesicles, as well as in isolated hepatocytes, the presence of chloride is an important requirement for maximal Na^+-dependent bile acid uptake. Therefore a more complex model with 2 Na^+/1 Cl^-, 1 TC stoichiometry

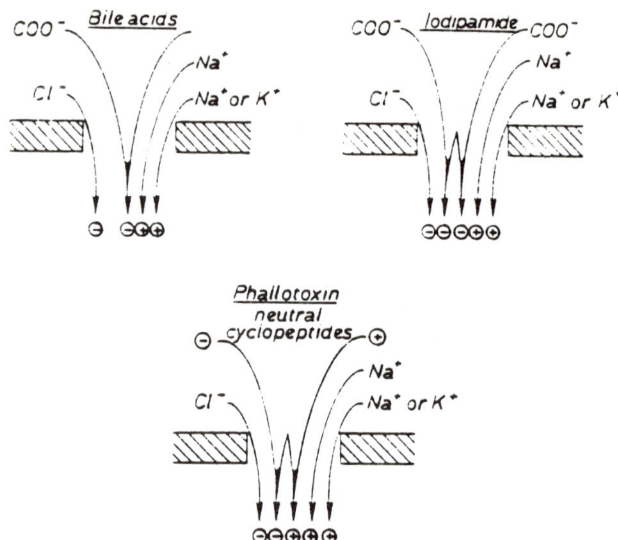

Fig. 2 Working hypothesis on the different electrogenicity of the hepatocellular uptake of bile acids and foreign substrates by co-transport with Na^+. Bile acid uptake is electroneutral, but replacement of Na^+ or Cl^- inhibits the transport. Iodipamide transport is negatively electrogenic. Electroneutral phallotoxins are translocated by a positive electrogenic transport (from ref. 21)

was described[3,21] which is electroneutral in the case of bile acid transport, but results in a negative or positive charge with other substrates (Fig. 2). Thus, this hypothetical system could introduce a high degree of transport flexibility and provide a potential explanation for the transport of differently charged substances by the same transport system.

2. Broad substrate specificity: surprisingly, the spectrum of substrates of the Na^+-dependent bile acid transport system includes diverse classes of endogenous substances (organic anions and cations, cyclic peptides etc.) and xenobiotics[22–26]. The explanation could be a unique carrier protein with multiple binding or transport sites. An alternative possibility is a transport system constituted by different binding proteins with overlapping substrate specificities[2,3,27].

Na^+-independent uptake of bile acids

The molecular substrate and function of this transport system is less clear than of the Na^+-dependent system. A carrier-mediated transport with exchange of hydroxyl/bile acid was described[28]. However, the prerequisite of an alkaline pH gradient also drives the cholate uptake in protein-free liposomes; therefore this cholate transport represents non-ionic diffusion rather than a carrier-mediated process[29]. In any case, pH gradient-dependent transport appears to be of minor significance for cholate uptake across sinusoidal membrane.

Intracellular transport of bile salts

The transcellular pathway by which bile acids are translocated from the sinusoidal uptake system to the bile canaliculus is under controversial discussion. Two mechanisms have been proposed:

1. Transcellular transport in solution bound to proteins (for review see refs 3 and 6).
2. Transcellular transport by intracellular vesicles (for review see refs 4–6).

Evidence for the first mechanism stems from the isolation and characterization of several cytoplasmic binding proteins with overlapping substrate specificity for bile acids and other organic anions. Such cytosolic proteins with high-affinity binding sites are ligandin and other glutathione-S-transferases, two proteins designated 'Y' and 'Z', and two proteins termed 'bile acid binder I and II'. The significance of each specific protein within this group for transcellular transport is unclear as yet. Protein binding of bile salts may serve to reduce the effective cytosolic free concentration of bile salts to low level. The very short transit time ($\sim$ 2 min) is compatible with movement by this transport mechanism.

Evidence for vesicular acid transport stems from morphological studies: proliferation of Golgi and demonstration of pericanalicular vesicle during bile secretion. Furthermore, kinetic studies have shown that vesicles derived from the endoplasmic reticulum or Golgi exhibit saturable taurocholate uptake. With immunohistochemical methods the 54 kD bile salt-binding polypeptide was localized in the sinusoidal membrane as well as in the endoplasmic reticulum. Therefore it was suggested that this polypeptide is involved in the transport of bile acids from the sinusoidal membrane to the endoplasmic reticulum and Golgi for vesicle formation in these organelles. However, the very short transit time and the separation in time of biliary secretion of bile acids from vesicle-mediated lipid secretion argue against a major role of vesicular transport.

Canalicular secretion of bile salts

Canalicular secretion is the rate-limiting step in overall transport of bile salts from blood into bile. Intracellular bile salt concentrations in the normal hepatocyte are of order of 0.2 mmol/l, but may in reality be much lower in free solution due to the presence of cytosolic bile salt-binding proteins. Bile salt concentration in hepatic bile is of the order of 20 mmol/l. Bile salts are thus secreted against a high concentration gradient.

Kinetic studies in vesicles of highly purified canalicular plasma membranes[30–32] have demonstrated that transport through the canalicular membrane is carrier-mediated with saturation kinetic, specificity and competition between different bile salts. In contrast to the major transport system in the sinusoidal membrane the canalicular bile salt transport is Na^+ independent. The energy for pumping bile salts against a high concentration gradient derives, at least in part, from the intracellular negative membrane potential of -30 to -40 mV.

In order to understand canalicular secretion on a molecular level the carrier protein was identified and characterized by several groups[12,33,34]. Using photoaffinity labelling of liver snips with a photolabile derivative of taurocholate a single bile salt-binding polypeptide with an apparent molecular weight of 100–110 kD was localized in the bile canalicular membrane (Fig. 1B). In the absence of Ca^{2+} there is no effect on the uptake of bile salts, whereas their. secretion is completely prevented. Accordingly under Ca^{2+} deprivation the labelling of the sinusoidal polypeptides is unchanged, whereas labelling of the canalicular polypeptide is missing.

The canalicular bile salt-binding protein could be solubilized by octyl-glucoside and purified by anion exchange and lectin affinity chromatography[34,35]. It is a glycoprotein which is sialylated; its molecular weight decreases by deglycosylation from 100 to 48 kD. A monospecific antibody against the purified protein inhibits taurocholate transport into canalicular but not into basolateral vesicles[34,35]. Kinetic studies demonstrated that the anion transport inhibitor DIDS inhibits both photoaffinity labelling and taurocholate transport. By incorporation of the 100 kD polypeptide in artificial proteoliposomes the taurocholate transport system could be reconstituted with properties of the native system such as trans-stimulation, inhibition by DIDS and potential sensitivity[36,37].

Recently different ATP-binding proteins and ATP-dependent transport systems have been identified in the canalicular membrane. Therefore photoaffinity labelling with the ATP-derivative $[^{35}S]$ATPγS was performed. Using this method several proteins could be identified in the canalicular but not sinusoidal membrane[37]. Immunoprecipitation with a monoclonal antibody (Fig. 3a,b) against a 110 kD polypeptide demonstrated that the bile salt-binding protein, labelled with the photolabile analogue of taurocholate, and the 100 kD ATP-binding protein, labelled with $[^{35}S]$ATP, were identical with respect to migration distance in SDS-gel electrophoresis and isoelectric point in two-dimensional electrophoresis (IEF followed by SDS PAGE)[37].

Kinetic studies with canalicular membrane vesicles demonstrated ATP-stimulated taurocholate uptake[37]. This uptake was saturable with respect to ATP concentration with an apparent K_m value of 800 μmol/l (Fig. 4A,B). The stimulation of taurocholate uptake was specific for ATP. Other nucleotides, i.e. GTP, UTP, CTP, as well as ATP analogues, had no effect. Vanadate inhibits ATP-dependent taurocholate transport. This suggests that γ-phosphate transfer from ATP is involved in the process of bile salt transport. Finally, the canalicular ATP-dependent taurocholate transport system was reconstituted in proteoliposomes[37]. Solubilized canalicular membrane proteins mediated ATP-dependent taurocholate transport and a significantly higher specific transport activity was obtained when the purified 110 kD glycoprotein was used for reconstitution (Table 1). Thus, it can be concluded with strong evidence that the ATP-dependent transport of taurocholate through the canalicular membrane is mediated by the 110 kD glycoprotein as carrier.

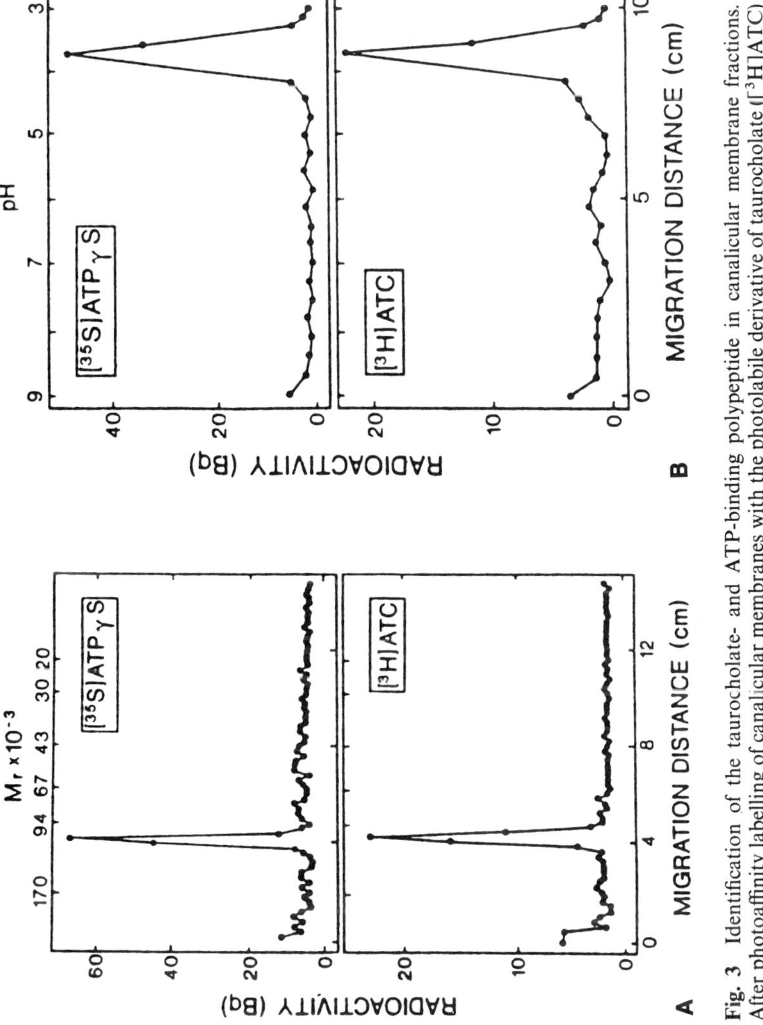

Fig. 3 Identification of the taurocholate- and ATP-binding polypeptide in canalicular membrane fractions. After photoaffinity labelling of canalicular membranes with the photolabile derivative of taurocholate ([^{3}H]ATC) and ATP ([^{35}S]ATPγS) immunoprecipitation with the monoclonal antibody (mAb Be 9,2). (**A**) SDS-Polyacrylamide gel electrophoresis; (**B**) two-dimensional electrophoresis: isoelectric focusing followed by SDS-polyacrylamide gel electrophoresis. Identical properties of the taurocholate- and ATP-binding polypeptides (from ref. 37)

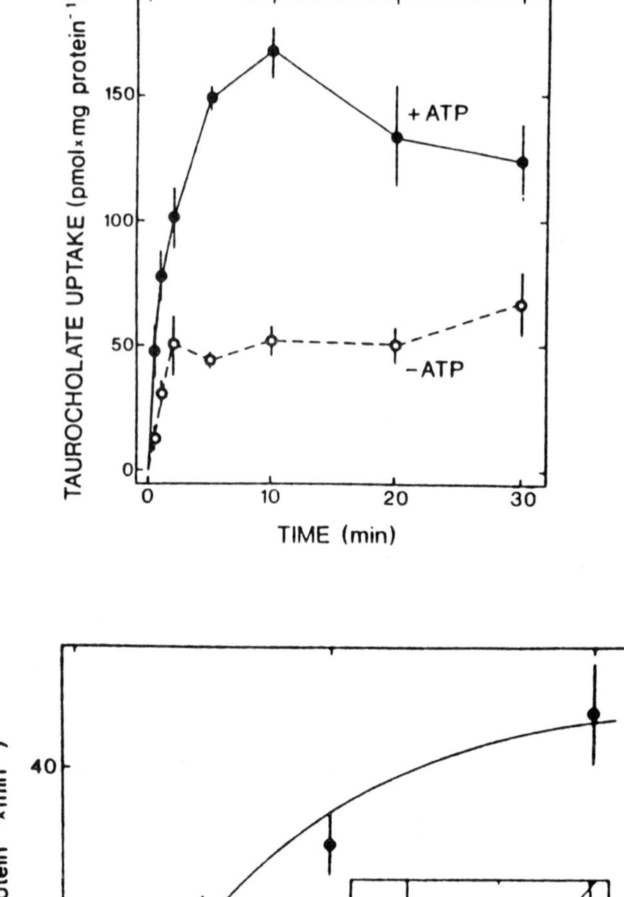

Fig. 4 Taurocholate uptake by canalicular membrane vesicles. (**A**) Time-course of uptake with and without ATP; (**B**) ATP-dependence of uptake (saturation kinetic) (from ref. 37).

Table 1 Reconstitution of the ATP-dependent taurocholate transport system in proteoliposome vesicles using purified gp110 or canalicular membrane proteins (pmol per mg protein)

Protein addition	+ATP	−ATP	ATP-dependent transport
Canalicular membrane proteins	239 ± 8	56 ± 5	183 ± 4
Purified gp110	569 ± 40	76 ± 34	493 ± 17

Proteoliposome vesicles containing all canalicular membrane proteins (50 µg) or purified gp110 (10 µg) were incubated with 5 µmol/l [^{3}H]taurocholate at 37°C for 30 min. ATP-dependent transport was calculated from the difference in radioactivity taken up into proteoliposomes in the presence or absence of 1 mmol/l ATP. Data are expressed as mean values ± SD; $n = 5$

BILE SALT-INDEPENDENT BILE FLOW

This fraction is defined by extrapolation of the regression line between bile acid output and bile flow to zero bile acids. This means canalicular bile flow at low bile acid secretion, absence of bile acids or in addition to the bile acid-dependent bile flow. But this is merely an operational definition. Direct proof for the existence of a bile salt-independent bile flow is still lacking. The size of this fraction may be overestimated, since bile acids stimulate larger volumes of water secretion per molecule at levels below their critical micellar concentrations. Also the solutes that are responsible for this fraction of bile flow have not been clearly identified. But in spite of these objections, most of the evidence supports the real existence of bile salt-independent fraction of bile flow. Possible candidates as solutes providing osmotic filtration in the absence of bile salt are:

1. inorganic ions, such as HCO_3^- and Cl^-;
2. organic ions, such as oxidized glutathione and its conjugates.

Inorganic ions

In canalicular membrane vesicles a Cl^-/HCO_3^- exchanger[38] and a chloride channel[39] could be demonstrated. Secretion of HCO_3^- by this exchanger and exit of Cl^- through the Cl^- channel driven by the membrane potential are an attractive hypothesis. The HCO_3^--rich hypercholeresis after ursodeoxycholic and its inhibition by either amiloride or carbonic anhydrase inhibitors supports the role of HCO_3^- as a determinant of bile salt-independent bile flow. But it is unclear whether the source of HCO_3^- are the hepatocytes or bile ducts, or both. At present it remains to be shown whether these ion transporters play a direct role in the bile secretory process or whether they are secondarily linked to the secretion process as regulators of cell volume or intracellular pH (for review see ref. 6).

Glutathione

There is strong evidence that glutathione contributes to bile salt-independent bile flow by carrier-mediated transport into bile providing a driving force for osmotic filtration (for review see refs 1–6). Glutathione, the tripeptide of glutamate, cysteine and glycine, is synthesized within hepatocytes. In rat liver the ratio between the reduced (thiol) GSH and oxidized (disulphide) GSSG is approximately $1:300$[40]. GSH is predominantly released in the sinusoidal blood. The efflux occurs down a concentration gradient (> 100 in:out) by a carrier-mediated transport system.

In contrast to GSH, GSSG and GS conjugates are preferentially, if not exclusively, excreted into the bile canaliculi[41]. The gradient between intracellular concentration of GSSG and its concentration in biliary space is $1:50$. The biliary secretion of GSSG against this high concentration gradient occurs by an active, energy-consuming carrier-mediated transport[42,43].

From previous experiments it was concluded that the canalicular GSSG transport is electrogenic and is driven by the membrane potential with negative charge on the inside[43]. But recently ATP-dependency was demonstrated by several groups[44–47] (Fig. 5A,B). The ATP-dependent transport of GSSG and GS conjugates follows Michaelis–Menten kinetics. Competitive inhibition of GSSG transport was demonstrated with various GS-conjugates and glucuronides (Fig. 6), but not with GSH and sulphates[47]. Taurocholate also competitively inhibits ATP-dependent transport of GSSG and GS conjugates. However, the high K_i value of taurocholate and the finding that cholate, even in high concentration of $0.4\,\text{mmol/l}$, has no inhibitory effect indicate that the carrier for GSSG and GS conjugates is not identical to the canalicular carrier for bile salts[47].

The existence of two distinct transport systems for bile acids and GSSG is underlined by observations in mutant Wistar rats with inherited conjugated hyperbilirubinaemia. Canalicular transport of GSSG, GS conjugates and glucuronides is defective in this mutant, whereas the canalicular secretion of bile acids is normal[46]. The defect is phenotypically similar to that seen in mutant Corriedale sheep and the Dubin–Johnson syndrome in humans.

A variety of drugs, including vinblastine, vincristine, daunomycin and verapamil, are secreted via a common multi-drug transporter in the biliary space[48,49]. The transport is ATP-dependent. Kinetic data[47], and its intact function in the mutant rat[46], demonstrate that this multi-drug system is clearly distinct from the transport systems both for bile acids and for GSSG, GS conjugates and glucuronides.

In summary at least three different ATP-dependent export carriers exist in the canalicular membrane: (1) for bile salts (GP 110); (2) for GS conjugates and glucuronides, such as cysteinyl-leukotrienes and BSP; and (3) for a variety of hydrophobic, mostly basic drugs, such as vincristine and verapamil (Fig. 7).

MODIFICATION OF BILE COMPOSITION DURING DUCTULAR PASSAGE

Primary canalicular bile is modified during passage along the epithelial cell of bile ductules and ducts by secretory and absorptive processes (for reviews

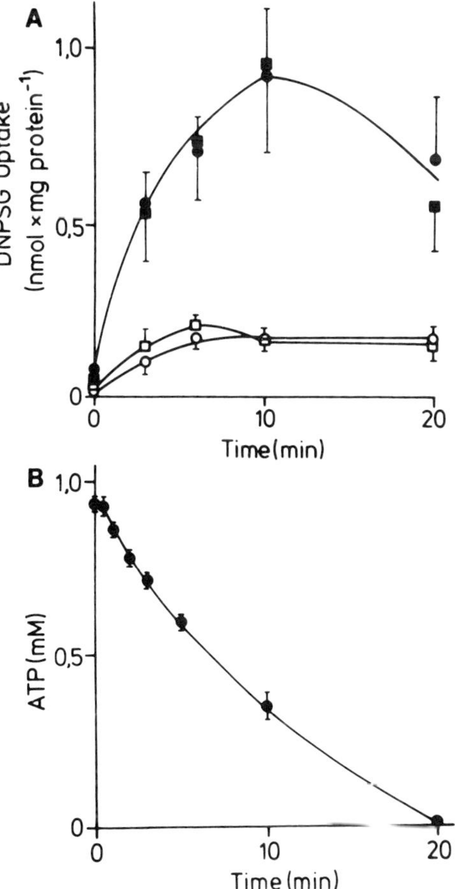

Fig. 5 (A) Time-course of S-(2,4-dinitrophenyl)-glutathione (DNPSG) in canalicular membrane vesicles. Effect of ATP and valinomycin-induced potassium diffusion potential. $\bigcirc$, no additions; $\square$, + valinomycin; $\bullet$ +1 mmol/l ATP; $\blacksquare$, +1 mmol/l ATP + valinomycin. (B) ATP concentration as a function of time during transport of DNPSG across canalicular membrane (from ref. 47)

see ref. 50).

Secretion by ductular epithelia concerns water, HCO_3^- and IgA. The amount of water secreted by ductular epithelia under normal conditions is about 150 ml/day; but this amount is highly variable. Experimental studies suggest that water reabsorption in the ductular and ductal system can also take place induced by fasting or bile stasis. The secretion of water and HCO_3^- is stimulated by secretin. Therefore secretin choleresis is accompanied by a pH increase in bile and a decreased bile acid concentration.

A ductular reabsorption of bile salts was shown using fluorescent bile salt derivatives. This process might play a role in the hypercholeresis induced by ursodeoxycholic acid, since the reabsorbed bile acid – probably by non-ionic

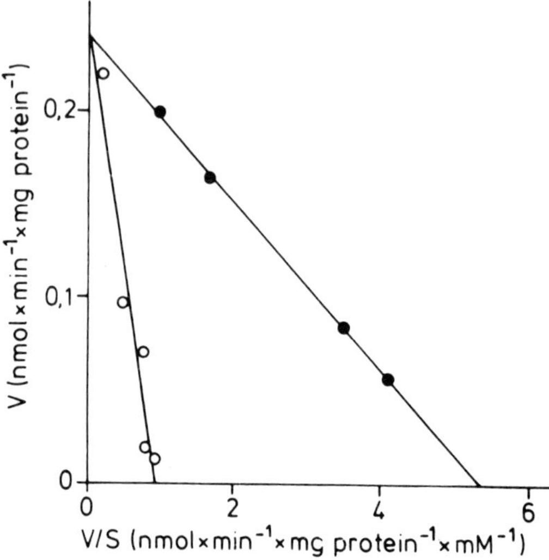

Fig. 6 Competitive inhibition of GSSG uptake in canalicular membrane vesicles by a glucuronide. Eadie–Hofstee plot of DNPSG uptake in (●) absence and (○) presence of 2 mmol/l naphthylglucuronide (from ref. 47)

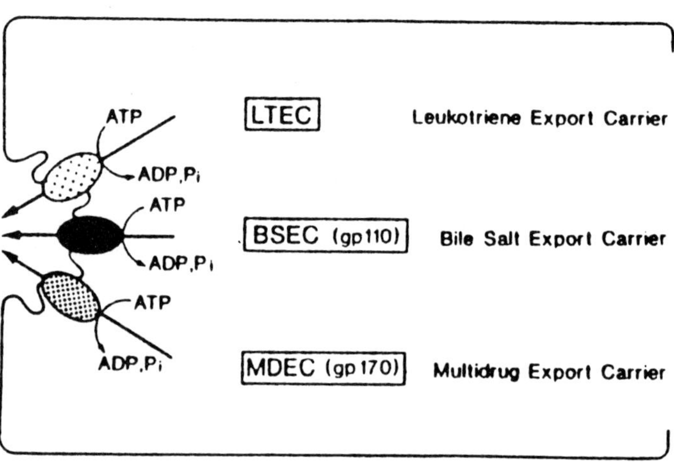

Fig. 7 ATP-dependent primary-active export carriers in the canalicular membrane involved in the hepatobiliary elimination of bile salts, cysteinyl leukotrienes (+ GSSG, BSP and glucuronides), and hydrophobic drugs (from ref. 37)

diffusion – is taken up and resecreted by the hepatocytes, thereby increasing bile flow and bicarbonate secretion. This 'cholehepatic shunt pathway' may be the basis for choleresis by side-chain shortened bile acids, e.g. 23-nor-ursodeoxycholate and nor-chenodeoxycholate.

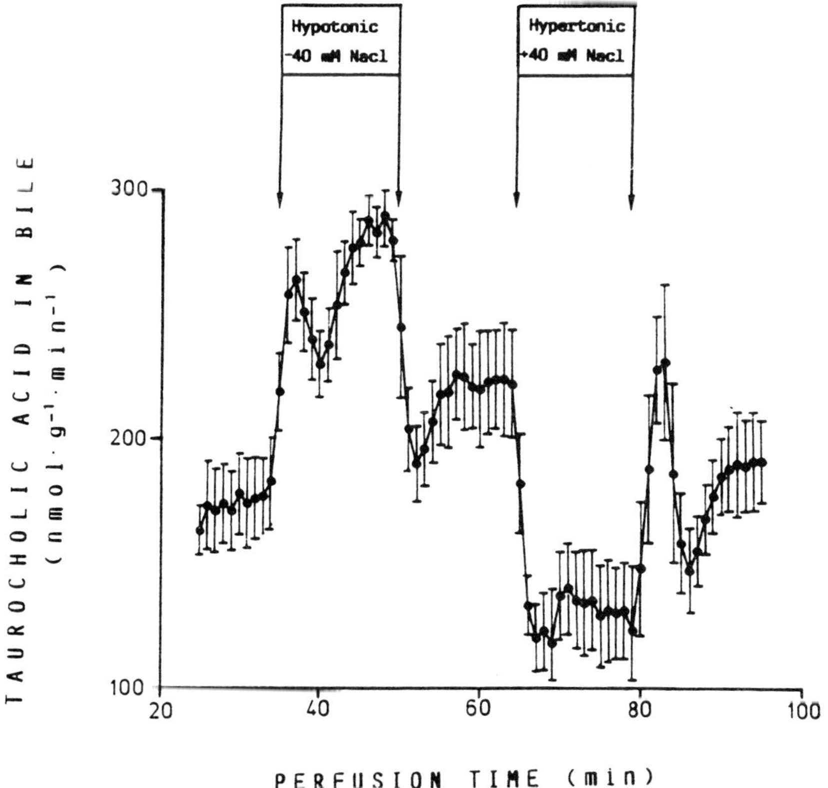

Fig. 8 Effect of aniso-osmotic exposure with cell volume swelling and shrinkage, respectively, on biliary taurocholate excretion. Single-pass perfused rat liver. Taurocholate concentration in the influent perfusion 100 μmol/l. Osmolarity changes by addition or removal of NaCl from the influent perfusate (from ref. 51)

REGULATION OF BILE FLOW

With the exception of secretin little is known about regulation of bile flow by metabolites, hormones or the nervous system. Although there are several experimental or clinical observations about the influence of metabolites, such as amino acids and glucose, of the hormones insulin, glucagon and thyroxin and of mediator substances such as gastrin and the prostaglandins (for review see ref. 4), no systematic investigation of bile flow regulation exists. The majority of these observations are of a rather anecdotal character.

Recently, it was shown in the experimental model of the isolated perfused liver that cell volume alterations represent a new principle controlling liver metabolism and bile flow. Alterations of cell volume act like a second or third messenger mediating hormone effects[51].

Bile flow is markedly stimulated by exposure of the liver to hyposmotic

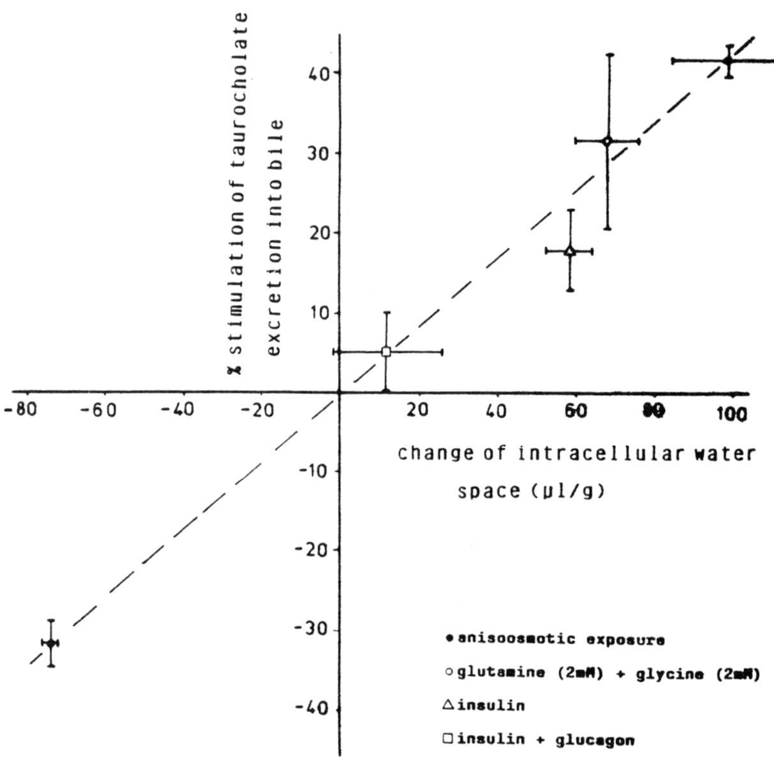

Fig. 9 Relationship between taurocholate excretion into bile and cell volume. Single-pass perfused rat liver with taurocholate concentration 100 µmol/l in the influent perfusate. Taurocholate excretions (hormones and amino acids absent) 185 ± 9 nmol/min per g liver. Data on taurocholate excretion under the influence of various effectors on cell volume are given as percentage hereof (from ref. 51)

perfusion medium with the consequence of increasing cell volume. This increase of bile flow is not only the result of an increased water shift according to higher osmotic gradient, but is induced by a remarkable stimulation of taurocholate secretion (Fig. 8). The mechanism of this effect is unclear as yet. Conversely, shrinkage of cell volume decreases biliary excretion of taurocholate and bile flow. Also isotonic cell swelling – induced by supply of amino acids, such as glutamine or glycine, or by hormones, such as insulin – stimulates taurocholate excretion and bile flow. This effect is counteracted by vasopressin and glucagon, which are known to reverse insulin-induced cell swelling. There is a roughly linear relationship between biliary taurocholate excretion and cell volume change under the influence of anisotonicity, amino acids and insulin (Fig. 9). These effects can also be shown in the absence of added bile acids, but are less pronounced. These data suggest that metabolites and hormones regulate bile flow and bile salt secretion via alterations of cell volume.

References

1. Coleman R. Biochemistry of bile secretion. Biochem J. 1987;244:249–61.
2. Meier PJ. Transport polarity of hepatocytes. Sem Liv Dis. 1988;8:293–307.
3. Frimmer M, Ziegler K. The transport of bile acids in liver cells. Biochim Biophys Acta. 1988;947:75–99.
4. Erlinger S. Bile flows. In Arias IM, Jakoby WB, Popper H, Schachter D, Schafritz DA, editors. The liver: biology and pathobiology. New York: Raven Press; 1988:643–61.
5. Meier PJ. The bile salt secretory polarity of hepatocytes. J Hepatol. 1989;9: 124–9.
6. Sellinger M, Boyer JL. Physiology of bile secretion and cholestasis. In Popper H, Schaffner F, editors. Progress in liver diseases, vol. IX. Philadelphia: WB Saunders; 1990:237–60.
7. Kramer W, Bickel U, Buscher HP, Gerok W, Kurz G. Bile-salt-binding polypeptides in plasma membranes of hepatocytes revealed by photoaffinity labelling. Eur J Biochem. 1982;129:13–24.
8. von Dippe P, Drain P, Levy D. Synthesis and transport characteristics of photoaffinity probes for the hepatocyte bile acid transport system. J Biol Chem. 1983;258:8890–5.
9. von Dippe P, Levy D. Characterization of the bile acid transport system in normal and transformed hepatocytes. J Biol Chem. 1983;258:8896–901.
10. Ziegler K, Frimmer M, Müllner S, Fasold H. 3′-Isothiocyanatobenzamido-^{3}H-cholate, a new affinity label for the uptake of both bile acids and phalloidin. Biochim Biophys Acta. 1984;773:11–22.
11. Ziegler K, Frimmer M, Fasold H. Further characterization of membrane proteins involved in the transport of organic anions in hepatocytes. Comparison of two different affinity labels. Biochim Biophys Acta. 1984;769:117–29.
12. Fricker G, Schneider S, Gerok W, Kurz G. Identification of different transport systems: for bile salts in sinusoidal and canalicular membranes of hepatocytes. Biol Chem Hoppe-Seyler. 1987;368:1143–5.
13. Kurz G, Müller M, Schramm U, Gerok W. Identification and function of bile salt binding polypeptides of hepatocyte membrane. In: Petzinger E, Kinne KH, Sies H, editors. Hepatic transport in organic substances. Berlin: Springer Verlag; 1989:267–78.
14. von Dippe P, Ananthanarayanan M, Drain P, Levy D. Purification and reconstitution of the bile acid transport system from hepatocyte sinusoidal plasma membranes. Biochim Biophys Acta. 1986;862:352–60.
15. von Dippe P, Levy D. Reconstitution of the immunopurified 49-kDa Sodium-dependent bile acid transport derived from hepatocyte sinusoidal plasma membranes. J Biol Chem. 1990;265:14812–16.
16. Ananthanarayanan M, von Dippe P, Levy D. Identification of the hepatocyte Na$^+$-dependent bile acid transport protein using monoclonal antibodies. J Biol Chem. 1988;263:8338–43.
17. Hagenbuch B, Lübbert H, Stieger B, Meier PJ. Expression of the hepatocyte Na$^+$/bile acid cotransporter in *Xenopus laevis* oocytes. J Biol Chem. 1990;265:5357–60.
18. Stremmel W, Potter BJ, Berk PD. Studies of albumin binding to rat liver plasma membranes. Implications for the albumin receptor hypothesis. Biochim Biophys Acta. 1983;756:20–7.
19. Weisiger RA. Dissociation from albumin: a potentially rate-limiting step in the clearance of substances by the liver. Proc Natl Acad Sci. 1985;82:1563–7.
20. Horie T, Mizuma T, Kasai S, Awazu S. Conformational change in plasma albumin due to interaction with isolated rat hepatocyte. Am J Physiol. 1988;254:9465–70.
21. Petzinger E, Ziegler K, Frimmer M. Occurrence of a multispecific transporter for the hepatocellular accumulation of bile acids and various cyclopeptides. In: Paumgartner G, Stiehl A, Gerok W, editors. Bile acids and the liver. Lancaster: MTP Press; 1987:111–24.
22. Petzinger E, Joppen C, Frimmer M. Common properties of hepatocellular uptake of cholate, iodipamide and antamanide, as distinct from the uptake of bromosulfophthalein. Naunyn-Schmiedeberg's Arch Pharmacol. 1983;322:174–9.
23. Buscher HP, Fricker G, Gerok W, Kramer W, Kurz G, Müller M, Schneider S, Schramm U, Schreyer H. Hepatic transport systems for bile salts: localization and specificity. In: Paumgartner G, Stiehl A, Gerok W, editors. Bile acids and the liver. Lancaster: MTP Press; 1987:95–110.
24. Kröncke KD, Fricker G, Meier PJ, Gerok W, Wieland Th, Kurz G. α-amanitin uptake

into hepatocytes. Identification of hepatic membrane transport used by amatoxins. J Biol Chem. 1986;261:12562–7.

25. Zimmerli B, Valantinas J, Meier PJ. Multispecificity of Na$^+$ dependent taurocholate uptake in basolateral (sinusoidal) rat liver plasma membrane vesicles. J Pharmacol Exp Ther. 1989;250:301–8.

26. Meijer DK, Mol WEM, Müller M, Kurz G. Carrier-mediated transport in the hepatic distribution and elimination of drugs, with special reference to the category of organic cations. J Pharmacokinet Biopharm. 1990;18:35–70.

27. Berk PD, Potter BJ, Stremmel W. Role of plasma membrane ligand-binding proteins in the hepatocellular uptake of albumin-bound organic anions. Hepatology. 1987;7:165–76.

28. Blitzer BL, Terzakis Ch, Scott KA. Hydroxyl/bile acid exchange. A new mechanism for the uphill transport of cholate by basolateral liver plasma vesicles. J Biol Chem. 1986;261:12042–6.

29. Caflisch C, Zimmerli B, Reichen J, Meier PJ. Cholate uptake in basolateral rat liver plasma membrane vesicles and in liposomes. Biochim Biophys Acta. 1990;1021:70–6.

30. Inoue M, Kinne R, Tran T, Arias IM. Taurocholate transport by rat liver canalicular membrane vesicles. Evidence for the presence of an Na$^+$-independent transport system. J Clin Invest. 1984;73:659–63.

31. Meier PJ, Meier-Abt AS, Barrett C. Mechanisms of taurocholate transport in canalicular and basolateral rat liver plasma membrane vesicles. Evidence for an electrogenic canalicular organic anion carrier. J Biol Chem. 1984;259:10614–22.

32. Meier PJ, Meier-Abt AS, Boyer JL. Properties of the canalicular bile acid transport system in rat liver. Biochem J. 1987;242:465–9.

33. Buscher HP, Fricker G, Gerok W, Kramer W, Kurz G, Müller M, Schneider S. Membrane transport of amphiphilic compounds by hepatocytes. In: Greten H, Windler E, Beisiegel U, editors. Receptor-mediated uptake in the liver. Heidelberg: Springer Verlag; 1986:189–99.

34. Ruetz S, Fricker G, Hugentobler G, Winterhalter K, Kurz G, Meier PJ. Isolation and characterization of the putative canalicular bile salt transport system of rat liver. J Biol Chem. 1987;262:11324–30.

35. Sippel CJ, Ananthanarayanan M, Suchy FJ. Isolation and characterization of the canalicular membrane bile acid transport protein of rat liver. Am J Physiol. 1990;258:728–37.

36. Ruetz S, Hugentobler G, Meier PJ. Functional reconstitution of the canalicular bile salt transport system of rat liver. Proc Natl Acad Sci, USA. 1988;85:6147–51.

37. Müller M, Ishikawa T, Berger U, Klünemann C, Lucka L, Schreyer A, Kannicht Ch, Reutter W, Kurz G, Keppler D. ATP-dependent transport of taurocholate across hepatocyte canalicular membrane mediated by a 110-Kda glycoprotein binding ATP and bile salt. J Biol Chem. 1991;266: 18920–6.

38. Meier PJ, Knickelbein R, Moseley RH, Dobbins JW, Boyer JL. Evidence for carrier-mediated chloride/bicarbonate exchange in canalicular rat liver plasma membrane vesicles. J Clin Invest. 1985;75:1256–63.

39. Sellinger M, Weinman SA, Henderson RM, Zweifach A, Boyer JL, Graf J. Properties of an anion channel in rat liver canalicular membranes. Ann NY Acad Sci. 1989;574:57–9.

40. Akerboom Th, Bilzer M, Sies H. The relationship of biliary glutathione disulfide efflux and intracellular glutathione disulfide content in perfused rat liver. J Biol Chem. 1982;257:4248–52.

41. Akerboom Th, Inoue M, Sies H, Kinne R, Arias IM. Biliary transport of glutathione disulfide studied with isolated rat liver canalicular-membrane vesicles. Eur J Biochem. 1984;141:211–15.

42. Inoue M, Kinne R, Tran T, Arias IM. Glutathione transport across hepatocyte plasma membrane. Analysis using isolated rat-liver sinusoidal membrane vesicles. Eur J Biochem. 1984;138:491–5.

43. Akerboom T, Bilzer M, Sies H. Competition between transport of glutathione disulfide (GSSG) and glutathione-S-conjugates from perfused rat liver into bile. Competition between biliary output of GSSG and S-conjugate. FEBS Lett. 1982;140:73–6.

44. Kobayashi K, Sogame Y, Hayashi K, Nicotera P, Orrenius S. ATP stimulates the uptake of S-dinitrophenylglutathione by rat liver plasma membrane vesicles. FEBS Lett. 1988; 240: 55–8.

45. Kobayashi K, Sogame Y, Hara H, Hayashi K. Mechanism of glutathione-S-conjugate transport in canalicular and basolateral rat liver plasma membranes. J Biol Chem. 1990;265:7737–41.

46. Kitamura T, Jansen P, Hardenbrook C, Kamimoto Y, Gatmaitan Z, Arias IM. Defective

ATP-dependent bile canalicular transport of organic anions in mutant (TR) rats with conjugated hyperbilirubinemia. Proc Natl Acad Sci. USA. 1990;87:3557–61.

47. Akerboom Th, Narayanaswami V, Kunst M, Sies H. ATP-dependent S-(2,4-dinitrophenyl) glutathione transport in canalicular plasma membrane vesicles from rat liver. J Biol Chem. 1991;266:13147–52.
48. Kamimoto Y, Gatmaitan Z, Hsu J, Arias IM. The function of GP 170, the multidrug resistance gene product, in rat liver canalicular membrane vesicles. J Biol Chem. 1989;264:11693–8.
49. Arias IM. Multidrug resistance genes, p-glycoprotein and the liver. Hepatology. 1990;12: 159–65.
50. Tavolini N. The intrahepatic biliary epithelium: an area of growing interest in hepatology. Sem Liv Dis. 1987;7:280–92.
51. Hallbrucker C, Lang F, Gerok W, Häussinger D. Cell swelling increases bile flow and aurocholate excretion into bile in isolated perfused rat liver. Biochem J. 1992;281:593–5.
52. Hagenbuch B, Stieger B, Foguet M, Lübbert H, Meier PJ. Functional expression cloning and characterization of the hepatocye Na$^+$/bile acid cotransport system. Proc Natl Acad Sci USA. 1991;38:10629–33.

2
Ontogenesis of hepatic bile salt transport

F. J. SUCHY and M. ANANTHANARAYANAN

The vectorial transport of bile acids, the major determinant and motive force for generation of bile secretion, is critically dependent upon the polarized distribution of specific transport proteins on the plasma membrane. The ontogenic expression of hepatic bile salt transport has been under study in our laboratory at the cellular and molecular level. A key concept from this work in a rat model is that the sinusoidal (basolateral) and canalicular carriers for bile acids are expressed and inserted into the plasma membrane at very specific times during perinatal development.

The significance of these observations can be considered in the context of our current understanding of hepatobiliary function during development. Bile acid concentrations are significantly lower in the biles of several neonatal mammals including the human, reflecting a small bile acid pool size and an immaturity of hepatic transport mechanisms[1]. In the intact newborn rabbit and dog, and in the isolated perfused suckling rat liver, basal rates of bile flow and bile salt secretion, as well as the response to infusion of exogenous bile salts, are markedly decreased in comparison with adult animals[2-4]. Moreover, bile salt secretion rates appear to be reduced to an even greater extent than rates of uptake, supporting the concept that decreased canalicular bile salt secretion is the primary factor limiting bile formation by the immature liver[1].

Well-characterized preparations of basolateral and canalicular plasma membrane vesicles have been used in our work to study the pre- and postnatal expression of bile acid transport activity. The vesicle technique allows the determination of membrane transport apart from age-related variables such as organ perfusion, volume distribution, lobular geometry, and biliary modification of canalicular secretions encountered with intact or perfused livers. Moreover, the vesicle studies in large part overcome problems observed with isolated hepatocytes including the loss of cell polarity and developmental differences in cell size, metabolism, and intracellular compartmentation.

Recent studies have employed a strategy to identify and isolate the

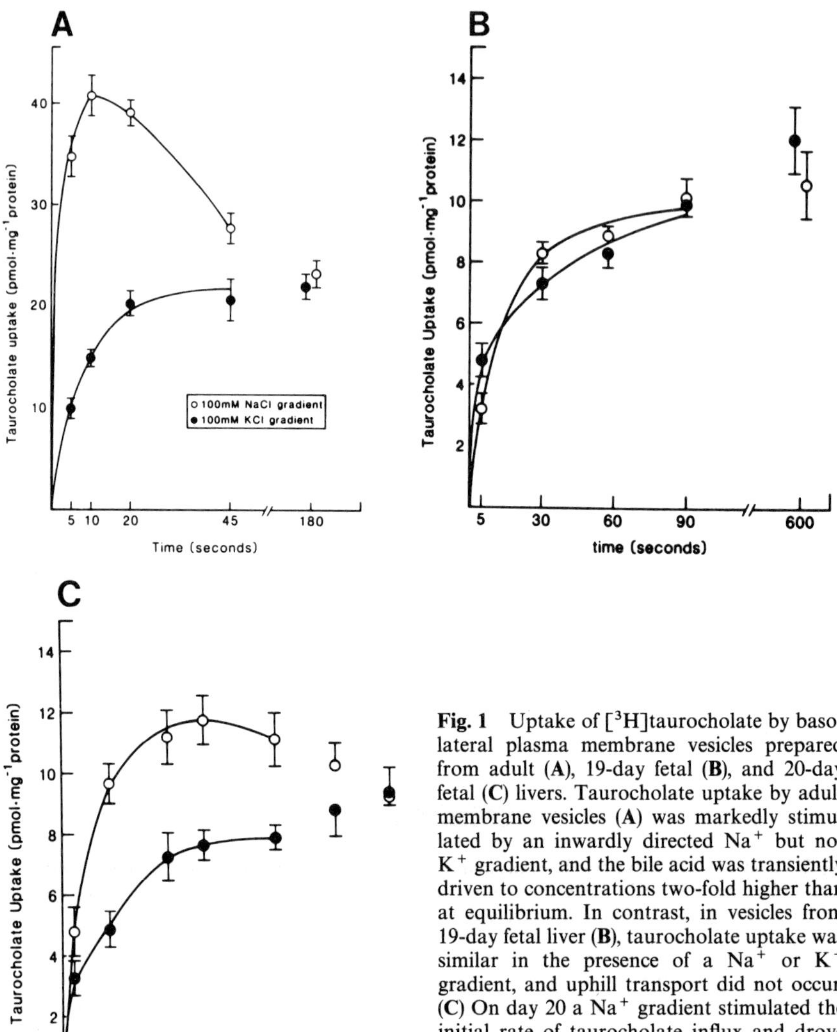

Fig. 1 Uptake of [³H]taurocholate by basolateral plasma membrane vesicles prepared from adult (**A**), 19-day fetal (**B**), and 20-day fetal (**C**) livers. Taurocholate uptake by adult membrane vesicles (**A**) was markedly stimulated by an inwardly directed Na^+ but not K^+ gradient, and the bile acid was transiently driven to concentrations two-fold higher than at equilibrium. In contrast, in vesicles from 19-day fetal liver (**B**), taurocholate uptake was similar in the presence of a Na^+ or K^+ gradient, and uphill transport did not occur. (**C**) On day 20 a Na^+ gradient stimulated the initial rate of taurocholate influx and drove the substrate above equilibrium (from ref. 5, with permission)

transport protein which mediates the basolateral, Na^+-dependent uptake of bile acids based upon the timing for ontogenic expression of this transport activity in fetal rat liver. As reported by several laboratories, we have demonstrated previously that an inwardly directed, transmembrane Na^+-gradient was found to provide the driving force for uphill transport of taurocholate by basolateral plasma membrane vesicles prepared from adult rat liver (Fig. 1A). In contrast, taurocholate uptake by vesicles from 19-day fetal liver was similar in the presence of a sodium or potassium gradient and accumulation of substrate above its equilibrium concentration was not

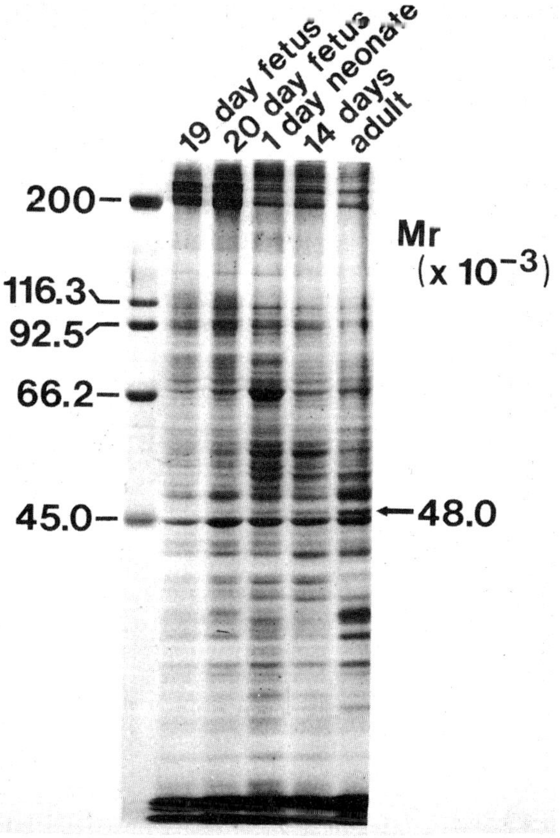

Fig. 2 Analysis of basolateral liver plasma membranes from fetal, neonatal, and adult rats by SDS–polyacrylamide gel electrophoresis. A protein of M_r 48 000 was absent on fetal day 19, barely detectable on day 20, and thereafter increased progressively with postnatal development (from ref. 7, with permission)

observed, suggesting that the transport mechanism was not present or functional (Fig. 1B)[5]. However, Na⁺-dependent transport activity was abruptly expressed just 24 h later on fetal day 20 (Fig. 1C). After the expression of Na⁺-bile acid cotransport in perinatal liver, there was a progressive increase in the initial rate of Na⁺-dependent uptake and peak intravesicular accumulation of taurocholate during postnatal development which was associated with an increase in the V_{max} for the transport process[5,6]. Analysis of basolateral plasma membranes by SDS polyacrylamide gel electrophoresis revealed that a protein of apparent molecular weight 48 000 was absent from fetal rat liver on day 19 of gestation, barely detectable on day 20, and thereafter increased progressively with postnatal development[7]. Monospecific, polyclonal antibodies directed against this developmentally regulated polypeptide inhibited Na⁺-dependent taurocholate transport by isolated rat hepatocytes and were used to deplete an extract of basolateral membrane proteins of the 48-kD peptide prior to reconstitution into synthetic proteoliposomes. The presence of the 48-kD protein was essential for functional reconstitution of Na^+-dependent taurocholate transport[7]. In preliminary studies with the Meier group in Zurich who have recently cloned a cDNA for the Na^+-dependent bile acid transporter, the anti-48 kD antibody recognized the primary translation product of mRNA produced from this clone. Northern blot analysis showed that message levels for the transporter closely paralleled the expression of transport activity and the amount of carrier protein within the membrane[8].

The postnatal ontogenesis of taurocholate transport has also been studied using canalicular plasma membrane vesicles[9]. Transport of bile acids across the hepatocyte canalicular membrane is mediated, in large part, via a Na^+-independent carrier mechanism which is driven by the negative intracellular electrical potential[10]. Decreased rates of bile flow and bile salt secretion in neonatal animals suggest that mechanisms for the canalicular transport of bile acids are poorly developed at birth. Therefore canalicular plasma membrane vesicles prepared by a Ca^{2+} precipitation method from developing (7 and 14 days old) and adult rat liver were used to directly examine the postnatal ontogenesis of taurocholate transport. The initial rate of 50 μmol/l taurocholate influx was 2-fold higher in canalicular vesicles from adult compared with vesicles from 7- and 14-day-old animals. Taurocholate uptake by vesicles derived from 14-day-old and adult but not 7-day-old animals was markedly inhibited by the anion transport inhibitor 4,4'-diisothiocyano-2,2'-stilbene disulphonic acid (DIDS). DIDS-sensitive taurocholate uptake was 21.6 ± 5.6 (SE) at 14 days compared with 58.1 ± 8.1 pmol/mg protein per 5 s in the adult, $p \leqslant 0.01$. Kinetic studies were performed by preloading these predominantly 'right-side out' vesicles with taurocholate (25–800 μmol/l) and measuring the initial rate (5 s) of efflux into bile salt-free medium. Computer analysis of the DIDS-sensitive portion of efflux revealed saturable kinetics with a similar V_{max} (2.72 ± 0.36 vs 1.97 ± 0.17 nmol/mg protein per min, $p = $ n.s.) but a 3-fold higher K_m (0.35 ± 0.09 vs 0.11 ± 0.02 mmol/l, $p \leqslant 0.05$) in 14-day vs adult canalicular vesicles. In contrast, efflux from 7-day vesicles increased linearly with increasing concentrations of TC and was not inhibited by DIDS.

Western blots of canalicular membranes, probed with an antibody against the 100 kD bile acid transport protein[11] showed that the amount of immunoreactive carrier protein in the membranes of the 14-day-old and adult rats was similar but was only 37% of the adult level at 7 days of age. Moreover, the radioactivity associated with the 100 kD protein, covalently labelled with $[^3H]H_2DIDS$ and immunoprecipitated from solubilized membranes, was 28% on day 7 of that measured in the adult. The protein was localized exclusively by indirect immunofluorescence microscopy to the canalicular domain of the neonatal hepatocyte. We conclude from these studies that, similar to the ileal brush border membrane, the canalicular bile acid transport system is not functional in the neonate but can be detected at a much reduced level using immunochemical methods. Maturation of transport activity involves primarily an increased insertion of the protein into the canalicular membrane, but final biochemical modification of the transporter may be required for functional expression.

Ontogenic changes in hepatic structure and synthetic pathways for bile acids may be required before maturation of membrane carriers for bile acids is achieved. It has been well documented that the canalicular membrane is morphologically immature in the fetal and neonatal rat liver and does not assume the typical adult pattern of microvilli until 10 days of postnatal age[12]. Low concentrations of cytosolic binding peptides for bile acids and evidence for enhanced efflux of bile acids across the basolateral (sinusoidal) membrane of the developing hepatocyte would indicate that the process of vectorial transport to the apical membrane is extremely inefficient[13,14]. Studies using microelectrode techniques have demonstrated that a 'mature' transmembrane potential in excess of $-40\,mV$ was achieved in suckling mouse and rat livers by 7 and 14 days of age, respectively[15,16]. Thus, available data would indicate that bile acid transport is probably not limited by the driving force provided by the transmembrane electrical potential at least during the period examined in our studies. The factors regulating the expression of bile acid transport proteins in liver and intestine remain poorly defined, but may include the expanding bile acid pool and the response to the rapidly changing hormonal milieu.

References

1. Suchy FJ, Bucuvalas JC, Novac DA. Determinants of bile formation during development: ontogeny of hepatic bile acid metabolism and transport. Sem Liver Dis. 1987;7:77–84.
2. Shaffer EA, Zahavi I, Gall DG. Digest. Postnatal development of hepatic bile formation in the rabbit. Dig Dis Sci. 1985;30:558–62.
3. Tavoloni N, Jones NJT, Berk PD. Postnatal development of bile secretory physiology in the dog. J Pediatr Gastroenterol Nutr. 1985;4:265–7.
4. Tavolini N. Bile secretion and its control in the newborn puppy. Pediatr Res. 1986;20: 203–8.
5. Suchy FJ, Bucuvalas JC, Goodrich AL, Moyer MS, Blitzer BL. Taurocholate transport and Na^+-K^+-ATPase activity in plasma membrane vesicles from fetal and neonatal rat liver. Am J Physiol. 1986;251:G655–73.
6. Suchy FJ, Courchene SM, Blitzer BL. Taurocholate transport by basolateral plasma membrane vesicles isolated from developing rat liver. Am J Physiol. 1985;248:G648–54.
7. Ananthanarayanan M, Bucuvalas JC, Schneider B, Sippel CJ, Suchy FJ. An ontogenically regulated, 48-kDa protein is a component of the Na^+-dependent bile acid transport system of the hepatocyte basolateral membrane. Am J Physiol. (In press).
8. Boyer JL, Hagenbuch B, Ananthanarayanan M, Suchy FJ, Stieger B, Meier PJ. Phylogenic and ontogenic expression of the hepatic Na^+/bile acid cotransport system. Hepatology (abstract, in press).
9. Novak DA, Sippel CJ, Ananthanarayanan M, Suchy FJ. Postnatal expression of canalicular membrane taurocholate transport. Am J Physiol. 1991;260:G743–51.
10. Meier PJ, St. Meier-Abt A, Barrett C, Boyer JL. Mechanisms of taurocholate transport in canalicular and basolateral rat liver plasma membrane vesicles. J Biol Chem. 1984;159: 10614–22.
11. Sippel CJ, Ananthanarayanan M, Suchy FJ. Isolation and characterization of the canalicular membrane bile acid transport protein of rat liver. Am J Physiol. (Gastrointest Liver Physiol.) 1990;258:G728–37.
12. DeWolf-Peters C, DeVos R, Desmet V. Electron microscopy and histochemistry of canalicular differentiation in fetal and neonatal rat liver. Tissue Cell. 1977;4:379–88.
13. Stolz A, Sugiyama Y, Kuhlenkamp J, Osadchey B, Yamada T, Belknap W, Balistreri W, Kaplowitz N. Cytosolic bile acid binding protein in rat liver: radioimmunoassay, molecular

forms, developmental characteristics and organ distribution. Hepatology. 1986;6:433–9.
14. Belknap WM, Zimmer-Nechmias L, Suchy FJ, Balistreri WF. Bile acid efflux from suckling rat hepatocytes. Pediatr Res. 1989;23:364–7.
15. Chapman LM, Wondergem RJ. Transmembrane potential and intracellular potassium ion activity in fetal and maternal liver. Cell Physiol. 1984;121:7–12.
16. Erdman C, Wunderlich M. Das Membrane Potential von Leberzellen der Ratte in verschiedenen Lebensaltern. Acta Biol Med Germ. 1970;25:239–42.

3
Bile acid metabolism in children

R. J. VONK, F. KUIPERS, M. J. SMIT, H. ELZINGA,
C. M. A. BIJLEVELD, B. G. WOLTHERS, M. RAUTENSCHLEIN
and F. STELLAARD

Bile acids are of crucial importance for the maintenance of hepatic excretory function and for efficient intraluminal fat digestion and absorption. Conservation in the enterohepatic circulation maintains adequate concentrations of bile acids at the sites of their physiological actions. Faecal excretion of bile acids that have escaped enterohepatic cycling is essential for maintenance of cholesterol balance: the loss is compensated for by hepatic *de novo* synthesis of bile acids from cholesterol. Proper functioning of the enterohepatic circulation therefore requires a well co-ordinated sequence of metabolic (bile acid synthesis, bile acid conjugation) and transport processes (uptake and secretion of bile acids by the liver, intestinal bile acid absorption). It has become clear that in early life bile acid transport is underdeveloped at various levels of the enterohepatic circulation (see Chapter 2). Hepatic bile acid synthesis in the fetal/neonatal period is low and shows marked qualitative differences when compared to the adult situation. This period of physiological immaturity of the enterohepatic circulation is often referred to as 'physiological cholestasis'[1,2]. Considering the facts that (a) most newborns lose a large proportion of ingested fat in stool – fat malabsorption is particularly severe in premature infants; and (b) hepatotoxic products of fetal/neonatal bile acid synthesis may be involved in initiating or exacerbating cholestasis, it is of importance to have an understanding of bile acid metabolism in early life. In addition, altered bile acid metabolism, as cause or consequence of disease, may contribute to malabsorption phenomena often observed in children with disorders of liver and/or intestinal tract (e.g. benign recurrent intrahepatic cholestasis, cystic fibrosis). Analysis of bile acid metabolism in these cases may provide insight into the aetiology of the disease[3] or, alternatively, may be used to evaluate effects of treatment[4].

The development of novel analytical techniques in recent years has been the key to our present understanding of bile acid physiology in health and disease. However, further studies are required to gain insight into the various regulatory mechanisms involved in bile acid metabolism, especially with regard to the role of nutritional factors. Because of the distinct species differences in bile acid synthetic pathways that exist between humans and the commonly used experimental animals, methods have been developed that allow investigation of human bile acid metabolism *in vitro*, by using human hepatocytes in primary culture, and *in vivo*, by employing mass spectrometric techniques for quantification and structure identification as well as for metabolic tracer studies.

BILE ACID METABOLISM

Cholic acid ($3\alpha,7\alpha,12\alpha$-trihydroxy-5β-cholanoic acid) and chenodeoxycholic acid ($3\alpha,7\alpha$-dihydroxy-5β-cholanoic acid), the major primary bile acids in humans, are synthesized in the liver from cholesterol. The reactions involved are saturation of the double bond, epimerization of the 3β-hydroxyl group, introduction of α-hydroxyl groups at positions C_{12} and/or C_7, and oxidation of the side-chain of the cholesterol molecule. The sequence of these reactions, catalysed by enzymes present in endoplasmic reticulum, cytosol, mitochondria or peroxisomes, has been studied extensively. The major pathways have been defined with a high degree of certainty; details can be found in recent reviews[5,6]. After conjugation with glycine or taurine, the primary bile acids are secreted into the bile and enter the gallbladder for temporary storage. With meal-stimulated contraction of the bladder, the bile acids enter the intestine, where they participate in lipid digestion and absorption[7]. The primary bile acids may be reabsorbed from the intestine or transformed by intestinal microorganisms into secondary bile acids such as deoxycholic acid ($3\alpha,12\alpha$-dihydroxy-5β-cholanoic acid) and lithocholic acid (3α-monohydroxy-5β-cholanoic acid). The secondary bile acids can also be absorbed to some extent to participate in the enterohepatic circulation along with the primary bile acids. Consequently, the circulating bile acid pool contains a mixture of bile acid species, each with specific physicochemical and physiological properties[8].

The major pathway of bile acid synthesis in humans is initiated by 7α-hydroxylation of cholesterol (Fig. 1). Activity of cholesterol 7α-hydroxylase, a microsomal P-450 enzyme, is rate-limiting in the synthetic pathway leading to both cholic acid and chenodeoxycholic acid. Activity of the enzyme is controlled by a feedback inhibition mechanism in which bile acids returning to the liver during enterohepatic circulation inhibit their own production[5,6]. In addition, enzyme activity is subject to diurnal variation, which is independent of the regulation by bile acid feedback[5,6]. Recent studies in rats have established that cholesterol 7α-hydroxylase activity is regulated primarily at a pretranslational level[9,10]. In addition to this major pathway, in which changes in the cholesterol-nucleus precede side-chain oxidation, an alternative route may exist for the formation of chenodeoxycholic acid. This route, which appears to exist in experimental animals[11,12] as well as in humans[13], involves initial 26-hydroxylation of cholesterol by mitochondria. The resulting 26-hydroxycholesterol is subsequently converted to chenodeoxycholic acid with the monohydroxy bile acids 3β-hydroxy-5-cholenoic acid and lithocholic acid as intermediates (Fig. 1). Thus, changes in the side-

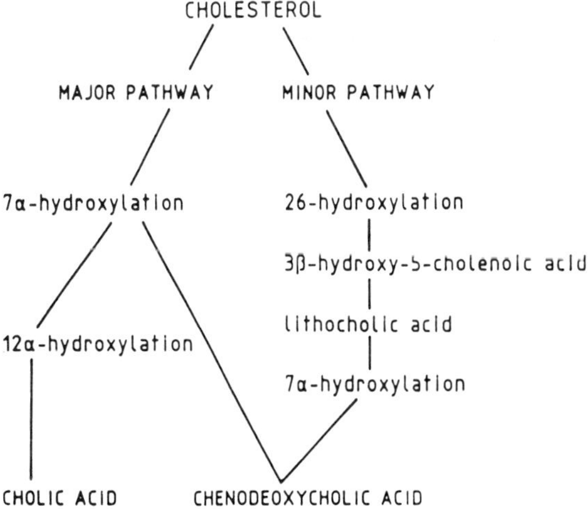

Fig. 1 Schematic overview of pathways in bile acid synthesis

chain precede modification of the nucleus in this biosynthetic pathway. The importance of this pathway is probably limited under normal conditions in humans: (a) cholic acid synthesis rate is higher than that of chenodeoxycholic acid in healthy subjects[14,15], and (b) the activity of cholesterol 26-hydroxylase, as assessed by determination of 26-hydroxycholesterol in serum, does not respond to treatment with the bile acid sequestrant colestipol[16]. However, the pathway appears to be of quantitative importance during the fetal/neonatal period (see below), as well as in children and adults with cholestatic liver disease[17–19].

As mentioned previously, the ontogeny of human bile acid metabolism has received considerable attention in recent years because of the specific nutritional problems encountered in newborns (in particular those of low birth weight), and the increasing recognition that abnormalities in bile acid synthetic pathways due to specific enzyme deficiencies may play a role in the aetiology of certain forms of cholestasis in newborns (see Chapter 15).

It is well established that fasting plasma levels of the primary bile acids are transiently elevated in normal neonates and infants during the first year of life[20,21]. In addition, the peak postprandial concentration of plasma bile acid is higher in infants than in older children[21]. These phenomena probably reflect the immaturity of hepatic bile acid transport and/or conjugation systems ('physiological cholestasis').

Meal-stimulated intraluminal bile acid concentrations are extremely low in premature infants when compared to full-term neonates[22,23]. A gradual but slight increase in intraluminal bile acid concentrations was found upon comparison of term newborns, infants (2–10 months), older children and adults (see ref. 21). Watkins *et al*[22] determined pool sizes and synthesis rates of cholic acid and chenodeoxycholic acid in premature infants between 32 and 36 weeks of gestation, using a stable isotope dilution technique with sampling of duodenal fluid. Pool size and synthesis rate of both primary bile acids were reduced 3–4-fold in the prematures when compared to full-term infants. Values obtained in this latter group were, in turn, about 3–5 times lower than those found in older infants[21] and approximately half of those estimated in adults[24], when expressed in terms of body surface area. Watkins *et al.*[23] also found that the bile acid pool, as well as the intraluminal bile acid concentrations, were significantly greater in preterm infants fed human milk as compared to those fed different infant formulas, while bile acid synthesis rates were comparable in the experimental groups. This suggests that human milk feeding influences intestinal and hepatic bile acid metabolism independent of developmental factors.

In addition to the marked quantitative differences in bile acid metabolism during the fetal/neonatal period, there are a number of striking qualitative differences, as revealed by detailed analysis of bile acid composition of fetal gallbladder bile[25,26], meconium[27–30], urine of newborns[31], and amniotic fluid[32]. The main message that emerges from these studies is that the bile acids found in the human fetus and newborn are remarkably diverse – more than 30 species have been identified until now – and, as a consequence, that the sequence of events in bile acid synthesis outlined previously is highly oversimplified.

Analysis of fetal gallbladder bile by 'state-of-the-art' analytical techniques[25,26] revealed the presence of cholic acid and chenodeoxycholic acid as early as the 14th week of gestation. Unlike the situation in the full-term infant and in adults, chenodeoxycholic acid appears to be the predominant bile acid synthesized and secreted by the fetal liver. This observation, together with the presence of 3β-hydroxy-5-cholenoic acid in fetal bile[25,26] and, in a relatively high proportion, in meconium[27] and in amniotic fluid[33], indicates that the 'alternative pathway' for the formation of chenodeoxycholic acid is of quantitative importance in early life. The monohydroxylated intermediates of this pathway, 3β-hydroxy-5-cholenoic acid and lithocholic acid, as well as their sulphated and glucuronidated derivatives, are potent cholestatic agents in experimental animals[33–37]. Potential means of the neonate to cope with these endogenous hepatotoxins are discussed elsewhere in this volume (see Chapter 4).

Besides the 'conventional' bile acids, a relatively large proportion of bile acids in fetal bile and meconium comprises metabolites usually not found in the adult situation. The presence of relatively high proportions of hyocholic acid ($3\alpha,6\alpha,7\alpha$-trihydroxy-5β-cholanoic acid) and several 1β-hydroxycholanoic acid isomers in fetal bile indicates that C-6 and C-1 hydroxylation are important pathways in fetal bile acid metabolism. In addition, Setchell *et al.*[25] provided evidence for the existence of a C-4 hydroxylation pathway by the identification in fetal bile of $3\alpha,4\beta,7\alpha$-trihydroxy-5β-cholanoic acid and $3\alpha,4\beta$-dihydroxy-5β-cholanoic acid. C-1 and C-6 hydroxylated bile acid species have also been identified in meconium[27]. Lester and associates[28–30] have established that, in addition to the described C_{24} bile acids, meconium contains a complex mixture of bile acids with 20 to 22 carbon atoms with a shortened side-chain. The origin and biosynthetic pathways of these compounds are unknown[30]; the finding that short-chain bile acids are present in meconium as glucuronide (and possibly sulphate) conjugates suggests that they are secreted by the fetal liver into bile. After intravenous injection in rats of radiolabelled hydroxyetianic acid, a monohydroxy C_{20} bile acid, the compound is rapidly secreted into bile as a mixture of carboxyl- and hydroxyl-linked glucuronides[38]; unlike the C_{24} monohydroxy bile acids mentioned previously, hydroxyetianic acid is a choleretic agent[39].

NEW APPROACHES IN HUMAN BILE ACID RESEARCH

Although much has been learned about human bile acid metabolism in the past two decades, many questions remain to be answered, in particular those concerning the metabolic adaptations that occur in response to disease and nutrition. A number of recently developed techniques that are used in our laboratory to address those questions will be discussed briefly in this section.

Human hepatocytes in primary culture

To gain further insight into the biochemical background of regulatory processes involved in human bile acid metabolism, procedures for isolation and culture of human hepatocytes have been developed in our laboratory, in collaboration with the 'Human Liver Group Groningen'. Hepatocytes are isolated from partly resected donor livers in the case of partial liver transplantation in children (transplantation programme Academic Hospital Groningen; head Prof. Dr M. J. H. Slooff). The livers are perfused with and stored in University of Wisconsin preservation solution for 3–40 h prior to the start of cell isolation. The isolation procedure is based on a calcium-free preperfusion followed by a collagenase perfusion[40]. When necessary, viable cells are separated from non-viable cells by centrifugation in a 36% Percoll solution at 100 g. The cells are cultured on six-well cluster plates as described[41] for up to 7 days. Initial studies were aimed at investigating the interactions of drugs with bile acid synthesis. It was found[41] that the antimycotic drug ketoconazole dose-dependently inhibited bile acid synthesis in cultured hepatocytes, giving half-maximal inhibition at a drug concentration of $10\,\mu\text{mol/l}$ in rat hepatocytes and at only $1\,\mu\text{mol/l}$ in human hepatocytes. Impaired bile acid synthesis was caused by inhibition of the activity of cholesterol 7α-hydroxylase. Bile acid synthesis was also potently inhibited by the immunosuppressive drug cyclosporin A; in this case the effect appeared to be mediated by inhibition of mitochondrial 26-hydroxylation of cholesterol[42].

Easy sampling of duodenal bile

Duodenal intubation to collect bile is a cumbersome procedure, especially for use in children. In addition, it is not easily applicable in longitudinal studies when serial samples are required to evaluate time-dependent effects of a certain treatment. To overcome this problem we have developed a simple, well-tolerated method for the collection of duodenal juice[43] making

Table 1 Bile acid composition (%) in duodenal juice obtained by Entero-Test from patients with cystic fibrosis without overt hepatic complications, patients with active Crohn's disease, and patients with benign recurrent intrahepatic cholestasis (BRIC) during a symptom-free period

Disease	n	CA	CDCA	DCA	LCA
Cystic fibrosis	19	56 ± 10	40 ± 9	4 ± 4	tr
Crohn's disease	5	62 ± 8	37 ± 7	2 ± 2	tr
BRIC	11	40 ± 21	36 ± 9	23 ± 19	tr

CA = cholic acid; CDCA = chenodeoxycholic acid; DCA = deoxycholic acid; LCA = lithocholic acid; tr = trace amounts.

use of the commercially available Entero-Test (HDC Corp., Mountain View, CA). Entero-Test, originally developed for diagnosis of enteral parasites, consists of an encapsulated thread, which is swallowed by a fasting subject with water while the end of the thread is taped at a corner of the mouth. The capsule dissolves in the stomach and the thread passes into the duodenum. After 4 h the thread is withdrawn and stored at 4°C until analysis. The adsorbed duodenal juice is eluted and can be used for analysis of bile acid pool composition[43] and/or determination of pancreatic enzyme activities (Smit *et al.*, unpublished results). The procedure is easily applicable, well tolerated and can be performed at home. A small version of the Entero-Test is available for use in children. In addition, a home-made version for use in newborns has been developed. The method has been used in our laboratory to study effects of dietary components, e.g. calcium[44], and the effects of various hepatic and gastrointestinal disorders on bile acid pool composition. Table 1 shows bile acid pool composition in paediatric patients with cystic fibrosis without hepatic complications, Crohn's disease, and benign recurrent intrahepatic cholestasis (BRIC) in a symptom-free period. All three disorders are associated with increased faecal bile acid loss due to malabsorption[4,45,46]; yet the duodenal bile acid composition of BRIC patients is characterized by increased amounts of deoxycholic acid, whereas deoxycholic acid is low in cystic fibrosis and Crohn patients. This, to our opinion, is an indication for a specific localization of defective bile acid absorption in BRIC, presumably in the small intestine.

GC–MS and GC–IRMS for metabolic studies

Determination of the kinetics of primary bile acids (poolsize, fractional turnover rate, synthesis rate) after dilution of the pool with stable isotope-labelled bile acids (i.e. the non-radioactive isotopes ^{13}C and ^{2}H) has become a well-established procedure[3,14,15,21–24,47–49], also for use in children[3,15,21–23]. In this procedure the decay of isotopic enrichment of the bile acids after oral administration of ^{13}C- or ^{2}H-labelled marker bile acids, measured by gas liquid chromatography–mass spectrometry and selected ion monitoring, is used for the calculation of the kinetic parameters. Recent developments in methodology (e.g. extraction procedures, capillary gas chromatography) allow determination of the isotopic enrichments in serum[14,15,47–49], which

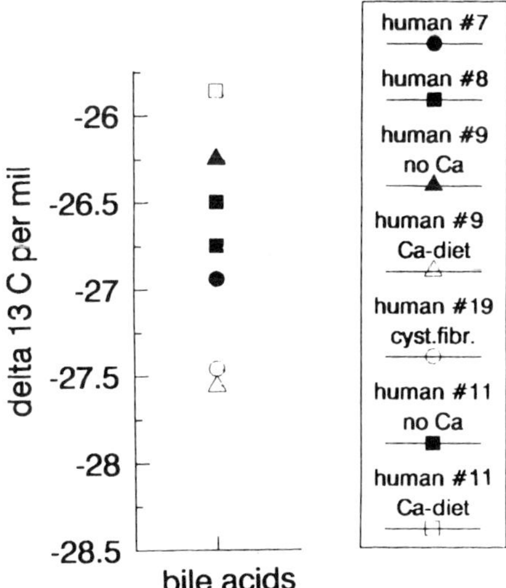

Fig. 2 Isotopic ratio (in delta $^{13}C_{PBD}$) of bile acids in duodenal juice obtained by Entero-Test

makes serial bile collections redundant and also allows studies to be performed on an outpatient basis. By making a proper choice of marker bile acids it is possible to determine the kinetics of the three major bile acids in humans, i.e. cholic, chenodeoxycholic and deoxycholic acids, simultaneously[49].

Isotope ratio mass spectrometry (IRMS), traditionally used for the measurement of natural variations in the $^{13}C/^{12}C$ ratio, is a technique that has not found an application in bile acid research so far. However, the recent development of a continuous-flow introduction method, in which the eluate of a gas chromatograph is directly introduced into the isotope ratio mass spectrometer after on-line combustion (GC-C-IRMS)[50], offers a number of interesting possibilities. In $^{13}C/^{12}C$ IRMS each compound is combusted to CO_2, of which the ratio is subsequently measured. This offers two advantages towards the achievement of high precision and accuracy: the ratio is measured by a triple Faraday cup, adjusted for the simultaneous recording of masses 44 ($^{12}C^{16}O_2$), 45 ($^{13}C^{16}O_2$) and 46 ($^{12}C^{16}O^{18}O$), and one can always use the same working standard gas (CO_2) to calibrate. GC-C-IRMS allows accurate determination of enrichments orders of magnitude lower than with GC-MS. In Figs 2 and 3 some preliminary results of studies employing this technique are shown. Figure 2 shows the natural variation in the $^{13}C/^{12}C$ ratio of bile acids in human bile sampled by Entero-Test. The scale is in delta $^{13}C_{PDB}$ values, i.e. the relative difference of the measured ratio compared to that of an international standard (PDB = Pee Dee belemnite limestone) given in parts per thousand. No differences between the three major bile acids (cholic, chenodeoxycholic and deoxycholic acids) were seen within a single subject. The values obtained from seven analyses in five different subjects fell within a relatively small range. No consistent effect of calcium supplementation (35.5 mmol/day for 2 weeks), which leads to a 50% increase

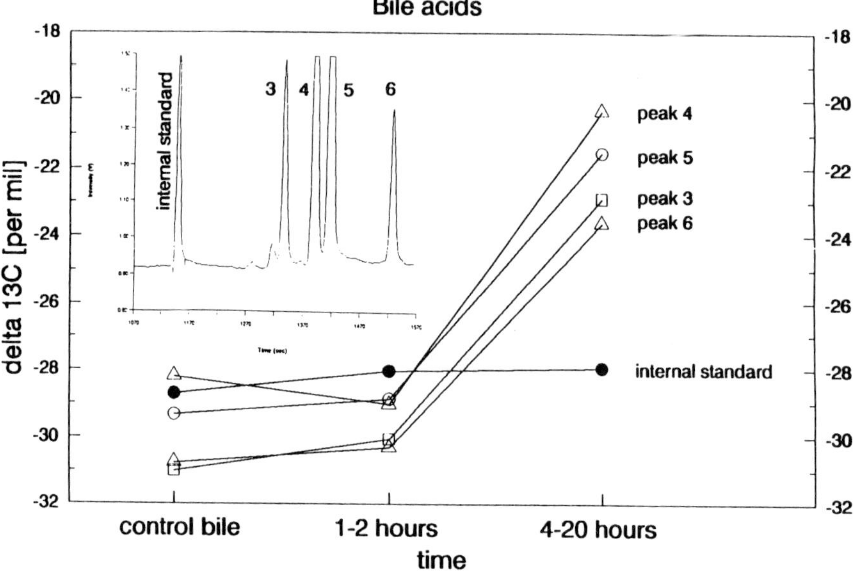

Fig. 3 Isotopic ratio (in delta $^{13}C_{PBD}$) of biliary bile acids in a rat with chronic bile diversion before and after intravenous administration of 50 μg of ^{13}C-labelled cholesterol in an ethanolic solution. Bile was collected from 1 to 2 h and from 4 to 20 h after injection. Insert shows a representative chromatogram ($^{12}C^{16}O_2{}^+$ ion current, m/z 44). Peak numbers are: 3 = α-muricholic acid, 4 = chenodeoxycholic acid, 5 = cholic acid, 6 = β-muricholic acid, internal standard = coprostanol

in faecal bile acid excretion[44], was observed. The value obtained from a cystic fibrosis patient fell within the same range as those from the healthy subjects. These data indicate that the natural variation in the $^{13}C/^{12}C$ ratio of the cholesterol precursor pools of these subjects was very similar, probably as a result of similar dietary habits. Intravenous injection of a small amount of ^{13}C-labelled cholesterol (50 μg) into a rat with chronic bile diversion resulted in a marked increase in delta $^{13}C_{PDB}$ values of all four primary bile acids (α-muricholic, β-muricholic, chenodeoxycholic and cholic acids) within a few hours. The fact that a similar increase was found for all bile acids does not favour the existence of separate cholesterol precursor pools for the formation of the individual bile acid species that depend to a varying degree upon *de novo* cholesterol synthesis. However, it should be kept in mind that long-term bile diversion markedly alters hepatic cholesterol and bile acid metabolism in comparison to the physiological situation. Although the presented results are preliminary, it is our opinion that GC-C-IRMS provides a promising tool for unravelling metabolic pathways involved in bile acid metabolism in health and disease.

Acknowledgements

Studies from our laboratory presented herein are supported by the Groningen Institute for Drug Studies (GIDS) and the Netherlands Heart Foundation.

References

1. Lester R. Physiologic cholestasis. Gastroenterology. 1980;78:864–5.
2. Balistreri WF, Heubi JE, Suchy FJ. Immaturity of the enterohepatic circulation in early life: factors predisposing to physiologic maldigestion and cholestasis. J Pediatr Gastroenterol Nutr. 1983;2:346–54.
3. Bijleveld CMA, Vonk RJ, Kuipers F, Havinga R, Boverhof R, Koopman BJ, Wolthers BG, Fernandes J. Benign recurrent intrahepatic cholestasis; altered bile acid metabolism. Gastroenterology. 1989;97:427–32.
4. Nagakawa M, Colombo C, Setchell KDR. Comprehensive study of the biliary bile acid composition of patients with cystic fibrosis and associated liver disease before and after UDCA administration. Hepatology. 1990;12:322–34.
5. Bjorkhem I. Mechanisms of bile acid biosynthesis in mammalian liver. In Danielsson H, Sjovall J, editors. Sterols and bile acids. Amsterdam: Elsevier; 1985:231–77.
6. Danielsson H, Wikvall K. Biosynthesis of bile acids. In Fears R, Sabine JR, editors. Cholesterol 7α-hydroxylase (7α-monooxygenase). Boca Raton: CRC Press; 1986:9–19.
7. Carey MC, Small DM, Bliss CM. Lipid digestion and absorption. Ann Rev Physiol. 1983;45:651–77.
8. Hofmann AF. Chemistry and enterohepatic circulation of bile acids. Hepatology, 1984;4:45–145.
9. Jelinek DF, Andersson S, Slaughter CA, Russell DW. Cloning and regulation of cholesterol 7α-hydroxylase, the rate-limiting enzyme in bile acid biosynthesis. J Biol Chem. 1990;265:8190–7.
10. Sundseth SS, Waxman DJ. Hepatic P-450 cholesterol 7α-hydroxylase. Regulation in vivo at the protein and mRNA level in response to mevanolate, diurnal rhythm, and bile acid feedback. J Biol Chem. 1990;265:15090–5.
11. Kok E, Burstein S, Javitt NB, Gut M, Byon GY. Bile acid synthesis. Metabolism of 3β-hydroxy-5-cholenoic acid in the hamster. J Biol Chem. 1981;256:6155–9.
12. Mitropoulos KA, Myant NB. The formation of lithocholic acid, chenodeoxycholic acid, and other bile acids from 3β-hydroxychol-5-enic acid in vitro and in vivo. Biochim Biophys Acta. 1967;144:430–9.
13. Anderson KE, Kok E, Javitt NB. Bile acid synthesis in man: metabolism of 7α-hydroxy-cholesterol-^{14}C and 26-hydroxycholesterol-[3]H. J Clin Invest. 1972;51:112–17.
14. Stellaard F, Sackmann M, Sauerbruch T, Paumgartner G. Simultaneous determination of cholic acid and chenodeoxycholic acid pool sizes and fractional turnover in human serum using ^{13}C-labeled bile acids. J Lipid Res. 1984;25:1313–19.
15. Koopman BJ, Kuipers F, Bijleveld CMA, van der Molen JC, Nage GT, Vonk RJ, Wolthers BG. Determination of cholic acid and chenodeoxycholic acid pool sizes and fractional turnover rates by means of stable isotope dilution technique, making use of deuterated cholic acid and chenodeoxycholic acid. Clin Chim Acta. 1988;175:143–56.
16. Van Doormaal JJ, Smit N, Koopman BJ, van der Molen JC, Wolthers BG, Doorenbos H. Hydroxycholesterols in serum from hypercholesterolemic patients with and without bile acid sequestrant therapy. Clin Chim Acta. 1989;181:273–80.
17. Bremmelgaard A, Sjovall J. Bile acid profiles in urine of patients with liver diseases. Eur J Clin Invest. 1979;9:341–8.
18. Back P. Identification and quantitative determination of urinary bile acids excreted in cholestasis. Clin Chim Acta. 1973;44:199–207.
19. Nemeth A, Strandvik B. Excretion of tetrahydroxylated bile acids in children with alpha-1-antitrypsin deficiency. Scand J Lab Invest. 1984;44:387–92.
20. Suchy FJ, Balistreri WF, Heubi JE. Physiologic cholestasis: elevation of the primary serum bile acids in normal infants. Gastroenterology. 1980;79:1057.

21. Heubi JE, Balistreri WF, Suchy FJ. Bile salt metabolism in the first year of life. J Lab Clin Med. 1982;100:127–36.
22. Watkins JB, Szczepanik P, Gould JB, Klein P, Lester R. Bile salt metabolism in the human premature infant. Gastroenterology. 1975;69:706–13.
23. Watkins JB, Jarvenpaa AL, Szczepanik-van Leeuwen P, Klein PD, Rassin DK, Gaull G, Rassin NCR. Feeding the low-birth weight infant: V. Effects of taurine, cholesterol, and human milk on bile acid kinetics. Gastroenterology. 1983;85:793–800.
24. Vlahcevic ZR, Miller JR, Farrar JT, Swell L. Kinetics and pool size of primary bile acids in man. Gastroenterology. 1971;61:85–90.
25. Setchell KDR, Dumaswala R, Colombo C, Ronchi M. Hepatic bile acid metabolism during early development revealed from the analysis of human fetal gallbladder bile. J Biol Chem. 1988;263:16637–44.
26. Colombo C, Zuliani G, Ronchi M, Breidenstein J, Setchell KDR. Biliary bile acid composition of the human fetus in early gestation. Pediatr Res. 1987;21:197–200.
27. Back P, Walter K. Developmental pattern of bile acid metabolism as revealed by bile acid analysis of meconium. Gastroenterology. 1980;78:671–6.
28. Pyrek J St, Lester R, Adcock EW, Sanghvi AT. Constituents of human meconium. I. Identification of 3-hydroxyetianic acids. J Steroid Biochem. 1983;18:341–51.
29. Pyrek J St, Sterzycki R, Lester R, Adcock EW. Constituents of human meconium. II. Identification of steroidal acids with 21 and 22 carbon atoms. Lipids. 1982;17:241–9.
30. Lester R, Pyrek J St, Little JM, Adcock EW. Diversity of bile acids in the fetus and newborn infants. J Pediatr Gastroenterol Nutr. 1983;2:355–64.
31. Back P. Urinary bile acids. In: Setchell KDR, Kritchevsky D, Nair PP, editors. The bile acids, vol. 4. New York: Plenum; 1988:405–40.
32. Nagakawa M, Setchell KDR. Bile acid metabolism in early life: studies of amniotic fluid. J Lipid Res. 1990;31:1089–98.
33. Javitt NB, Emerman S. Effects of sodium taurolithocholate on bile flow and bile acid excretion. J Clin Invest. 1968;47:1002–14.
34. Miyai K, Richardson AL, Mayr W, Javitt NB. Subcellular pathology of rat liver in cholestasis and choleresis induced by bile salts. I. Effects of lithocholic, 3β-hydroxy-5-cholenoic, cholic, and dehydrocholic acids. Lab Invest. 1977;36:249–58.
35. Oelberg DG, Chari MV, Little JM, Adcock EW, Lester R. Lithocholate glucuronide is a cholestatic agent. J Clin Invest. 1984;73:1507–14.
36. Yousef IM, Tuchweber B, Vonk RJ, Masse D, Audet M, Roy CC. Lithocholate cholestasis-sulfated glycolithocholate-induced intrahepatic cholestasis in rats. Gastroenterology. 1981;80:233–41.
37. Van der Meer R, Vonk RJ, Kuipers F. Cholestasis and the interactions of sulfated glyco- and taurolithocholate with calcium. Am J Physiol. 1988;254:G644–9.
38. Kuipers F, Radominska A, Zimniak P, Little JM, Havinga R, Vonk RJ, Lester R. Defective biliary secretion of bile acid 3-O-glucuronides in rats with hereditary conjugated hyperbilirubinemia. J Lipid Res. 1989;30:1835–45.
39. Little JM, Pyrek J St, Lester R. Hepatic metabolism of 3-alpha-hydroxy-5-beta-etianic acid (3-alpha-hydroxy-5-beta-androstan-17-beta-carboxylic acid) in the adult rat. J Clin Invest. 1983;71:73–80.
40. Sandker GW, Weert B, Slooff MJH, Groothuis GMM. Preservation of isolated rat and human hepatocytes in UW solution. Transplant Proc. 1990;22:2204–5.
41. Princen HMG, Huijsmans CMG, Kuipers F, Vonk RJ, Kempen HJM. Ketoconazole blocks bile acid synthesis in hepatocyte monolayer cultures and *in vivo* in rat by inhibiting cholesterol 7α-hydroxylase. J Clin Invest. 1986;78:1064–71.
42. Princen HMG, Meijer P, Wolthers BG, Vonk RJ, Kuipers F. Cyclosporin A blocks bile acid synthesis in cultured hepatocytes by specific inhibition of chenodeoxycholic acid synthesis. Biochem J. 1991;275:501–5.
43. Vonk RJ, Kneepkens CMF, Havinga R, Kuipers F, Bijleveld CMA. Enterohepatic circulation in man. A simple method for the determination of duodenal bile acids. J Lipid Res. 1986;27:901–4.
44. Van der Meer R, Welberg JWM, Kuipers F, Kleibeuker JH, Mulder NH, Termont DSML, Vonk RJ, de Vries HT, de Vries EGE. Effects of supplemental dietary calcium on the intestinal association of calcium phosphate and bile acids. Gastroenterology. 1990;99:653–9.

45. Fondacaro JD, Heubi JE, Kellogg FW. Intestinal bile acid malabsorption in cystic fibrosis: a primary mucosal cell defect. Pediatr Res. 1982;16:494–8.
46. Rutgeerts P, Ghoos Y, Vantrappen G. Bile acid studies in patients with Crohn's colitis. Gut. 1979;20:1072–7.
47. Stellaard F, Schubert R, Paumgartner G. Measurement of bile acid kinetics in human serum using stable isotope labeled chenodeoxycholic acid and capillary gas chromatography electron impact mass spectrometry. Biomed Mass Spectrom. 1983;10:187–91.
48. Stellaard F, Sackmann M, Berr F, Paumgartner G. Simultaneous determination of pool sizes and fractional turnover rates of deoxycholic acid in man by isotope dilution with ^{2}H and ^{13}C labels and serum sampling. Biochem Environ Mass Spectrom. 1987;14:609–11.
49. Berr F, Stellaard F, Pratschke E, Paumgartner G. Effects of cholecystectomy on the kinetics of primary and secondary bile acids. J Clin Invest. 1989;83:1541–50.
50. Rautenschlein M, Habfast K, Brand W. High-precision measurement of ^{13}C/^{12}C ratios by on-line combustion of GC eluates and isotope ratio mass spectrometry. In Chapman TE, Berger R, Reijngoud DJ, Okken A, editors. Stable isotopes in paediatric nutritional and metabolic research. Andover: Intercept; 1990:133–48.

4
Mechanism of resistance of the neonate to the experimental induction of cholestasis

P. ZIMNIAK, A. RADOMINSKA, F. KUIPERS, Y. C. AWASTHI, R. VONK and R. LESTER

'Physiological cholestasis' occurs in the newborn as the result of immaturity of the hepatic and intestinal mechanisms necessary to maintain adequate bile salt composition, secretion, and bile flow[1–12]. The associated phenomena have been well demonstrated in experimental animals and in humans, and their biological basis is presently being examined using the techniques of cell and molecular biology[13–16]. In contrast, it is less generally appreciated that neonatal animals are resistant to the experimental induction of cholestasis using such cholestatic agents as lithocholic acid. So, for example, in 2-week-old guinea pigs doses of lithocholic acid that are cholestatic in the adult animal failed to decrease bile flow, and the administered lithocholic acid was efficiently secreted into bile[17,18]. Similarly, in 2- and 3-week-old rats lithocholic acid was not cholestatic and, in contrast to adult animals, was not retained in the liver[19]. While the resistance to induction of cholestasis in the neonate has been observed, no satisfactory explanation of the observation has been advanced. On the contrary, the resistance to induction of cholestasis in animals maturationally susceptible to cholestasis presents something of an enigma.

In this review, two hypotheses are offered to provide an explanation for the observed neonatal resistance to the experimental induction of cholestasis. The first outlines a possible mechanism of resistance based on maturational differences in the metabolism of bile acid loads in the newborn. The second suggests, in analogy to the mutant GY rat, a mechanism related to potential differences in organic anion transport by the newborn. It should be emphasized that these hypotheses are based on studies in their preliminary stages, and that they are not intended to exclude other hypothetical mechanisms.

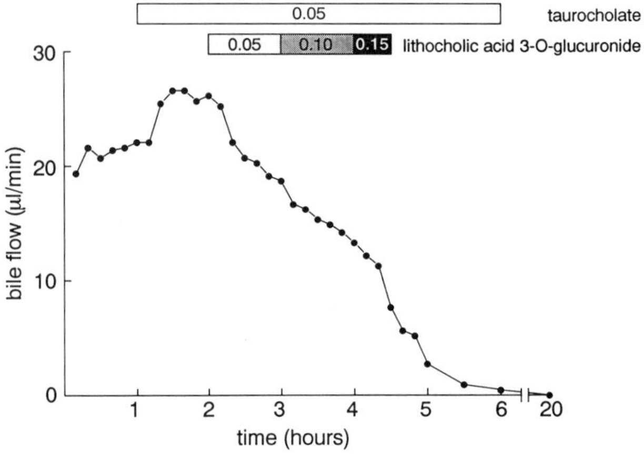

Fig. 1 Structures of lithocholic acid 3-*O*-glucuronide (**A**) and lithocholic acid carboxyl-linked glucuronide (**B**)

Fig. 2 Cholestatic properties of lithocholic acid 3-*O*-glucuronide. A rat prepared with an external biliary fistula was infused with taurocholate and increasing concentrations of lithocholic acid 3-*O*-glucuronide. The infusion protocol is shown as bars in the figure; the values indicate doses in μmol/min per 100 g body weight. (Adapted from ref. 23)

LITHOCHOLIC ACID GLUCURONIDATION IN THE DEVELOPING RAT

Lithocholic acid administered intravenously in milligram quantities to adult rats diminishes bile flow[20,21]. As much as one-third of the lithocholic acid administered which is secreted in bile is secreted in the form of the 3-*O*-glucuronide (Fig. 1)[22]. These observations are of importance: studies of the direct intravenous injection of lithocholic acid 3-*O*-glucuronide into adult rats prepared with an external biliary fistula establish that this derivative of lithocholic acid is, itself, a cholestatic agent (Fig. 2)[23]. Indeed, it is three to four times more potent as a cholestatic agent than the parent compound, and apparently is the most potent cholestatic bile acid thus far characterized[21]. The phase II conversion of lithocholic acid to its hydroxyl-linked glucuronide, unlike most phase II biotransformations, thus potentiates, rather than

40

diminishes, toxicity, perhaps by preventing further metabolism, e.g. hydroxylation.

The hydroxyl group of lithocholic acid is only one of two possible sites for glucuronidation of the molecule. Glucuronidation of lithocholic acid, and indeed of any bile acid, might also potentially occur at the C-24 carboxyl group (Fig. 1). In order to provide a definitive demonstration of the biosynthesis of the carboxyl-linked glucuronide of lithocholic acid, and to characterize its behaviour, it would be essential to establish reliable methods for its purification from biological material, as well as to synthesize chemically and to radiolabel the compound. While protected lithocholic acid carboxyl-linked glucuronide (preparations with acetylated hydroxyl and methylated carboxyl groups) had been synthesized[24], it had not been possible previously to obtain free lithocholic acid carboxyl-linked glucuronide.

This problem has now been overcome, and free, radiolabelled lithocholic acid carboxyl-linked glucuronide has been prepared (I. Panfil et al., submitted). The material is radiochemically pure and identical by HPLC–MS to lithocholic acid carboxyl-linked glucuronide prepared biosynthetically. The compound is relatively alkali-labile, and it is extremely susceptible to transesterification. Complete transesterification is observed in methanol after 7 days at $-25°C$. It can be anticipated that the identification of a compound with such properties in human biological samples would be extremely difficult, especially since methanol is commonly used in preparative and analytical procedures involving bile acids; thus, the failure to observe carboxyl-linked glucuronides in such samples thus far does not exclude it as a human metabolite. Lithocholic acid carboxyl-linked glucuronide has, moreover, now been identified *in vitro* in experimental animals as a product of microsomal lithocholic acid metabolism (I. Panfil et al., submitted). Furthermore, studies of lithocholic acid metabolism by human liver microsomes also demonstrate the formation of the carboxyl-linked glucuronide (unpublished observation). Such activities are only one-third the activity of the 6-O-glucuronidation of 6-hydroxylated bile acids by human liver microsomes. The formation of lithocholic acid carboxyl-linked glucuronide by human liver microsomes is, however, roughly equal to the formation of the 3-O-glucuronide.

As noted above, the 3-O-glucuronide of lithocholic acid is secreted in bile after intravenous injection and is a potent cholestatic agent (Fig. 2). Recent studies have demonstrated that the carboxyl-linked glucuronide of lithocholic acid is also rapidly secreted in bile after intravenous injection (unpublished observations). In contrast to the 3-O-glucuronide, however, the carboxyl-linked glucuronide of lithocholic acid is not a cholestatic agent. Thus, the positional isomerism of the glucuronide leads to a major difference in biological behaviour. If the neonatal experimental animal had a mechanism for the avoidance of the formation of the hydroxyl-linked glucuronide and the promotion of the formation of the carboxyl-linked glucuronide, it would have a potential means for resistance to the induction of cholestasis by lithocholic acid. This consideration led us to an examination of the development of the enzymes necessary for the formation of the two forms of lithocholic acid glucuronide (unpublished observations). In brief, microsomes from rats from 1 day to 62 days of age were incubated under appropriate conditions with lithocholic acid and UDP-glucuronic acid. The glucuronidated products were separated and the activities for hydroxyl- and carboxyl-linked lithocholic acid glucuronide formation were assessed. Hydroxyl-linked glucuronide formation was not measurable at birth and became measurable only after weaning. It increased thereafter to maximal values after 62 days. In contrast, carboxyl-linked glucuronide forming activity was present at birth and increased only two-fold during development. At 62 days hydroxyl-linked glucuronide formation was many-fold greater than carboxyl-linked glucuronide formation.

These developmental differences give an advantage to the neonate in resistance to the experimental induction of cholestasis with lithocholic acid. In sum, on the basis of these developmental enzymological studies, it would be predicted that while the adult synthesizes both glucuronide conjugates of lithocholic acid when given a load of lithocholic acid, the neonate lacks the enzymatic apparatus for the formation of the potent cholestatic 3-*O*-glucuronide and can be anticipated to form only the non-cholestatic carboxyl-linked glucuronide. The resistance of the neonate to induction of cholestasis by lithocholic acid may thus, in part, be due to the developmental enzymology of glucuronidation.

THE CANALICULAR TRANSPORT OF LITHOCHOLIC ACID GLUCURONIDES

A second potential explanation of neonatal resistance to induction of cholestasis by lithocholic acid relates to canalicular organic ion transport. Several proteins responsible for such transport have been characterized. The multidrug resistance gene products, P-glycoproteins, function as canalicular ATPases/transporters for positively charged, hydrophobic compounds, a number of which are commonly used chemotherapeutic agents. Similarly, a previously isolated and partially characterized taurocholate transporter may correspond to a 110 kD ATPase/transporter recently isolated from canalicular membranes, reconstituted, and shown to promote ATP-dependent uptake of taurocholate into liposomes. Until recently, however, little has been known about the mechanism of the canalicular transport of organic anions other than conventional conjugated bile acids. This conceptual hiatus has been important, since many of the most potent cholestatic agents appear to be transported by the putative organic anion transporter. It has now been shown that canalicular transport for a set of divalent organic anions is dependent on an ATPase with substrate specificity distinct from the other canalicular transporting ATPases mentioned above[25,26]. Both transport and enzymic (ATPase) activities for this mechanism have been demonstrated in canalicular membranes using suitable organic anion substrates including conjugated bilirubin and dinitrophenylglutathione[25,27–32]. A similar or identical ATPase has been isolated from human red blood cell plasma membranes and partially characterized[33–38]. A defect in the transport activity has been demonstrated in canalicular membranes from mutant rats with congenital conjugated hyperbilirubinaemia (variously designated GY, TR, and EHBR)[25,39–42].

In recent studies we have begun the molecular characterization of the canalicular organic anion transporter/ATPase. We have established that a polyclonal antibody directed against the transporter/ATPase of human red blood cells crossreacts with a protein (or proteins) in detergent extracts of mixed or canalicular, but not sinusoidal human and rat membranes[37,43]. Using SDS-PAGE and Western blotting techniques[43], a 28–30 kD protein(s) has been defined in rat liver canalicular membrane extracts subjected to affinity chromatography on dinitrophenylglutathione-Sepharose and ATP-Sepharose. Confirmation of this finding has been provided by synthesizing a photoaffinity probe for the organic anion transporter. The probe, azidonitrophenyl-[^{35}S]glutathione, was used to label the 28–30 kD protein band in both total membrane extracts and affinity chromatography-purified preparations. These studies were further corroborated by the application of 8-azido-ATP as a photoaffinity probe for the transporter/ATPase. The results suggest that the 28–30 kD protein(s) is a subunit or fragment of the organic anion transporter/ATPase with the antigenic properties and binding sites for both substrates (ATP and glutathione conjugates) preserved. Thus far, the methods used have not allowed for the identification of differences between transporters of mutant GY and control animals.

As has been shown both *in vivo*[40–42,44–46] and *in vitro*[25,30,41,42], the secretion of such organic divalent anions as bilirubin diglucuronide, dinitrophenyl-glutathione, and the divalent sulphates and glucuronides of bile acids, is defective in the GY rat. The 3-*O*-glucuronide of lithocholic acid is a divalent anion and, although uptake by the hepatocyte appears to be normal, it is defectively secreted into bile after intravenous administration to the GY rat. (It might be noted that the carboxyl-linked glucuronide of lithocholic acid is a monovalent anion, and is secreted at near normal rates by the GY rat (unpublished observations).) In addition, lithocholic acid 3-*O*-glucuronide is a potent cholestatic agent in control animals, but it fails to produce cholestasis in the GY rat when administered intravenously at comparable doses. Similar results were obtained with sulphated glycolithocholic acid, another divalent lithocholic acid conjugate which is poorly secreted in the GY mutant[39]. Sulphated glycolithocholic acid readily induces cholestasis in control rats, a process which coincides with the appearance of insoluble calcium-sulphated glycolithocholic acid precipitates in the bile[47,48], but fails to do so in the GY rat[48]. For these and other similar cholestatic agents the dictum would therefore appear to be: no secretion, no cholestasis. Thus an organism which had defective canalicular secretion of divalent organic anions might have a mechanism of resistance to the induction of cholestasis with lithocholic acid. Lithocholic acid 3-*O*-glucuronide would not be secreted into bile and would not produce cholestasis. Studies performed *in vivo* suggest that newborn animals have a defect for the canalicular secretion of organic anions similar to that found in the GY rat. These need to be confirmed by the characterization of the defect through work performed at the membrane and molecular level. If the defect is indeed shown to be functionally similar to that of the GY rat, it will be possible to hypothesize a similar resistance to the induction of cholestasis with lithocholic acid.

In summary, we propose two hypotheses to explain the resistance of the newborn animal to cholestasis induced with lithocholic acid. First, differences in enzymic development prevent the formation of the potent cholestatic agent, lithocholic acid 3-*O*-glucuronide, and promote the formation of the non-cholestatic carboxyl-linked glucuronide. Second, probable developmental retardation of the activity of the organic anion transporter prevents the secretion of lithocholic acid 3-*O*-glucuronide and, as an associated phenomenon, prevents its induction of cholestasis. These hypotheses are being tested by further experimental analysis.

References

1. de Belle RC, Vaupshas V, Vitullo BB, Haber LR, Shaffer E, Mackie GG, Owen H, Little JM, Lester R. Intestinal absorption of bile salts: immature development in the neonate. J Pediatr. 1979;94:472–6.
2. Lester R. Physiologic cholestasis. Gastroenterology. 1980;78:864–5.
3. Lester R, Smallwood RA, Little JM, Brown AS, Piasecki GJ, Jackson BT. Fetal bile salt metabolism. The intestinal absorption of bile salt. J Clin Invest. 1977;59:1009–16.
4. Little JM, Lester R. Ontogenesis of intestinal bile salt absorption in the neonatal rat. Am J Physiol. 1980;239:G319–23.
5. Little JM, Richey JE, Van Thiel DJ, Lester R. Taurocholate pool size and distribution in the fetal rat. J Clin Invest. 1979;63:1042–9.
6. Morris AI, Little JM, Lester R. Development of the bile acid pool in rats from neonatal life through puberty to maturity. Digestion. 1983;28:216–24.
7. Lester R. Bile acid metabolism in the newborn. J Pediatr Gastroenterol Nutr. 1983;2:335–6.
8. Lester R, Little JM, Adcock EW. Atypical bile acids and their possible role in neonatal diarrhea. In: Lebenthal E, editor. Chronic diarrhea in children. New York: Raven Press; 1984:365–9.
9. Lester R, Pyrek J St, Little JM, Adcock EW. Nature of bile acids in the fetus and newborn infant. J Pediatr Gastroenterol Nutr. 1983; Suppl. 2:S197–206.
10. Lester R, Pyrek J St, Little JM, Adcock EW. Diversity of bile acids in the fetus and newborn infant. J Pediatr Gastroenterol Nutr. 1983;2:355–64.
11. Watkins JB, Ingall D, Szczepanik P, Klein PD, Lester R. Bile-salt metabolism in the newborn. Measurement of pool size and synthesis by stable isotope technique. N Engl J Med. 1973;288:431–4.
12. Zimniak P, Lester R. Bile acid metabolism in the perinatal period. In: Lebenthal E, editor. Human gastrointestinal development. New York: Raven Press; 1989:561–80.
13. Ruetz S, Hugentobler G, Meier PJ. Functional reconstitution of the canalicular bile salt transport system of rat liver. Proc Natl Acad Sci USA. 1988;85:6147–51.
14. Hagenbuch B, Lubbert H, Stieger B, Meier PJ. Expression of the hepatocyte Na$^+$/bile acid cotransporter in *Xenopus laevis* oocytes. J Biol Chem. 1990;265:5357–60.
15. Yousef IM, Tuchweber B, Weber A. Prevention of lithocholate-induced cholestasis by cycloheximide, an inhibitor of protein synthesis. Life Sci. 1983;33:103–10.
16. Yousef IM, Tuchweber B, Weber A, Roy CC. Contribution of the fluid phase endocytosis to bile flow in cholestasis and choleresis in rats. Proc Soc Exp Biol Med. 1988;189:147–51.
17. Lewittes M, Tuchweber B, Weber A, Roy CC, Yousef IM. Resistance of the suckling guinea pig to lithocholic acid-induced cholestasis. Hepatology. 1984;4:486–91.
18. Tuchweber B, Ducruet N, Perea A, Yousef IM, Weber AM. Development of bile secretory function in the neonatal guinea pig. Biol Neonate. 1990;58:279–90.
19. Tuchweber B, Perea A, Lee D, Yousef IM. Lithocholic acid-induced cholestasis in newborn rats. Toxicol Lett. 1983;19:107–12.
20. Miyai K, Mayr WW, Richardson AL. Acute cholestasis induced by lithocholic acid in the rat. Lab Invest. 1975;32:527–35.
21. Oelberg DG, Lester R. Cellular mechanisms of cholestasis. Annu Rev Med. 1986;37:297–317.

22. Little JM, Zimniak P, Shattuck KE, Lester R, Radominska A. Metabolism of lithocholic acid in the rat: Formation of lithocholic acid 3-*O*-glucuronide in vivo. J Lipid Res. 1990;31:615–22.
23. Oelberg DG, Chari MV, Little JM, Adcock EW, Lester R. Lithocholate glucuronide is a cholestatic agent. J Clin Invest. 1984;73:1507–14.
24. Radominska-Pyrek A, Zimniak P, Chari M, Golunski E, Lester R, Pyrek JS. Glucuronides of monohydroxylated bile acids: specificity of microsomal glucuronyltransferase for the glucuronidation site, C-3 configuration, and side chain length. J Lipid Res. 1986;27:89–101.
25. Kitamura T, Jansen P, Hardenbrook C, Kamimoto Y, Gatmaitan Z, Arias IM. Defective ATP-dependent bile canalicular transport of organic anions in mutant (TR-) rats with conjugated hyperbilirubinemia. Proc Natl Acad Sci. USA. 1990;87:3557–61.
26. Oude Elferink RPJ, Ottenhoff R, Radominska A, Hofmann AF, Kuipers F, Jansen PLM. Inhibition of glutathione-conjugate secretion from isolated hepatocytes by dipolar bile acids and other organic anions. Biochem J. 1991;274:281–6.
27. Kobayashi K, Sogame Y, Hayashi K, Nicotera P, Orrenius S. ATP stimulates the uptake of S-dinitrophenylglutathione by rat liver plasma membrane vesicles. FEBS Lett. 1988;240:55–8.
28. Oude Elferink RPJ, Ottenhoff R, Liefting WGM, Schoemaker B, Groen AK, Jansen PLM. ATP-dependent efflux of GSSG and GS-conjugate from isolated rat hepatocytes. Am J Physiol Gastrointest Liver Physiol. 1990;258:G699–706.
29. Kobayashi K, Sogame Y, Hara H, Hayashi K. Mechanism of glutathione S-conjugate transport in canalicular and basolateral rat liver plasma membranes. J Biol Chem. 1990;265:7737–41.
30. Ishikawa T, Mueller M, Kluenemann C, Schaub T, Keppler D. ATP-dependent primary active transport of cysteinyl leukotrienes across liver canalicular membrane. Role of the ATP-dependent transport system for glutathione S-conjugates. J Biol Chem. 1990;265:19279–86.
31. Kobayashi K, Komatsu S, Nishi T, Hara H, Hayashi K. ATP-dependent transport for glucuronides in canalicular plasma membrane vesicles. Biochem Biophys Res Commun. 1991;176:622–26.
32. Awasthi YC, Singhal SS, Gupta S, Ahmad H, Zimniak P, Radominska A, Lester R, Sharma R. Purification and characterization of an ATPase from human liver which catalyzes ATP hydrolysis in presence of the conjugates of bilirubin, bile acids and glutathione. Biochem Biophys Res Commun 1991;175:1090–6.
33. Awasthi YC, Singh SV, Ahmad H, Wronski LW, Srivastava SK, LaBelle EF. ATP dependent primary active transport of xenobiotic-glutathione conjugates by human erythrocyte membrane. Mol Cell Biochem. 1989;91:131–6.
34. LaBelle EF, Singh SV, Srivastava SK, Awasthi YC. Dinitrophenyl glutathione efflux from human erythrocytes is primary active ATP-dependent transport. Biochem J. 1986;238:443–9.
35. LaBelle EF, Singh SV, Ahmad H, Wronski L, Srivastava SK, Awasthi YC. A novel dinitrophenylglutathione-stimulated ATPase is present in human erythrocyte membranes. FEBS Lett. 1988;228:53–6.
36. Sharma R, Gupta S, Ahmad H, Ansari GAS, Awasthi YC. Stimulation of a human erythrocyte membrane ATPase by glutathione conjugates. Toxicol Appl Pharmacol. 1990;104:421–8.
37. Sharma R, Gupta S, Singh SV, Medh RD, Ahmad H, LaBelle EF, Awasthi YC. Purification and characterization of dinitrophenylglutathione ATPase of human erythrocytes and its expression in other tissues. Biochem Biophys Res Commun. 1990;171:155–61.
38. Singhal SS, Sharma R, Gupta S, Ahmad H, Zimniak P, Radominska A, Lester R, Awasthi YC. The anionic conjugates of bilirubin and bile acids stimulate ATP hydrolysis by S-(dinitrophenyl) glutathione ATPase of human erythrocyte. FEBS Lett. 1991;281:255–57.
39. Kuipers F, Enserink M, Havinga R, van der Steen AB, Hardonk MJ, Fevery J, Vonk RJ. Separate transport systems for biliary secretion of sulfated and unsulfated bile acids in the rat. J. Clin Invest. 1988;81:1593–9.
40. Kuipers F, Radominska A, Zimniak P, Little JM, Havinga R, Vonk RJ, Lester R. Defective biliary secretion of bile acid 3 O glucuronides in rats with hereditary conjugated hyperbilirubinemia. J Lipid Res. 1989;30:1835–45.
41. Oude Elferink RPJ, Ottenhoff R, Liefting W, De Haan J, Jansen PLM. Hepatobiliary

transport of glutathione and glutathione conjugate in rats with hereditary hyperbilirubinemia. J Clin Invest. 1989;84:476–83.

42. Takikawa H, Sano N, Narita T, Uchida Y, Yamanaka M, Horie T, Mikami T, Tagaya O. Biliary excretion of bile acid conjugates in a hyperbilirubinemic mutant Sprague-Dawley rat. Hepatology. 1991;14:352–60.

43. Zimniak P, Ziller III SA, Panfil I, Radominska A, Wolters H, Kuipers F, Sharma R, Saxena M, Moslen MT, Vore M, Vonk R, Awasthi YC, Lester R. Identification of an anion-transport ATPase that catalyzes glutathione conjugate-dependent ATP hydrolysis in canalicular plasma membranes from normal rats and rats with conjugated hyperbilirubinemia (GY mutant). Arch Biochem Biophys (In press).

44. Yousef IM, Tuchweber B, Vonk RJ, Masse D, Audet M, Roy CC. Lithocholate cholestasis-sulfated glycolithocholate-induced intrahepatic cholestasis in rats. Gastroenterology. 1981;80:233–41.

45. Jansen PL, Peters WH, Lamers WH. Hereditary chronic conjugated hyperbilirubinemia in mutant rats caused by defective hepatic anion transport. Hepatology. 1985;5:573–9.

46. Jansen PL, Groothuis GM, Peters WH, Meijer DKF. Selective hepatobiliary transport defect for organic anions and neutral steroids in mutant rats with hereditary-conjugated hyperbilirubinemia. Hepatology. 1987;7:71–6.

47. Van der Meer R, Vonk RJ, Kuipers F. Cholestasis and the interactions of sulfated glyco- and taurolithocholate with calcium. Am J Physiol. 1988;265:G644–9.

48. Kuipers F, Hardonk MJ, Vonk RJ, Van der Meer R. Bile secretion of sulfated glycolithocholic acid is required for its cholestatic action in rats. Am J Physiol. (In press).

Section 2
Pathology and Pathophysiology of Cholestasis

5
Pathophysiology of cholestasis

S. ERLINGER

INTRODUCTION

For the clinician, cholestasis refers to pruritus and/or jaundice with conjugated hyperbilirubinaemia, increased serum alkaline phosphatase, 5'-nucleotidase and γ-glutamyl transferase activities, and fat malabsorption. For the pathologist, as described by Dr Desmet in Chapter 6, cholestasis refers to the presence of bile pigments in liver cells and bile canaliculi ('bilirubinostasis') and to alterations of hepatocytes possibly related to accumulation of bile salts ('cholate stasis'). For the physiologist, cholestasis is defined by decreased canalicular bile flow into the duodenum.

Cholestasis may be due to obstruction of extrahepatic bile ducts, obstruction of intrahepatic bile ducts or altered bile secretion by the hepatocytes (Fig. 1). My purpose is to review the major cellular mechanisms that have been implicated in the initiation or perpetuation of this syndrome. Most of them have been proposed on the basis of experimental observations in animals.

REVERSE POLARITY OF THE HEPATOCYTE

The hepatocyte is a highly polarized cell with the basolateral membrane facing the blood sinusoids and the canalicular membrane limiting the bile

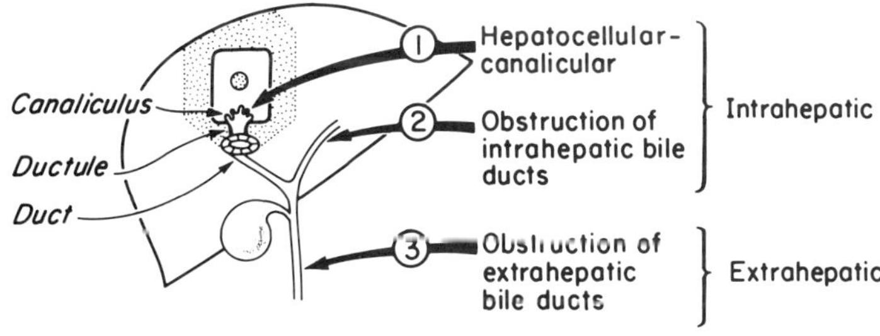

Fig. 1 Types of cholestasis

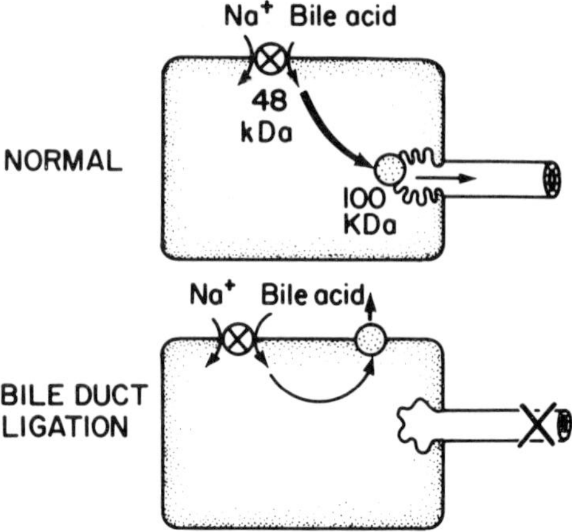

Fig. 2 Reverse polarity of hepatocytes in rats with bile duct ligation. The canalicular 100 kD carrier is 'mislocated' on the sinusoidal membrane after bile duct ligation

canaliculi. The vectorial transport of substrates from blood to bile, responsible for bile secretion, is made possible by the asymmetrical distribution of transporters between these two membranes[1].

The transporters on the sinusoidal membrane allow the uptake from blood into the hepatocyte. In particular, a 48 kD protein carrier is responsible for the uptake of conjugated bile acids. Transporters on the canalicular membrane allow the secretion from the hepatocyte into the canalicular lumen. Several have been identified: for example, the multidrug resistance protein (or gp 170), the ATP-dependent organic anion carrier[2], and the carrier(s) for bile acids. One of these is a 100 kD protein[3]. Recently, an ATP-dependent transport system has also been identified[4]: its relationship to the 100 kD carrier is not yet clear.

In *obstructive cholestasis* there is probably regurgitation of bile at various places in the biliary system. Regurgitation could occur between hepatocytes through the intercellular junctions, or across the biliary epithelium. Bile pigments are sometimes visible within biliary epithelial cells. In addition to regurgitation, a displacement of the 100 kD canalicular carrier from the canalicular membrane to the basolateral membrane has been demonstrated in rats with bile duct ligation[5]. This could result in reverse secretion of bile acids, after their uptake, from the hepatocyte into blood rather than into bile. This reverse polarity could account, in part, for cholestasis (Fig. 2).

INHIBITION OF BASOLATERAL Na$^+$,K$^+$-ATPase

In rats with oestrogen-induced cholestasis, an inhibition of Na$^+$,K$^+$-ATPase activity in the plasma membrane has been demonstrated[6]. Such an inhibition could result in a decreased uptake of bile acids by the hepatocyte. Thus, interestingly, a defect in uptake could lead to a decreased secretion.

The mechanism of the decrease in enzyme activity has not been fully

Table 1 Drugs and conditions associated with inhibition of hepatic Na$^+$,K$^+$-ATPase

Oestrogens
Androgenic steroids
Chlorpromazine
Tricyclic antidepressants
Endotoxin
Hypothyroidism, antithyroid drugs

elucidated. The most widely accepted explanation is a decrease in membrane fluidity related to an increase in cholesterol content of the plasma membrane[7].

Several drugs or chemicals have been shown experimentally to inhibit Na$^+$,K$^+$-ATPase. A non-exhaustive list is given in Table 1. Among the drugs known to induce cholestasis in clinical practice, oestrogens, androgens and chlorpromazine are possible candidates.

INCREASED PERMEABILITY OF THE PARACELLULAR PATHWAY

In oestrogen-induced cholestasis in the rat, in spite of the decrease in bile flow, there is an increase in the biliary clearance of sucrose[8]. Sucrose is thought to obtain access into bile mostly through the paracellular pathway. (A transcellular pathway is also very likely, but represents a minor component.) During oestrogen-induced cholestasis the bile to plasma ratio of sucrose increases, resulting in an increased clearance. This indicates that the sugar gains access more easily into canalicular bile, and suggests an increased permeability of the paracellular pathway.

The theory is that substances usually secreted into canalicular bile, such as bile acids or bilirubin, will regurgitate into plasma after secretion. Indeed, ultrastructural lesions of the tight junction area have been observed in various models of experimental cholestasis.

It is at present unknown whether these changes are primary (and therefore likely to initiate cholestasis) or secondary (and therefore responsible only for the perpetuation of cholestasis). There is evidence for the second possibility[9].

CYTOSKELETON ALTERATIONS

Another possibility is that alterations in the cytoskeleton may alter secretory mechanisms and induce cholestasis. Microtubules appear to be important in the intracellular transport of bile acids[10,11]. Alterations of microtubules, by drugs or toxins for example, may lead to cholestasis. Microfilaments are also important for normal bile secretion. Microfilament poisons, such as cytochalasin B and phalloidin[12] are known to inhibit bile secretion. For example, the effects of phalloidin administration on bile flow in the rat are shown in Fig. 3. In parallel, phalloidin induces a marked thickening of the pericanalicular microfilament network in hepatocyte

The mechanism of cholestasis induced by microfilament dysfunction is not

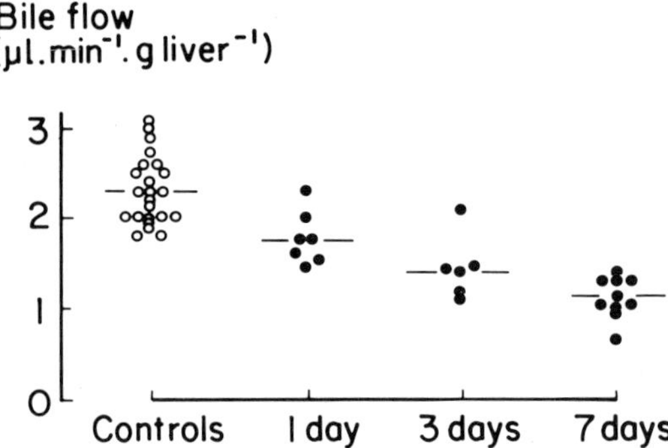

Fig. 3 Influence of phalloidin administration on bile flow in rats

known. Microfilaments may serve to maintain the shape of the cell and the normal structure of the bile secretory apparatus. A disturbance of this structure may lead to cholestasis. Alternatively, it has been proposed that they may have a contractile function: in this view contractions of the bile canaliculus would be essential to maintain a normal bile flow[13]. Cholestasis due to alterations of microfilaments would represent a 'motility' disorder[13]. This view has not yet received universal acceptance.

ALTERED INTRACELLULAR CALCIUM HOMEOSTASIS

More recently, a theory based on alterations of intracellular calcium homeostasis has been proposed.

Monohydroxylated bile acids, such as lithocholate and its conjugates, are potent cholestatic agents in the rat. Lester and his co-workers[14] observed that these bile acids had a high affinity for calcium, and they proposed that they could interfere with normal calcium homeostasis in hepatocytes. To test this hypothesis we measured intracellular ionized calcium in suspensions of isolated rat hepatocytes using the fluorescent indicator Quin2. We observed[15], as did Lester and his co-workers, that lithocholate and taurolithocholate increased cytosolic ionized calcium concentration in a dose-dependent fashion. This effect occurred at concentrations of the bile acids of the order of 10–100 µmol/l. When the experiments were repeated in the absence of extracellular calcium (after incubation with the calcium chelator EGTA), the increase in intracellular calcium was still observed, indicating that the increase was not related to an increase in calcium influx from the outside. Further experiments clearly indicated that the two bile acids acted on the same intracellular pool as vasopressin, i.e. the smooth endoplasmic reticulum. The effect was confirmed on isolated endoplasmic reticulum vesicles and was not observed on isolated mitochondria[16]. We proposed that lithocholate and taurolithocholate specifically induce a permeabilization of the smooth endoplasmic reticulum to calcium ions. This results in an increase in cytosolic calcium and in a depletion of endoplasmic reticulum stores. This depletion, by depriving the cell of an essential regulatory calcium pool, could impair a

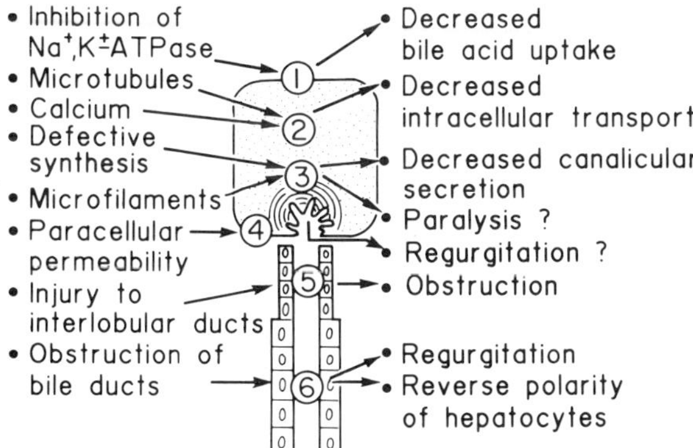

Fig. 4 Summary of mechanisms of cholestasis

number of intracellular transport processes and play a role in lithocholate-induced cholestasis.

This view has been challenged recently by the observation that 2,5-di(*tert*-butyl-1,4-benzohydroquinone (tBuBHQ), which induces a depletion of the endoplasmic reticulum calcium pool, did not induce cholestasis in the isolated perfused liver[17]. Further studies are needed to clarify this issue. It is possible that the effect of monohydroxylated bile acids on intracellular calcium plays a role in the toxicity of these compounds on the hepatocyte, but is not directly responsible for cholestasis.

DECREASED CANALICULAR SECRETION OF BILE ACIDS

A rare, but interesting, possibility is the decreased canalicular secretion of bile acids observed in the inborn errors of bile acid metabolism discussed in Chapter 15 of this book. In these conditions there is a defective synthesis and secretion of normal bile acids, which result in cholestasis, together with accumulation of an abnormal metabolite, potentially toxic for the hepatocyte. Administration of primary bile acids (cholate and chenodeoxycholate) may correct cholestasis.

SUMMARY

A summary of these mechanisms is represented in Fig. 4. It is important to note that each of these processes has been identified in different situations. In a given case it is possible that several of these mechanisms may apply. We are still lacking a unifying theory which would include all these alterations.

References

1. Meier PJ. The bile salt secretory polarity of hepatocytes. J Hepatol. 1989;9:124 9.
2. Kitamura T, Jansen P, Hardenbrook C, Kamimoto Y, Gatmaitan Z, Arias IM. Defective

ATP-dependent bile canalicular transport of organic anions in mutant (TR-) rats with conjugated hyperbilirubinemia. Proc Natl Acad Sci USA. 1990;87:3557–61.
3. Ruetz S, Hugentobler G, Meier PJ. Functional reconstitution of the canalicular bile salt transport system of the rat. Proc Natl Acad Sci USA. 1988;85:6147–51.
4. Nishida T, Gatmaitan Z, Che M, Arias IM. Rat liver canalicular membrane vesicles contain an ATP-dependent bile acid transport system. Proc Natl Acad Sci USA. 1991;88:6590–4.
5. Fricker G, Landmann L, Meier PJ. Extrahepatic obstructive cholestasis reverses the bile salt secretory polarity of rat hepatocytes. J Clin Invest. 1989; 84:876–85.
6. Keeffe EB, Scharschmidt BF, Blankenship NM, Ockner RK. Studies of relationship among bile flow, liver plasma membrane Na^+,K^+-ATPase, and membrane microviscosity in the rat. J Clin Invest. 1979;64:1590–8.
7. Davis RA, Kern F, Showalter R, Sutherland E, Sinenski M, Simon FR. Alteration of hepatic Na^+,K^+-ATPase and bile flow by estrogen: effects on liver surface membrane lipid structure and function. Proc Natl Acad Sci USA. 1978;75:4130–4.
8. Forker EL. The effect of estrogen on bile formation in the rat. J Clin Invest. 1969;48:654–63.
9. Jaeschke H, Trummer E, Krell H. Increase in biliary permeability subsequent to intrahepatic cholestasis by estradiol valerate in rats. Gastroenterology. 1987;93:533–8.
10. Dubin M, Maurice M, Feldmann G, Erlinger S. Influence of colchicine and phalloidin on bile secretion and hepatic ultrastructure in the rat. Possible interaction between microtubules and microfilaments. Gastroenterology. 1980;79:646–54.
11. Crawford JM, Berken CA, Gollan JL. Role of the hepatocyte microtubular system in the excretion of bile salts and biliary lipid: implications for intracellular vesicular transport. J Lipid Res. 1988;29:144–56.
12. Dubin M, Maurice M, Feldmann G, Erlinger S. Phalloidin-induced cholestasis in the rat: relation to changes in microfilaments. Gastroenterology. 1978;74:450–5.
13. Phillips MJ, Poucell S, Oda M. Biology of disease. Mechanisms of cholestasis. Lab Invest. 1986;54:593–608.
14. Anwer MS, Engelking LR, Nolan K, Sullivan D, Zimniak P, Lester R. Hepatotoxic bile acids increase cytosolic Ca^{++} activity of isolated rat hepatocytes. Hepatology. 1988;8:887–91.
15. Combettes L, Dumont M, Berthon B, Erlinger S, Claret M. Release of calcium from the endoplasmic reticulum by bile acids in rat liver cells. J Biol Chem. 1988;263:2299–303.
16. Combettes L, Berthon B, Doucet E, Erlinger S, Claret M. Characteristics of bile acid-mediated Ca^{2+} release from permeabilized liver cells and liver microsomes. J Biol Chem. 1989;264:157–67.
17. Farrell GC, Duddy SK, Kass GEN, Llopis J, Gahm A, Orrenius S. Release of Ca^{2+} from the endoplasmic reticulum is not the mechanism for bile acid-induced cholestasis and hepatotoxicity in the intact rat liver. J Clin Invest. 1990;85:1255–9.

6
Pathology of paediatric cholestasis

V. J. DESMET

The histopathological features of the liver in cholestasis of the neonate and young child can be divided into: 'basic' features of histological cholestasis, which are found to a variable extent in most cholestatic conditions of the neonate; and histological changes which are helpful in identifying a particular aetiology.

BASIC FEATURES OF HISTOLOGICAL CHOLESTASIS IN NEONATES AND CHILDREN

Features of histological cholestasis in general

Preliminary note

It is useful first to consider two important concepts in the histopathology of cholestasis.

Histological cholestasis: bilirubinostasis and cholate stasis. The classical light microscopic features indicating cholestasis consist of the microscopically visible accumulation of bile pigment in liver tissue: as pigment granules in parenchymal cells, as intercellular bile plugs and subsequently also as pigment inclusions in Kupffer cells. These changes used to be referred to as 'histological cholestasis' (Fig. 1).

In recent years it has been proposed that this term be replaced by 'bilirubinostasis'[1], because the only bile constituent which is recognized corresponds to bile pigment (bilirubin) and it is by no means the only, and even not the most reliable, histological indicator of a cholestatic condition.

Indeed, several chronic cholestatic diseases are characterized by so-called 'cholate stasis'[2]. This term refers to a typical change in periportal (or in cirrhotic stages: periseptal) parenchymal cells. The hepatocytes appear swollen and pale, with coarse granules in their cytoplasm (Fig. 2). Staining with Shikata's orcein stain, or with Victoria Blue, reveals positive granules, indicating accumulation of copper binding protein (metallotheonein), rhodanine staining reveals positive granules corresponding to lysosomal copper

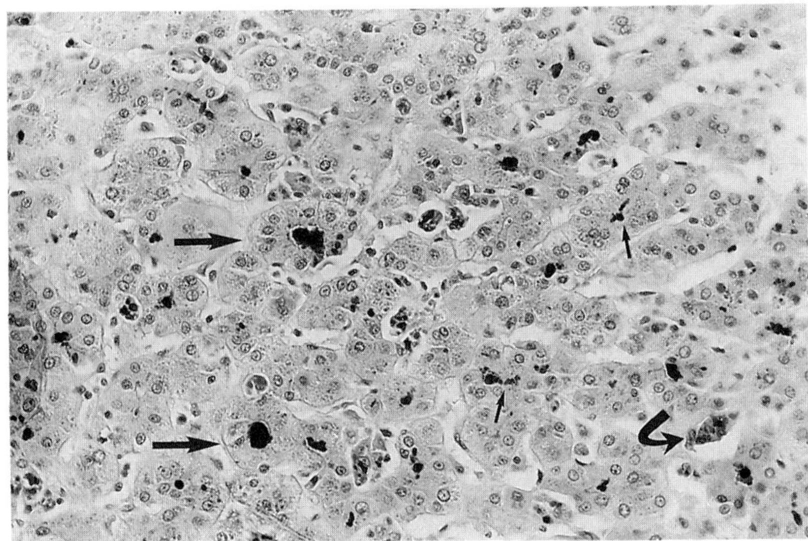

Fig. 1 Liver biopsy from infant with EHBDA, showing bilirubinostasis in acinar zone 3 (centrolobular parenchyma). The picture includes hepatocellular bilirubinostasis (pigment inclusions in hepatocytes), canalicular bilirubinostasis: bile plugs (small arrows) and bile concrements in cholestatic liver cell rosettes (large arrows), and Kupffer cell bilirubinostasis (pigment granules in hypertrophic Kupffer cells) (curved arrow). Haematoxylin and eosin, × 200

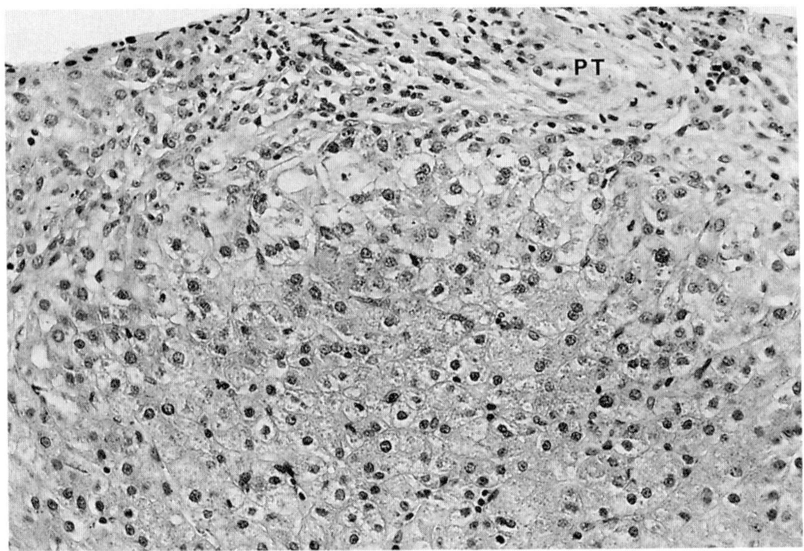

Fig. 2 Liver biopsy from child with EHBDA, featuring light microscopic appearance of (early stage) of periportal cholate stasis. The upper part shows part of a portal tract (PT). Note the swollen, clear appearance and some coarse granularity of the periportal parenchymal cells as compared to the rest of the parenchyma. Haematoxylin and eosin, × 325

accumulation. Mallory bodies appear in these hepatocytes, and eventually also bilirubin inclusions. The 'cholate stasis' is less marked in early stages of chronic cholestasis, but becomes more prominent with time along the sequence of staining results mentioned above, resulting in the full-blown picture.

Complete versus incomplete block in bile secretion. Chronic cholestasis, or chronic arrest of bile secretion, may be due to extrahepatic occlusion of larger bile ducts: *extrahepatic cholestasis* or *mechanical cholestasis.*

The occlusion may be abrupt and complete (for instance, impacted stone in common bile duct, malignant tumour of large bile ducts), or variably incomplete (for instance, bile duct stricture, annular pancreas).

Intrahepatic cholestasis refers to cholestatic conditions in which the disease primarily affects the intrahepatic bile ducts and/or the liver parenchymal cells themselves.

The diseases of the intrahepatic bile ducts associated with chronic cholestasis usually involve progressive occlusion or destruction of increasing numbers of intrahepatic bile duct branches, thus corresponding to 'incomplete' obstruction for a variable time period during their course. Typical examples of such diseases are primary biliary cirrhosis (PBC) and primary sclerosing cholangitis (PSC).

In conditions of intrahepatic cholestasis due to primary disturbance of the bile secreting parenchymal cells, it is unknown whether the arrest in bile secretory function of individual hepatocytes is complete or incomplete.

Presumably it is complete in the most affected hepatocytes. However, in many instances of intrahepatic cholestasis due to parenchymal disease, not all hepatocytes are involved to a similar extent, and classical features of cholestasis are often restricted to acinar zone 3 parenchymal cells.

The distinction between complete and incomplete arrest in bile secretion is useful in explaining the variable appearance of 'bilirubinostasis'.

Bilirubinostasis with appearance of intercellular bile plugs is an early and constant feature in all forms of complete secretory block, be it parenchymal disease (for instance, drug-induced cholestasis) or extrahepatic obstruction (for instance, extrahepatic bile duct atresia).

In contrast, bilirubinostasis is not a constant feature, and in fact is usually absent for very long time periods in diseases characterized by incomplete block to bile secretion, whether due to extrahepatic or to intrahepatic bile duct disease.

The practical implications for the diagnostic histopathologist are two-fold:

1. In diseases with incomplete obstruction of extra- and/or intrahepatic bile ducts, his or her diagnosis of chronic cholestasis must be based on histological changes amongst which bilirubinostasis, the 'classical' feature of cholestasis, is totally absent.
2. When in the later course of such diseases 'bilirubinostasis' still appears, it should be taken as a warning sign. It may indicate a complication, such as superimposed drug-induced disease. In terminal stages it may be an ominous sign, as it may indicate the imminent completeness of the

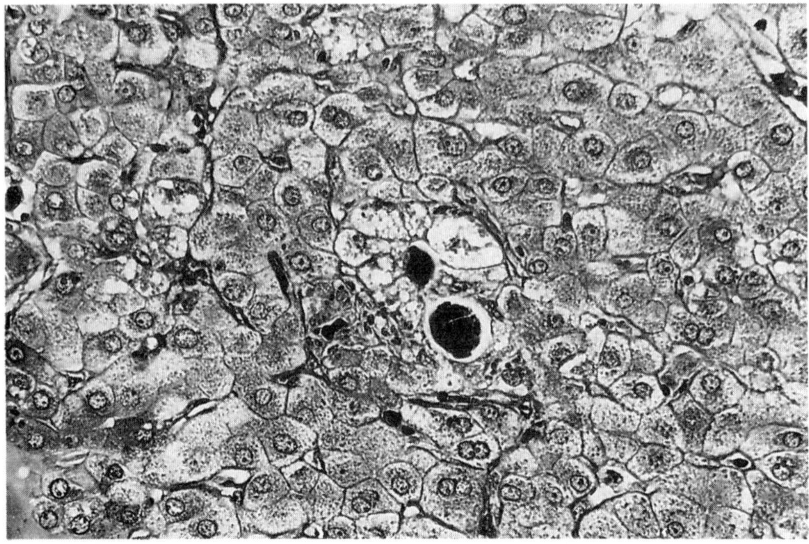

Fig. 3 Liver biopsy from child with EHBDA, showing feathery degeneration of parenchymal cells, arranged in a tubular fashion around a central dilated lumen containing an inspissated bile concrement (cholestatic liver cell rosette). Masson's trichrome; × 325

occlusion of intrahepatic bile duct radicles or the superimposed functional bile secretory failure of decompensating parenchymal cells.

Parenchymal changes

Besides bilirubinostasis and cholate stasis discussed above, the main parenchymal changes in chronic cholestasis comprise: feathery degeneration, xanthomatous and pseudoxanthomatous cells and cholestatic liver cell rosettes[3].

Feathery degeneration refers to swollen, hydropic hepatocytes with a thread-like reticular appearance of their bile-stained cytoplasm (Fig. 3). Such cells may be seen singly or in groups throughout the parenchyma (for the latter see 'pseudoxanthomatous cells').

Xanthomatous cells usually occur in clusters in portal tracts or in the parenchyma. They appear as foamy, vacuolated cells, and correspond to lipid-laden histiocytes (reflecting the hyperlipidaemia in chronic cholestasis). They are to be differentiated from mineral oil granulomas.

Pseudoxanthomatous cells correspond to groups of parenchymal cells displaying a foamy or reticulated clear cytoplasm, often with variable degree of bilirubin impregnation; they probably correspond to a variant or a stage of 'feathery degeneration'. A clear distinction between xanthomatous and pseudoxanthomatous cells is not always possible[4].

Cholestatic liver cell rosettes correspond to a transformation of liver parenchymal cell plates into tubular structures; in light microscopy they appear as glandular structures lined by four or more hepatocytes around a

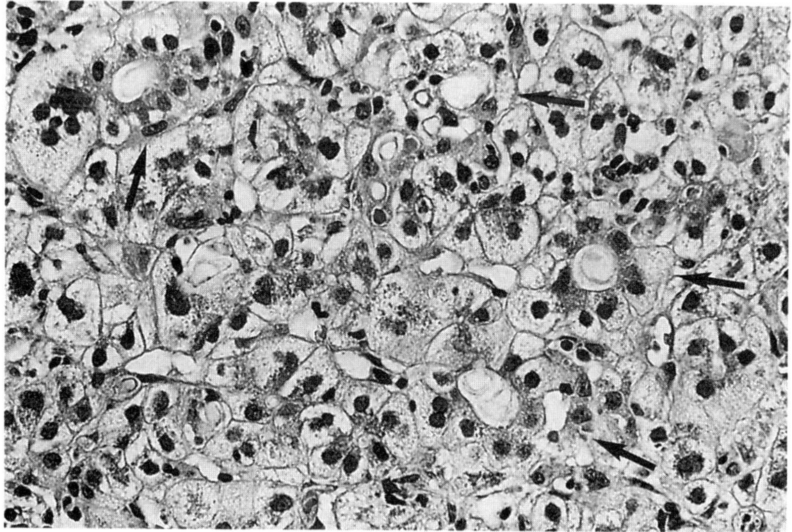

Fig. 4 Liver biopsy from child with EHBDA, showing cholestatic liver cell rosettes (arrows); some of the dilated lumina contain some biliary material. Haematoxylin and eosin, × 325

central lumen of variable diameter (Figs 3 and 4). The apical cell membranes are often more clearly delineated. The lumen may be empty, or may contain eosinophilic or bilirubin-stained material with variable degree of inspissation. Part or all of the lining hepatocytes may show features of feathery degeneration.

Cholestatic liver cell rosettes have been studied by computer-assisted three-dimensional reconstruction methods[5], and were shown to correspond to hepatocellular tubules in continuity with bile ductules. Furthermore, hepatocytes in cholestatic liver cell rosettes display 'bile duct type' cytokeratins, indicating a phenotypic shift of the involved parenchymal cells to bile duct type cells[6].

Ductular metaplasia of acinar zone 1 hepatocytes. Immunostaining of liver sections with polyclonal cytokeratin antibodies or tissue polypeptide antigen (TPA) antibodies appears to be a sensitive technique for identifying chronic states of low-grade cholestasis. Periportal (and periseptal) hepatocytes show increased expression of non-hepatocyte cytokeratins and of TPA, even before features of cholate stasis are recognizable in light microscopy[7].

Periportal and architectural changes in chronic cholestasis

Complete and incomplete blockade in bile secretion, especially when caused by diseases of extra- and intrahepatic bile ducts, is associated with '*ductular reaction*'. This term refers to an increased number of ductular profiles in the periphery of the portal tract, gradually extending into the periportal parenchyma. The increase in number of ductular structures is accompanied by oedema and infiltration by neutrophil polymorphonuclear leucocytes

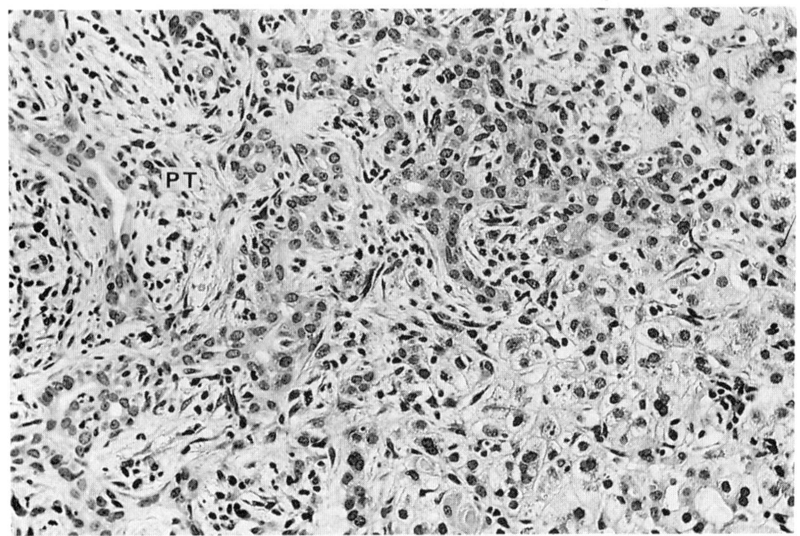

Fig. 5 Liver biopsy from child with EHBDA, showing marked ductular reaction. The left upper corner shows a portal tract (PT), surrounded by irregular ductular profiles extending into the surrounding parenchyma. The ductular structures are accompanied by inflammatory infiltration and fibrosis. Haematoxylin and eosin, × 200

(cholangiolitis) and fibrosis (Fig. 5).

The increment in ductular structures is due to active proliferation (mitoses!) of pre-existing ductules (especially in complete mechanical obstruction) and to ductular metaplasia of acinar zone 1 hepatocytes (predominant in cases of chronic incomplete obstruction to bile flow)[8].

The cholangiocytes lining the ductules may show signs of reabsorption of bile constituents, reflected in: vacuolization of the cytoplasm, accumulation of lipofuscin and bilirubin inclusions, leading in some instances to formation of inspissated bile concrements in the lumen[8].

The periportal extension of the 'ductular reaction' with its accompanying inflammatory infiltrate in periportal parenchymal areas showing features of cholate stasis and loss of parenchymal cells creates an irregular portal–parenchymal interface, which has been termed *'biliary piecemeal necrosis'*[1,2].

The 'ductular reaction' and inflammation may subside in isolated portal tracts, resulting in periportal fibrosis containing sequestrated parts of liver cell plates in the periphery of the expanded portal tract (indicated by the term *'fibrosing piecemeal necrosis'*)[9].

The irregular outline of the portal–parenchymal interface in case of vigorous 'ductular reaction' is referred to as *'ductular piecemeal necrosis'*[9].

The progressive wedge-shaped extensions of the 'ductular reaction' eventually lead to fibrous linkage of adjacent portal tracts (portal–portal septa). This stage of *biliary fibrosis*[9] is a potentially reversible lesion, since the basic intrahepatic vascular relationships are preserved.

With ongoing cholestasis, portal–central septa also ensue, accompanied

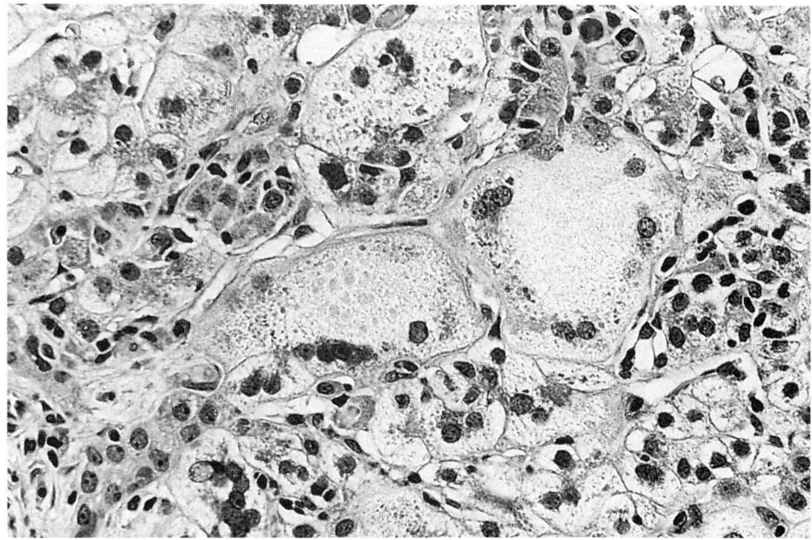

Fig. 6 Liver biopsy from child with EHBDA; parenchymal giant cells and infiltrating inflammatory cells. Haematoxylin and eosin, × 325

by nodular parenchymal regeneration, resulting in some instances in the final irreversible stage of (secondary) *biliary cirrhosis*[9].

Features of histological cholestasis specific for the neonatal age

In addition to the general features of cholestasis, two further changes often characterize the histological picture in neonatal cholestatic liver disease: parenchymal giant cells and extramedullary haematopoiesis.

Parenchymal giant cells

The multinucleated giant cells in neonatal cholestasis are of parenchymal nature, and seem to result from syncytial fusion of several mononucleated parenchymal cells[7]. The number of nuclei and their location inside the cytoplasm is variable. Giant cells often contain pigment granules which correspond to bilirubin, lipofuscin or haemosiderin, or a combination of these pigments (Fig. 6).

The biological significance of parenchymal giant cells is unknown. Since giant cell transformation of liver parenchymal cells may occur in a variety of different conditions, it is considered a non-specific reaction of the infant's hepatocytes to various types of injury, and appears to be more age-specific than disease-specific[7].

Parenchymal giant cells may appear necrotic and surrounded by neutrophils[10].

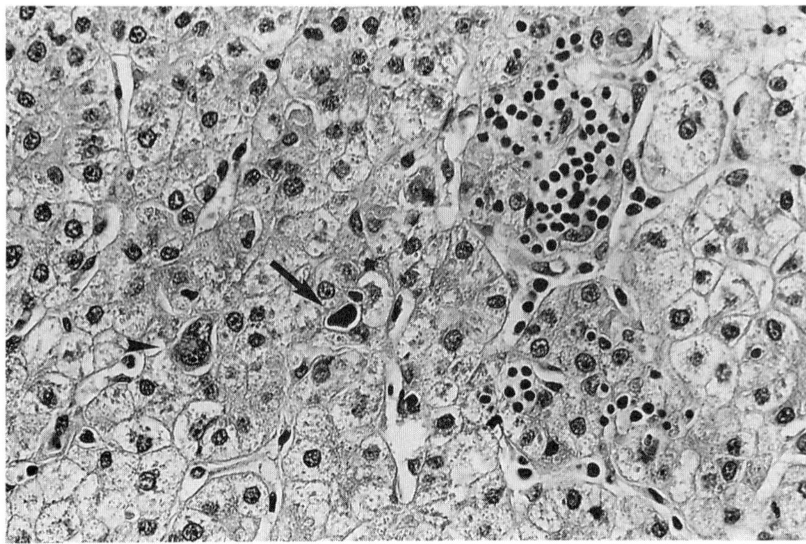

Fig. 7 Liver biopsy from child with EHBDA, revealing inspissated bile plugs (arrow) and extramedullary haematopoiesis: foci of erythropoiesis in the right part of the picture, and a megakaryocyte (arrowhead). Haematoxylin and eosin, × 200

Extramedullary haematopoiesis

Foci of extramedullary haematopoiesis, comprising clusters of erythrocyte precursor cells, myeloid precursor cells and megakaryocytes or a combination of these, are often observed in cholestatic liver specimens from young infants (Fig. 7). They are not a reliable criterion for differentiating between intrahepatic forms of cholestasis ('neonatal hepatitis') and extrahepatic bile duct atresia[7].

HISTOLOGICAL CHANGES INDICATIVE OF A SPECIFIC AETIOLOGY

With regard to hepatic changes indicative of a specific aetiology, it is useful to subdivide the broad group of patients with 'neonatal cholestasis' into three main categories: 'neonatal hepatitis', paucity of interlobular bile ducts (PILBD), and extrahepatic bile duct atresia (EHBDA).

'Neonatal hepatitis syndrome'

The 'neonatal hepatitis syndrome' can be further subdivided into three subgroups: (1) idiopathic neonatal hepatitis or cryptogenic neonatal cholestasis; (2) intrauterine and perinatal infections, and (3) metabolic diseases[11,12].

Cryptogenic neonatal cholestasis

Cryptogenic neonatal cholestasis remains of unknown aetiology; it is also referred to as 'neonatal hepatitis' and '(neonatal) giant cell hepatitis'. The histopathological features correspond to the basic features of neonatal cholestasis mentioned above, eventually supplemented with some degree of parenchymal siderosis and intralobular fibrosis. The liver histology is not helpful in suggesting a particular aetiology. This category of neonatal cholestasis presumably represents a heterogeneous group of liver diseases with diverse, but still unrecognized, aetiology.

In general, the histological liver alterations in 'neonatal hepatitis' are more prominent in the parenchyma than in the portal tracts. Ductular proliferation is usually mild, if present at all, which helps to differentiate from extrahepatic cholestasis (EHBDA). The fibrosis is more intralobular in 'neonatal hepatitis', in contrast to the more periportal predominance of fibrosis in EHBDA[7].

Intrauterine and perinatal infections

Rather than being indicated with the vague term 'neonatal hepatitis', this category is more appropriately termed 'hepatitis in the neonate', since it concerns a group of diseases in which the aetiological infectious agent can be identified[11].

The histopathological picture includes features of neonatal cholestasis (like bilirubinostasis and parenchymal giant cells) and necro-inflammatory lesions in variable proportions. Histology and histochemistry may be helpful in identifying the causal agent. Examples include: characteristic nuclear inclusions in cytomegalovirus and herpes hepatitis, and immunohistochemical demonstration of hepatitis B surface antigen or hepatitis B core antigen in viral hepatitis B[7] (Fig. 8).

In patients with endotoxic/septic shock the liver biopsy may reveal a striking and characteristic cholangiolitis with ductular bilirubinostasis. The portal tracts are surrounded by dilated cholangioles which extend into the periportal area and contain bilirubin-stained, PAS-positive concretions; neutrophil polymorphs are present within and surrounding the ductules[13,14] (Fig. 9).

Metabolic disorders

Some metabolic diseases associated with cholestasis in the neonate are characterized by suggestive histological features.

1. *Galactosaemia* is characterized by severe histological bilirubinostasis, with bile plugs in pseudoglandular arrangements of hepatocytes and a constant fatty change[10,15,16]; the early stage is characterized by ductular proliferation around the portal tracts.
2. *Fructose intolerance* causes a similar picture, usually with less ductular proliferation and minor cholestasis.
3. *Tyrosinaemia* causes liver lesions which are similar to those of galactosaemia, including steatosis, bilirubinostasis, pseudoglandular transformation of liver cell plates, pericellular and periportal fibrosis; furthermore,

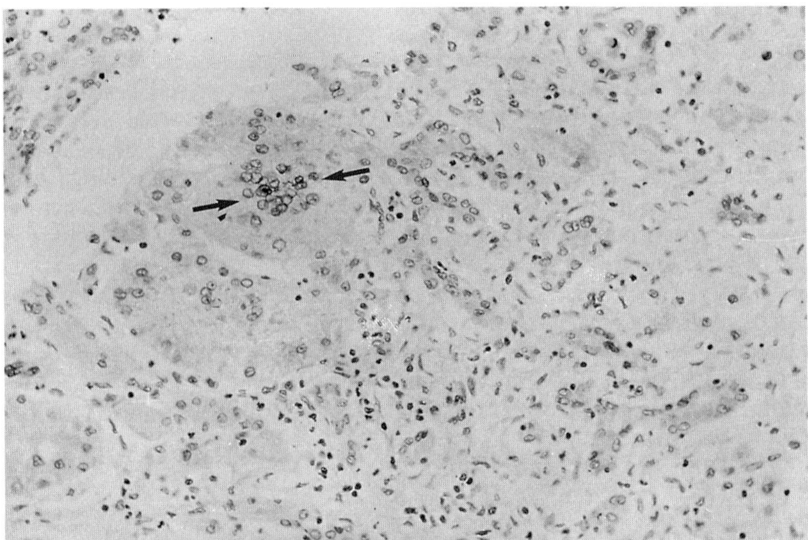

Fig. 8 Liver specimen from 10-month-old child who died from fulminant viral hepatitis B. The picture shows two large parenchymal giant cells, and collapsing mesenchymal framework containing a few duct-like structures and mild inflammatory infiltration. A few nuclei in one of the multinucleated parenchymal giant cells are immunoreactive for hepatitis B core antigen (arrows). Immunoperoxidase stain for hepatitis B core antigen, haematoxylin stain for nuclei, × 325

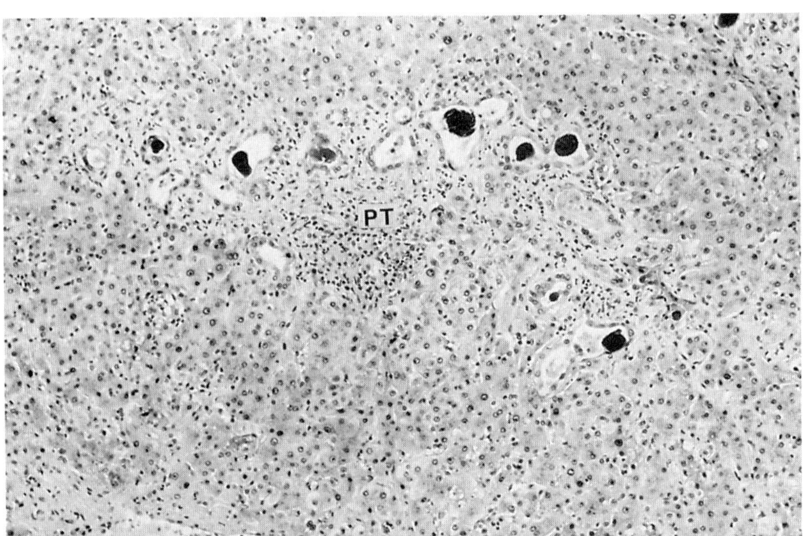

Fig. 9 Liver biopsy from patient with septicaemia. A portal tract (PT) is surrounded by dilated ductules containing dark bile concrements. Haematoxylin and eosin, × 80

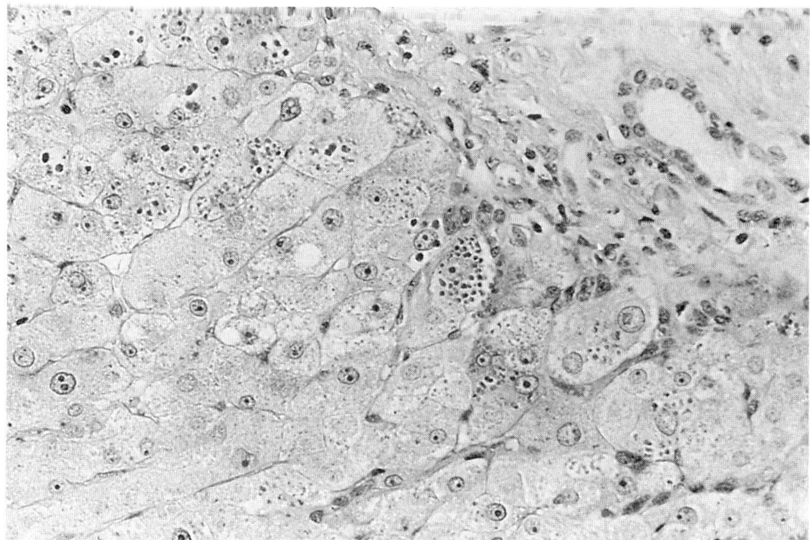

Fig. 10 Liver biopsy from patient with α_1-antitrypsin deficiency. The right upper corner shows the edge of a portal tract (with bile duct). The periportal hepatocytes contain variable numbers of PAS-positive, diastase-resistant inclusions of variable size. PAS-diastase stain, × 325

one finds variable parenchymal haemosiderosis, extramedullary haemato-poiesis, and variably sized foci of nodular regeneration. The nodules often show more striking fat accumulation than the adjacent parenchyma[16,17].

4. *α_1-Antitrypsin deficiency* may be associated with some periportal ductular reaction and parenchymal bilirubinostasis; this entity is identified histologically by the characteristic, periodic acid Schiff (PAS)-positive, diastase-resistant globular inclusions in periportal hepatocytes (Fig. 10). The inclusions can be shown to contain α_1-antitrypsin by immunohistochemical staining with specific polyclonal or monoclonal antibodies[18]. In 4–26% of cases paucity of interlobular bile ducts may be seen[19] (see overleaf).

5. *Byler syndrome* (synonyms: progressive intrahepatic cholestasis, familial intrahepatic cholestasis) is a rare, autosomal recessive form of intrahepatic cholestasis progressing to cirrhosis and death in infancy or early childhood[19]. The aetiology is unknown, but an abnormality in bile acid metabolism and secretion is suspected. The liver alterations include bilirubinostasis in the early stage, giant cell transformation in about 50% of patients, and bile duct paucity (see below) in 70% of cases. The histopathological changes further include duct destruction and ductular proliferation. Fibrosis develops both around the central veins and around portal tracts. The cirrhosis which characterizes the later stage is of the biliary type, with bilirubinostasis, cholate stasis and periportal increase in ductular structures[19].

6. *Long-term parenteral nutrition* may cause cholestatic jaundice. Initially, the liver biopsy reveals acinar zone 3 hepatocellular and canalicular

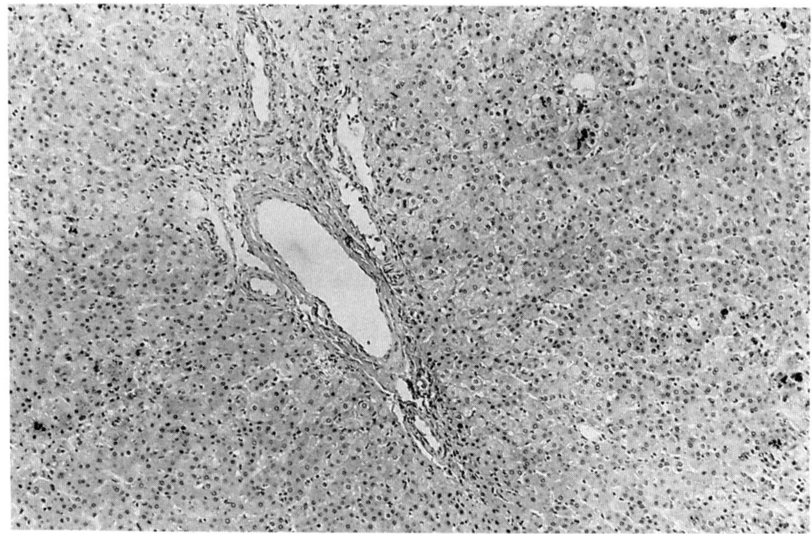

Fig. 11   Liver biopsy from child with paucity of interlobular bile ducts (non-syndromic form). The portal tract contains branches of the hepatic artery and portal vein, but the interlobular duct is missing. Note scattered areas with bilirubinostasis in the lobular parenchyma. Haematoxylin and eosin, × 80

bilirubinostasis. Periportal inflammation is variable and fatty change infrequent. With continuous therapy over 3 months, progressive periportal fibrosis and cirrhosis may develop[20,21].

Paucity of interlobular bile ducts (PILBD)

Paucity of interlobular bile ducts (PILBD) is defined as a decrease in the number of interlobular ducts in association with a patent extrahepatic biliary tree (Fig. 11). The most direct way to recognize PILBD is to establish the bile duct to portal space (BD/PS) ratio by counting the total number of interlobular bile ducts and portal spaces in a liver specimen. The normal BD/PS ratio in normal children[22] is between 0.9 and 1.8. However, in premature infants prior to 38 weeks after conception, a BD/PS ratio less than 0.9 may be normal[23].

For diagnosis of PILBD, earlier workers suggested the need of serial sectioning operative wedge biopsies of the liver[24,25]. However, the BD/PS ratio can reliably be established on needle biopsy specimens of the liver comprising a minimum of five portal spaces[19].

PILBD may be either syndromic or non-syndromic.

Syndromic paucity of interlobular bile ducts

Synonyms are: Alagille syndrome and arteriohepatic dysplasia[26]. In syndromic PILBD the histopathology of the liver varies with the age of the patient, making it possible to distinguish early and late changes[19]. In early liver biopsies (up to 3 months of age) the number of interlobular ducts may be normal; but the ducts may show signs of duct destruction with pyknosis of bile duct lining cells and lymphocytic infiltration of the biliary epithelium. The lobular parenchyma shows parenchymal giant cells and bilirubinostasis, and some copper accumulation in periportal hepatocytes. Late changes (in children older than 3 months) include duct paucity of variable degree, often associated with periportal fibrosis. Parenchymal bilirubinostasis may be found in younger children; parenchymal giant cells are absent. Ductular proliferation is reported only occasionally in syndromic PILBD[7,19]. The different findings between early and late biopsies indicate that syndromic PILBD does not represent an agenesis of interlobular ducts, but corresponds to an acquired destruction of the ducts.

The diagnosis of syndromic PILBD relies on the histological demonstration of duct damage and destruction (in early biopsies) or paucity of ducts (in later biopsies), in association with the typical clinical findings in Alagille syndrome[19].

Non-syndromic paucity of interlobular bile ducts

Non-syndromic PILBD may be an isolated hepatic abnormality or one component of a more complex systemic process with or without a specific aetiology[19]. However, non-syndromic PILBD lacks the well-defined extrahepatic anomalies of Alagille syndrome. As in Alagille syndrome, the histopathological lesions in the liver vary with the age of the patient.

In early biopsies (up to 3 months of age of the patient), a reduced BD/PS ratio may already be observed, associated with signs of necro-inflammatory destruction of the remaining ducts in more than 50% of patients. The portal tracts may appear enlarged with periportal fibrosis and inflammatory infiltrate. The lobular parenchyma shows parenchymal giant cell transformation, bilirubinostasis, extramedullary haematopoiesis, perisinusoidal fibrosis and mild to moderate copper accumulation in periportal hepatocytes[19].

After 90 days, lobular changes tend to be less prominent, with less or no giant cell transformation of hepatocytes and only mild or no bilirubinostasis. Perisinusoidal fibrosis and mild periportal copper accumulation persist. Duct paucity remains, although the BD/PS ratios are not necessarily the same as those observed in earlier biopsies, presumably due to an irregular distribution of the ductal changes[19]. Ductular proliferation has been described in occasional patients with non-syndromic PILBD[27].

The diagnosis of non-syndromic PILBD relies on the histological demonstration of bile duct destruction or established paucity of ducts in an infant lacking the associated features of the Alagille syndrome. As mentioned, non-syndromic PILBD may be associated with a number of disorders, including infections, α_1-antitrypsin deficiency, hypopituitarism, chromosomal anomalies, altered bile acid metabolism (such as trihydroxy coprostanic acidaemia), Byler disease, Norwegian cholestasis, and a number of miscellaneous disorders. Most cases, however, remain idiopathic[19].

In the experience of some authors, non-syndromic PILBD constitutes the most frequent diagnosis in infants with conjugated hyperbilirubinaemia in the first 28 days of life, and is more frequently observed than extrahepatic bile duct atresia[19].

The observations in PILBD emphasize the importance of a detailed study of interlobular bile ducts in liver biopsies from children with neonatal cholestasis. Microscopic analysis of interlobular bile ducts may be facilitated by immunohistochemical staining for cytokeratins or tissue polypeptide antigen, which allow a better and more contrasted visualization of the bile ducts present[28].

Extrahepatic bile duct atresia (EHBDA)

Like PILBD, EHBDA also does not correspond to a lack of formation of the extrahepatic bile ducts or some of their segments, but represents a necro-inflammatory destruction of biliary conduits which have been formed. The aetiology and pathogenesis of the disease remain unknown[7].

Equally important is the conept, which emerged in the course of the past 15 years, that the mysterious process of destructive cholangitis which occurs in EHBDA is not restricted to the extrahepatic segments of the biliary tree, but also affects the intrahepatic bile ducts. EHBDA thus represents a panbiliary disease[7,29].

In the classical form of EHBDA the destructive cholangiopathy destroys interlobular ducts of normal tubular shape. However, in some 20–25% of infants with EHBDA, the interlobular bile ducts still appear in their immature, embryonic shape; such ducts assume the form of cylindrical plates, or segments thereof, termed 'ductal plate malformation'[7,30]. These interlobular ducts in ductal plate configuration are subject to progressive destruction and involution, as is the case for the mature interlobular ducts in classical forms of EHBDA. This observation suggests that in EHBDA with ductal plate malformation of the interlobular ducts the causal agent of EHBDA has started early during fetal life, at a stage when most interlobular ducts were still in their immature, embryonic form. This might explain why infants with this form of EHBDA present advanced liver fibrosis as early as the first few weeks of postnatal life, thus justifying the label 'early severe EHBDA'[7,31].

Classical extrahepatic bile duct atresia

The histopathology of the liver in classical EHBDA changes with advancing age of the patient. In the early stage the picture corresponds to that of 'neonatal cholestasis' (cf. above), and is not diagnostic for EHBDA. Gradually, portal oedema and ductular proliferation set in, as a reaction to the extrahepatic obstruction (see p. 59 above). The ductular reaction is associated with progressive periductular fibrosis, and is soon characterized by the appearance of bilirubin concrements in the ductular lumina (ductular bilirubinostasis) (Fig. 12). With advancing age the lesion progresses to biliary fibrosis and eventually biliary cirrhosis.

The portal and periportal changes are the most reliable for a histological

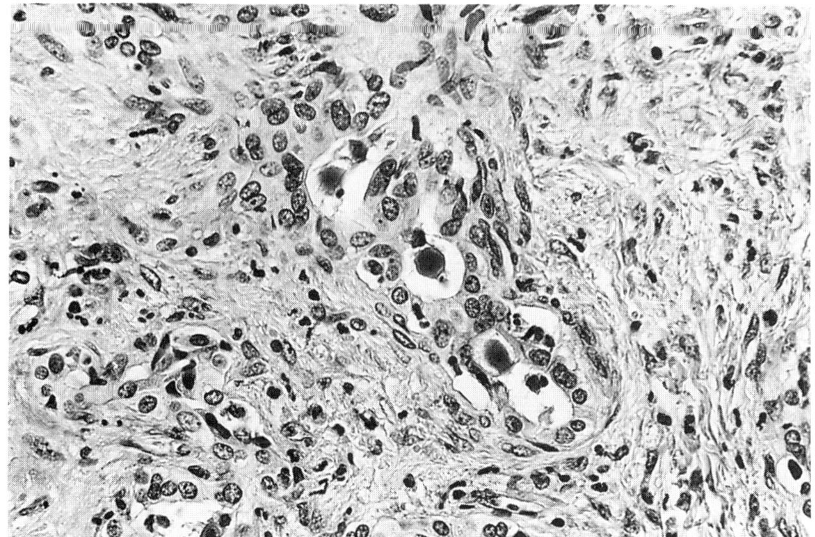

Fig. 12 Liver biopsy from child with EHBDA. Detail from the periphery of a portal tract, showing ductules with inspissated bile concrements (partly laminated) in the lumen. Haematoxylin and eosin, × 325

diagnosis of EHBDA. Since the ductular reaction takes some time to develop, some authors advise postponing diagnostic liver biopsy until the age of 6 weeks, at which time the ductular reaction should be well developed[32]. However, one should realize that there may be some variability in the speed of development of ductular reaction in different patients, so that liver biopsy may be diagnostic for EHBDA well before the age of 6 weeks[7].

Since the success of the hepatic porto-enterostomy or Kasai operation (and its variants) depends to a large extent on the younger age of the patient, the diagnosis of EHBDA should be established as early as possible.

Besides ductular reaction, ductular bilirubinostasis and periportal fibrosis, the alterations of the interlobular ducts also represent an important diagnostic hallmark.

In classical EHBDA the interlobular ducts have a normal, tubular shape, but show signs of necro-inflammatory destruction to a variable extent (Fig. 13). The appearance of the ductal lesions varies with the progression of the cholangiopathy. Interlobular ducts in an early stage of damage are characterized by irregularity of their lining epithelium, which shows vacuolization, nuclear pycnosis, atrophy and infiltration by inflammatory cells. A gradual thickening of the basement membrane occurs, associated with progressing atrophy and disappearance of the biliary epithelium. Finally, the duct disappears altogether. With increasing age of the patient one may find an increasing degree of intrahepatic ductopenia in EHBDA.

EHBDA is often characterized by hypoplasia of the portal vein branches. In later stages one may observe fusion between large preterminal portal

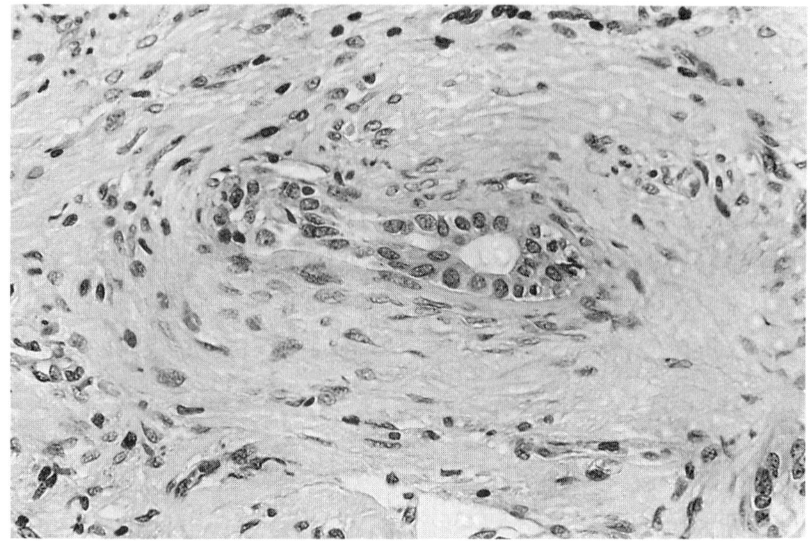

Fig. 13 Liver biopsy from child with EHBDA. Detail from a portal tract with interlobular bile duct; the latter shows epithelial irregularity, interepithelial lymphocytic infiltration, and beginning concentric periductal fibrosis. Haematoxylin and eosin, × 325

tracts, resulting in enlarged fibrous areas on cross-section. This picture suggests an abnormality in the pattern of branching of the portal vein[7].

'Early severe' extrahepatic bile duct atresia

In the 'early severe' variant of EHBDA, a variable number of interlobular ducts appear in the form of ductal plates (Fig. 14). Early severe EHBDA is characterized by the same main morphological alterations of the lobular parenchyma and periportal changes as observed in classical EHBDA, with the exception that giant cell transformation and extramedullary haemato-poiesis are usually lacking. The immature interlobular ducts (ductal plates or ductal plate remnants) show similar epithelial changes, progressive atrophy and finally disappearance of the ductal structures as in classical EHBDA.

In some instances double or even triple concentric rings of ductal plates (or ductal plate segments) may be observed in the portal tracts. This has been interpreted as a 'fetal type' of ductular reaction, caused by successive waves of concentric ductal plate formation[7].

The branches of the portal vein are often hypoplastic. Also in 'early severe' EHBDA there appears to exist an abnormality in the branching pattern of the portal vein, in the sense that too many and too narrow vessels are sprouting too closely together ('pollard willow' pattern). On cross-sectioning this arrangement results in grossly enlarged portal tracts (in fact, fusion of closely located portal tracts), containing several ductal plates arranged around hypoplastic central vessels.

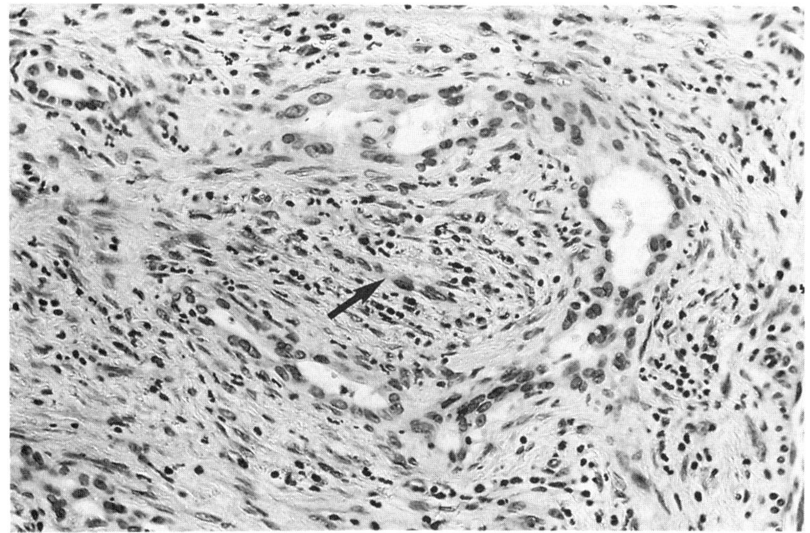

Fig. 14 Liver biopsy from child with EHBDA ('early severe' type). Detail from a portal tract containing an immature bile duct in cylindrical shape (ductal plate malformation). Note irregularity of the bile duct epithelial cells, occasional infiltrating inflammatory cells, and inflammation in the portal connective tissue. The centre is occupied by a collapsed, hypoplastic branch of the portal vein (arrow). Haematoxylin and eosin, × 200

Follow-up after hepatic portoenterostomy

Hepatic portoenterostomy relieves the extrahepatic obstruction in EHBDA and re-establishes bilio-intestinal continuity. However, the operation does not necessarily cure the destructive cholangiopathy which affects the intrahepatic bile ducts, and which has been termed 'the basic disease process'[7,33].

It appears that the 'basic disease process' may run a variable course in different patients: in some it is very active and persisting; in others it is slow and burns out after a variable time period. This variability in the activity, speed and duration of the destructive cholangiopathy may explain the diversity of lesions observed in follow-up liver biopsies of children who underwent a successful portoenterostomy followed by a favourable post-operative course[7].

The hepatic lesions observed in follow-up biopsies taken 4–5 years after portoenterostomy in 'clinically cured' patients include: mild periportal fibrosis; variable degrees of ductopenia associated with variable degrees of periportal fibrosis; a congenital hepatic fibrosis-like pattern (in patients who suffered from the 'early severe' variant of EHBDA); and biliary fibrosis.

These histological patterns are associated with variable degrees of lobular parenchymal changes indicating smouldering cholestasis: cholestatic liver cell rosettes, cholate stasis and periportal copper accumulation, and foci of periportal ductular reaction[7,34].

References

1. Bianchi L. Liver biopsy interpretation in hepatitis. Part I. Presentation of critical morphologic features used in diagnosis (Glossary). Pathol Res Pract. 1983;178:2–19.
2. Popper H. General pathology of the liver: light microscopic aspects serving diagnosis and interpretation. Semin Liver Dis. 1986;6:175–84.
3. Phillips MJ, Poucell S. Cholestasis: surgical pathology, mechanisms and new concepts. In: Farber E, Phillips MJ, Kaufman N, editors. Pathogenesis of liver diseases. International Academy of Pathology. Monograph no. 28. Baltimore: Williams & Wilkins; 1987:65–94.
4. International Group. Histopathology of the intrahepatic biliary tree. Liver. 1983;3:161–75.
5. Nagore N, Howe S, Scheuer PJ. The three-dimensional liver. In: Popper H, Schaffner F, editors. Progress in liver diseases. Vol. 9. Philadelphia: WB Saunders; 1990:1–10.
6. Van Eyken P, Sciot R, Desmet VJ. A cytokeratin immunohistochemical study of cholestatic liver disease: evidence that hepatocytes can express 'bile duct-type' cytokeratins. Histopathology. 1989;15:125–35.
7. Desmet VJ, Callea F. Cholestatic syndromes of infancy and childhood. In: Zakim D, Boyer TD, editors. Hepatology. A textbook of liver disease. Vol. 2, 2nd edition. Philadelphia: WB Saunders; 1990:1355–95.
8. Desmet VJ. Current problems in diagnosis of biliary disease and cholestasis. Semin Liver Dis. 1986;6:233–45.
9. Ludwig J. New concepts in biliary cirrhosis. Semin Liver Dis. 1987;7:293–301.
10. Thaler H. Leberkrankheiten. Histopathologie. Pathophysiologie. Klinik. Berlin: Springer Verlag; 1982.
11. Bujanover Y. Prognosis of neonatal cholestatic jaundice. J Pediatr Gastroenterol Nutr. 1987;6:163–7.
12. Balistreri WF. Interrelationship between the infantile cholangiopathies and paucity of the intrahepatic bile ducts. In: Balistreri WF, Stocker JT, editors. Pediatric hepatology. New York: Hemisphere; 1990:1–18.
13. Lefkowitch JH. Bile ductular cholestasis: an ominous histopathologic sign related to sepsis and 'cholangitis lenta'. Hum Pathol. 1982;13:19–24.
14. Desmet VJ. Liver reaction patterns in infections. In: Bianchi L, Maier K-P, Gerok W, Deinhardt F, editors. Infectious diseases of the liver. Dordrecht: Kluwer; 1990:31–47.
15. Scheuer PJ. Liver biopsy interpretation, 4th edn. London: Baillière Tindall; 1988.
16. Ishak KG, Sharp HL. Metabolic errors and liver disease. In: MacSween RNM, Anthony PP, Scheuer PJ, editors. Pathology of the liver, 2nd edn. Edinburgh: Churchill Livingstone; 1987.
17. Ishak KG. Pathology of inherited metabolic disorders. In: Balistreri WF, Stocker JT, editors. Pediatric hepatology. New York: Hemisphere; 1990:77–158.
18. Callea F, Brisigotti M, Faa G, Lucini L, Eriksson S. Identification of PiZ gene products in liver tissue by a monoclonal antibody specific for the Z mutant of alpha-1-antitrypsin. J Hepatol. 1991;12:372–6.
19. Kahn E. Paucity of interlobular bile ducts. Arteriohepatic dysplasia and nonsyndromic duct paucity. In: Abramowsky CR, Bernstein J, Rosenberg HS, editors. Perspectives in pediatric pathology. Transplantation pathology – hepatic morphogenesis. Basel: Karger; 1991:168–215.
20. Nayak NC. Nutritional liver disease. In: MacSween RNM, Anthony PP, Scheuer PJ, editors. Pathology of the liver. Edinburgh: Churchill Livingstone; 1987:265–80.
21. Suchy FJ, Mullick FG. Total parenteral nutrition-associated cholestasis. In: Balistreri WF, Stocker JT, editors. Pediatric hepatology. New York: Hemisphere; 1990:29–40.
22. Alagille D. Intrahepatic biliary atresia (hepatic ductular hypoplasia). In: Berenberg SR, editor. Liver disease in infancy and childhood. Baltimore: Williams & Wilkins; 1976:129–42.
23. Kahn E, Markowitz J, Aiges H, Daum F. Human ontogeny of the bile duct to portal space ratio. Hepatology. 1989;10:21–3.
24. Alagille D, Thomassin N. L'atrésie des voies biliaires intrahépatiques avec des voies biliaires extrahépatiques perméables chez l'enfant: à propos de 25 observations. Rev Med Chir Mal Foie. 1970;45:93–104.
25. Dommergues JP. L'atrésie des voies biliaires intrahépatiques avec voies biliaires extrahépa-

tiques perméables chez l'enfant: à propos de 23 observations. Ann Med Interne. 1972;123: 871–3.

26. Hashida Y, Yunis EJ. Syndromatic paucity of interlobular bile ducts: hepatic histopathology of the early and endstage liver. Pediatr Pathol. 1988;8:1–15.

27. Gathman H. Beitrag zur Diagnostik der Gallengangsatresie und Hypoplasie bei Kleinkindern. Acta Hepatogastroenterol. 1973;20:24–35.

28. Van Eyken P, Sciot R, Van Damme B, De Wolf-Peeters C, Desmet VJ. Keratin-immunohistochemistry in normal human liver. Cytokeratin pattern of hepatocytes, bile ducts and acinar gradient. Virchows Arch [A]. 1987;412:63–72.

29. Dahms BB. Biliary atresia: extrahepatic? Intrahepatic? Both? Neither? In: Abramowski CR, Bernstein J, Rosenberg HS, editors. Perspectives in pediatric pathology. Transplantation pathology. Hepatic morphogenesis. Vol. 14. Basel: Karger; 1991:VII.

30. Raweily EA, Gibson AAM, Burt AD. Abnormalities of intrahepatic bile ducts in extrahepatic biliary atresia. Histopathology. 1990;17:521–7.

31. Desmet VJ. Cholangiopathies: past, present and future. Semin Liver Dis. 1987;7:67–76.

32. Schweizer P, Mueller G. Gallengangsatresie. Cholestase-Syndrome im Neugeborenen- und Säuglingsalter. Stuttgart: Hippokrates Verlag; 1984.

33. Laurent J. Gauthier F, Bernard O, Hadchouel M, Odièvre M, Valayer M, Alagille D. Long-term outcome after surgery for biliary atresia. Study of 40 patients surviving more than 10 years. Gastroenterology. 1990;99:1793–7.

34. Callea F, Facchetti F, Lucini L, Favret M, Zorzi F, Guerini A, Bonetti M, Alberti D, Dessanti A, Caccia G. Liver morphology in anicteric patients at long-term follow-up after Kasai operation: a study of 16 cases. In: Ohi R, editor. Biliary atresia. Tokyo: Professional Postgraduate Services; 1987:304–10.

7
Lipid peroxidation in cholestasis

R. J. SOKOL

INTRODUCTION

Cholestatic liver disease is an important clinical problem in both children and adults. Neonatal cholestatic hepatobiliary disorders occur in from 1 in 5000 to 1 in 10 000 live births and include, among other diseases, extrahepatic biliary atresia, idiopathic neonatal hepatitis, syndromatic and non-syndromatic paucity of interlobular bile ducts, and various familial and metabolic cholestatic syndromes[1]. The progressive nature of many of these disorders is demonstrated by the fact that they are among the primary indications for hepatic transplantation in children[2]. In adults, cholestasis is a prominent feature of diseases such as primary biliary cirrhosis, primary sclerosing cholangitis, and obstructive biliary tract disease. These disorders, likewise, are responsible for a large percentage of adults referred for liver transplantation[3]. Currently, there is a lack of effective therapy for cholestatic disorders, although the use of ursodeoxycholic acid appears promising[4,5]. The development of new medical treatments for cholestasis relies on characterization of the underlying mechanisms by which the hepatocyte is injured, independent of what the initiating event leading to the cholestasis might be (e.g. structural, infectious, immunological, or metabolic abnormalities). Although there are a number of hypotheses as to why impaired bile flow leads to liver injury, most authorities believe that the accumulation of bile acids in the hepatocyte is the key factor involved[6]. In this regard it has been shown that the hydrophobic bile acids (e.g. the monohydroxy and the dihydroxy bile acids) are more hepatotoxic than the hydrophilic bile acids (trihydroxy bile acids and ursodeoxycholic acid)[7]. Previous investigators have postulated that the detergent properties of the hydrophobic bile acids alter plasma membrane or subcellular organelle membranes, leading to enzyme dysfunction, cell volume regulation abnormalities or intracellular release of toxic cations or enzymes[6-8]. The beneficial effect of ursodeoxycholic acid in human cholestatic disorders[4,5] and in several animal models of bile acid toxicity[9,10] supports the notion that substituting a more hydrophilic for the hydrophobic bile acids lessens hepatocellular injury. We have hypothesized that the difference in hepatotoxicity caused by the various bile acids may be related to the ability of the bile acids to lead to generation of free radicals within the hepatocyte, thereby causing injury and dysfunction. This chapter will outline the data base supporting the notion that free radicals and lipid peroxidation may be involved in the pathogenesis of cholestatic liver injury, and present preliminary data from our laboratory consistent with this hypothesis.

FREE RADICALS AND CHOLESTASIS

Several lines of evidence support the hypothesis that free radicals are generated in the liver during cholestasis and that peroxidation of membrane lipids might lead to hepatocyte dysfunction. Dahm et al.[11] have shown that the hydrophobic bile acids – lithocholic acid, chenodeoxycholic acid, and deoxycholic acid – stimulate release of superoxide from polymorphonuclear leucocytes that are primed with a phorbol ester (PMA). Lithocholic acid had the greatest stimulatory activity, causing eight-fold increases in superoxide at concentrations of 32–100 μmol/l. This concentration of bile acids is similar to that which may occur in plasma and, certainly, within hepatocytes during cholestasis. Cholic acid at similar concentrations produced minimal increases in superoxide generation from primed neutrophils. Thus, hydrophobic bile acids that may accumulate during cholestasis have the capacity to induce activated neutrophils to generate reactive oxygen species. Inasmuch as neutrophils are commonly visualized in portal tract inflammatory infiltrates in cholestatic liver (either human or bile duct-ligated rat)[12,13], it is possible that reactive oxygen species derived from neutrophils may be adding to hepatocyte injury. In addition, using millimolar concentrations of bile acids, DeLange and Glazer[14] were able to show, in an *in vitro* system, that bile acids may inhibit lipid peroxidation at low lipid concentrations, whereas at higher lipid concentrations bile acids may promote lipid peroxidation. Moreover, copper, which accumulates in the hepatocyte as a consequence of cholestasis[15], is a potent catalyser of the Haber–Weiss reaction in which H_2O_2 is converted to the hydroxyl free-radical[16]. The latter is a highly reactive oxygen species which rapidly reacts with and damages polyunsaturated fatty acids, thiol proteins and nucleic acids[16]. Therefore, if reactive oxygen species are generated in the cholestatic liver, the accumulated copper may promote formation of the most reactive oxygen species, the hydroxy free radical. Counterbalancing the generation of free radicals are the antioxidant enzymes, glutathione peroxidase, catalase, and superoxide dismutase[16]. Togashi et al.[17] have shown that CuZn–superoxide dismutase and catalase activities are reduced in the diseased human liver, possibly increasing the susceptibility of the liver to injury by oxygen-derived free radicals. In summary, bile acids in the presence of hepatic copper accumulation and depletion of antioxidant enzyme concentrations may combine to cause free radical injury to the liver during cholestasis.

There are several clinical lines of evidence to support this hypothesis. Lipid peroxides can be measured in the blood by the thiobarbituric acid reaction (TBARS[18]). Lemonnier et al.[19] measured plasma lipid peroxide levels in 40 children with chronic cholestasis, and found that mean levels were twice as high in children with extrahepatic biliary atresia and four times as high in those with paucity of interlobular bile ducts than in controls. This study is provocative, however; since elevated serum bilirubin can cause falsely high elevations of plasma lipid peroxides measured by TBARS, it may well be that the authors were measuring bilirubin rather than lipid peroxides[20]. It has been well demonstrated that the content of dietary fat influences the lipid composition of hepatocyte subcellular membrane fractions[21]. If increased polyunsaturated fatty acids, the substrate for lipid peroxidation[16], are ingested, an increased propensity towards lipid peroxidation would be present. In this regard, Deems *et al.*[22] have reported that the frequency of consumption of fats and oils in primary biliary cirrhosis patients correlated strongly with serum alkaline phosphatase and serum bilirubin levels, implying more severe liver injury. Similar findings have been reported for alcoholic liver disease wherein larger intake of lipids results in more severe liver disease[23]. We have developed an animal model to test the hypothesis that increased susceptibility to lipid peroxidation may worsen cholestatic liver injury[24]. Weanling rats were fed diets that were either vitamin E-deficient (E−) or vitamin E-sufficient (E+) combined with either normal lipid (11.9% calories as stripped corn oil), high lipid (35% calories as stripped corn oil), or n-3 fatty acid supplemented (fish oil supplementation) (11% of calories as stripped corn oil plus 24% of calories as stripped Menhaden oil). After 6 weeks of diet, rats underwent bile duct ligation and transection or similar sham surgery. Seventeen days later the rats were killed and liver and blood were removed. Serum total bilirubin was more elevated in vitamin E-deficient rats on either of the high-lipid diets (corn oil or Menhaden oil) compared to those on the normal lipid diet. In addition, significant lipid peroxidation was demonstrated in hepatic mitochondria from all bile duct-ligated groups compared to sham groups, and was significantly higher in the bile duct-ligated vitamin E-deficient groups receiving the high lipid diets. Thus, in our rat model the combination of vitamin E deficiency plus a high lipid intake (which was similar to the lipid intake in the average Western diet) led to oxidative alterations of mitochondrial lipids as well as increased liver injury during cholestasis. The importance of the vitamin E deficiency should be stressed inasmuch as most patients with chronic cholestasis develop a secondary deficiency of vitamin E caused by malabsorption of dietary tocopherol[25–29]. This study suggests that deficiency of vitamin E, the primary membrane-bound antioxidant, may lead to enhanced free radical damage in the cholestatic hepatocyte.

Additional support for our hypothesis was observed when we treated five children with chronic cholestasis and well-documented vitamin E deficiency with parenteral vitamin E for 2–3 years[30]. The correction of vitamin E deficiency was accompanied by a significant decrease in fasting serum cholylglycine blood concentrations over the period of study compared to the year prior to study. This suggests that there was ongoing free radical injury to the liver when the patients were vitamin E-deficient, and that correction of the vitamin E deficiency reduced this component of the liver injury. Taken together, these data indicate that free radical injury, particularly to membrane lipids, may be present during cholestasis, and that dietary manipulation of antioxidants and pro-oxidants may affect the degree of hepatic injury and lipid peroxidation during cholestasis. Based on these data, it will be important to determine if inhibition of free radical generation or scavenging of free radicals will be potential beneficial treatments in cholestatic liver disease.

BILE ACID TOXICITY STUDIES IN ISOLATED HEPATOCYTES

To test whether bile acid toxicity to the hepatocyte may involve the generation of free radicals we have performed the following studies in freshly isolated rat hepatocytes[31]. Hepatocytes were incubated with 100–200 μmol/l of taurocholic acid, taurochenodeoxycholic acid, taurolithocholic acid, or tauroursodeoxycholic acid. Over 4 h there was approximately a 60% loss of cell viability when taurolithocholic acid or taurochenodeoxycholic acid were incubated with the hepatocytes, whilst the other two bile acids were no different from controls with a loss of only 8–10% of viability over 4 h. There was increased generation of lipid peroxides (measured by the TBARS reaction) that either preceded or paralleled this loss of cell viability in the taurolithocholic acid and chenodeoxycholic acid-treated hepatocytes. In a separate set of experiments, inhibitors of free radical generation or chelators of iron were preincubated with hepatocytes for 30 min and the bile acids were then added to the hepatocyte suspension. α-Tocopheryl succinate (100–200 μmol/l), α-tocopherol (500 μmol/l), the antioxidant DPPD (100 μmol/l), superoxide dismutase (500 U/ml), catalase (1000 U/ml), the combination of superoxide dismutase plus catalase, deferoxamine (50 μmol/l), or apotransferrin (40 μmol/l), each inhibited the loss of cell viability by 90–100% and the lipid peroxidation by approximately 75–90% when hepatocytes were incubated with 200 μmol/l taurolithocholic acid for 4 h. The effect of these scavengers of reactive oxygen species and chelators of iron suggests that oxygen-derived free radicals were generated in our experimental system. The inhibition of lipid peroxidation that accompanied the protection against toxicity suggests that free radical pathways were involved in the pathogenesis of the hepatocyte toxicity and not merely a consequence of cell injury. These studies are now being expanded to pinpoint more clearly the source of the free radical species, the precise form of reactive oxygen that is involved in this toxicity, and whether the same results can be reproduced in an intact model of taurolithocholic acid toxicity.

FUTURE DIRECTIONS

Our data suggest that inhibitors or scavengers of oxygen free radicals may be of benefit in the treatment of cholestatic liver disease. If further studies support this hypothesis, then the development of antioxidants which would be non-toxic, reach the liver in sufficient concentrations to protect the hepatocyte from oxygen free radicals, and be amenable to oral therapy would be potential novel manoeuvres to reduce liver injury during cholestasis and prevent the progression to cirrhosis.

Acknowledgements

This work was supported in part by National Institutes of Health Grants R29-DK38446 and IP30AM34914, and the Abby Bennett Liver Research Fund.

References

1. Balistreri WF. Neonatal cholestasis: lessons from the past, issues for the future. Semin Liver Dis. 1987;7:61–6.
2. Whitington PF, Balistreri WF. Liver transplantation in pediatrics: indications, contraindications, and pretransplant management. J Pediatr. 1991;118:169–77.
3. Iwatsuki S, Shaw BW, Starzl TE. Current status of hepatic transplantation. Semin Liv Dis. 1983;3:173–80.
4. Leuschner U, Fischer H, Kurtz W, Guldutuna S, Hubner K, Hellstern A, Gatzen M, Leuschner M. Ursodeoxycholic acid in primary biliary cirrhosis: results of a controlled double-blind trial. Gastroenterology. 1989;97:1268–74.
5. Balistreri WF, A-Kader HH, Ryckman FC, Whitington PF, Heubi JE, Setchell KD. Biochemical and clinical response to ursodeoxycholic acid administration in paediatric patients with chronic cholestasis. In: Paumgartner G, Stiehl A, Gerok W, editors. Bile acids as therapeutic agents. Lancaster: Kluwer; 1991:323–33.
6. Greim H, Trulzsch D, Roboz J, Dressler K, Czygan P, Hutterer F, Schaffner F, Popper H. Mechanisms of cholestasis. Bile acids in normal rat livers and in those after bile duct ligation. Gastroenterology. 1972;63:837–45.
7. Scholmerich J, Becher MS, Schmidt K, Schubert R, Kremer B, Feldhaus S, Gerok W. Influence of hydroxylation and conjugation of bile salts on their membrane-damaging properties – studies on isolated hepatocytes and lipid membrane vesicles. Hepatology. 1984;4:661–6.
8. Combettes L, Dumont M, Berthon B, Erlinger S, Claret M. Release of calcium from the endoplasmic reticulum by bile acids in rat liver cells. J Biol Chem. 1988;263:2299–303.
9. Schölmerich J, Baumgartner U, Miyai K, Gerok W. Tauroursodeoxycholate prevents taurolithocholate-induced cholestasis and toxicity in rat liver. J Hepatol. 1990;10:280–3.
10. Galle PR, Theilmann L, Raedsch R, Otto G, Stiehl A. Ursodeoxycholate reduces hepatotoxicity of bile salts in primary human hepatocytes. Hepatology. 1990;12:486–91.
11. Dahm LJ, Hewett JA, Roth RA. Bile and bile salts potentiate superoxide anion release from activated, rat peritoneal neutrophils. Toxicol Appl Pharmacol. 1988;95:82–92.
12. Kountouras J, Billing BH, Scheuer PJ. Prolonged bile duct obstruction: a new experimental model for cirrhosis in the rat. Br J Exp Pathol. 1984;65:305–11.
13. Scheuer PJ. Liver biopsy interpretation, Baillière Tindall, London; 1980:36–59.
14. DeLange RJ, Glazer AN. Bile acids: antioxidants or enhancers of peroxidation depending on lipid concentration. Arch Biochem Biophys. 1990;276:19–25.
15. Sternlieb I. Copper and the liver. Gastroenterology. 1980;78:1615–28.
16. Halliwell B. Reactive oxygen species in living systems: source, biochemistry, and role in human disease. Am J Med. 1991;91(suppl 3C):14S–22S.
17. Togashi H, Shinzawa H, Wakabayashi H, Nakamura T, Yamada N, Takahashi T, Ishikawa M. Activities of free oxygen radical scavenger enzymes in human liver. J Hepatol. 1990;11:200–5.
18. Yagi K. A simple fluorometric assay for lipoperoxide in blood plasma. Biochem Med. 1976;15:212–16.
19. Lemonnier F, Cresteil D, Feneant M, Couturier M, Bernard O, Alagille D. Plasma lipid peroxides in cholestatic children. Acta Paediatr Scand. 1987;76:928–34.
20. Gutteridge JMC, Tickner TR. The thiobarbituric acid-reactivity of bile pigments. Biochem Med. 1978;19:127–32.
21. Kools AM, Straka JG, Hill HD, Whitmer DI, Holman RT, Bloomer JR. Modulation of hepatic ferrochelatase activity by dietary manipulation of mitochondrial phospholipid fatty acyl group. Hepatology. 1989;9:557–61.

22. Deems RG, Friedman LS, Friedman MI, Munoz SJ, Maddrey WC. Alkaline phosphatase and bilirubin levels are related to dietary fat intake in cholestatic liver disease. Gastroenterology. 1989;96(part 2):A591.
23. Nanji AA, French SW. Dietary factors and alcoholic cirrhosis. Alcoholism. 1986;10:271–3.
24. Sokol RJ, Devereaux M, Khandwala RA. Effect of dietary lipid and vitamin E on mitochondrial lipid peroxidation and hepatic injury in the bile duct-ligated rat. J Lipid Res. 1991;32:1349–57.
25. Sokol RJ, Heubi JE, Iannaccone S, Bove KE, Balistreri WF. Mechanism causing vitamin E deficiency during chronic childhood cholestasis. Gastroenterology. 1983;85:1171–82.
26. Sokol RJ, Balistreri WF, Hoofnagle JH, Jones EA. Vitamin E deficiency in adults with chronic liver disease. Am J Clin Nutr. 1985;41:66–72.
27. Munoz SJ, Heubi JE, Balistreri WF, Maddrey WC. Vitamin E deficiency in primary biliary cirrhosis; gastrointestinal malabsorption, frequency, and relationship to other lipid-soluble vitamins. Hepatology. 1989;9:525–31.
28. Sokol RJ, Kim YS, Hoofnagle JH, Heubi JE, Jones EA, Balistreri WF. Intestinal malabsorption of vitamin E in primary biliary cirrhosis. Gastroenterology. 1989;96:479–86.
29. Arria AM, Tarter RE, Warty V, Van Thiel DM. Vitamin E deficiency and psychomotor performance in adults with primary biliary cirrhosis. Am J Clin Nutr. 1990;52:383–90.
30. Sokol RJ, Heubi JE, McGraw C, Balistreri WF. Correction of vitamin E deficiency in children with chronic cholestasis. II. Effect on gastrointestinal and hepatic function. Hepatology. 1986;6:1263–9.
31. Sokol RJ, Devereaux MW, Khandwala R, O'Brian K. Protective effect of free radical inhibitors and scavengers against bile acid toxicity in isolated rat hepatocytes. (Abstract) Clin Res. 1992;40:10A.

8
Parameters of the antioxidant protective system in cystic fibrosis patients with cholestatic liver disease

B. M. WINKLHOFER-ROOB, D. H. SHMERLING, M. G. SCHIMEK and P. E. TUCHSCHMID

BACKGROUND

The pathogenesis of cholestatic liver disease (CLD) in cystic fibrosis (CF) patients is not fully elucidated[1,2]. Experimental studies and limited data of CLD patients suggest that antioxidant deficiencies may have adverse effects on hepatic function[3,4].

PATIENTS AND METHODS

This study was designed to determine whether CF patients with CLD more frequently exhibit antioxidant deficiencies compared with those without. Twelve CF patients with sonographic and laboratory evidence of CLD were compared with 24 without (NCLD) for plasma and erythrocyte α-tocopherol, plasma β-carotene, and erythrocyte glutathione peroxidase[5-7].

RESULTS

CLD patients showed significantly lower erythrocyte α-tocopherol than NCLD (Wilcoxon matched pair signed rank test; $W = 13$, one-sided, $\alpha = 0.05$). A higher proportion of CLD patients, although supplemented with α-tocopherol, was deficient for the ratio plasma α-tocopherol:cholesterol and for erythrocyte α-tocopherol, compared with NCLD (binomial fiducial limits; $1 - \alpha = 0.95$; $p = 0.30$ for CLD, $0 \leqslant \pi \leqslant 0.28$ for NCLD compared to $p = 0.70$ for CLD, $0.08 \leqslant \pi \leqslant 0.53$ for NCLD). The relationship between plasma α-tocopherol:cholesterol and γ-glutamyltransferase followed an inverse multiplicative model ($y = ax^b$, significant slope b, $\alpha = 0.05$), indicating severe α-tocopherol deficiency in advanced CLD. Also, β-carotene and glutathione peroxidase were lower in CLD patients compared with NCLD (Mann–Whitney test, one-sided, $\alpha = 0.05$, $U = 146$ and $U = 145$ respectively). Five CLD patients were deficient for two, and seven for all three antioxidants.

CONCLUSIONS

Advanced CLD is accompanied by severe α-tocopherol, β-carotene and glutathione peroxidase deficiency. The relationships however, may be two-fold:

1. CLD. causes antioxidant deficiencies due to bile acid deficiency (α-tocopherol, β-carotene) and, since the antioxidants act in concert against oxidative injury, other antioxidants (e.g. glutathione peroxidase) also may undergo increased consumption.
2. CLD may preferably occur or progress in patients with an impaired antioxidant defence system.

Prospective studies are required to confirm a direct contribution of a long-lasting lack of antioxidant protection to the development and progression of CLD in CF patients.

References

1. Roy CC, Weber AM, Morin CL *et al*. Abnormal biliary lipid composition in cystic fibrosis: effect of pancreatic enzymes. N Engl J Med. 1977;297:1301–5.
2. Gaskin KJ, Waters DLM, Howman-Giles R, *et al*. Liver disease and common-bile-duct stenosis in cystic fibrosis. N Engl J Med. 1988;318:340–6.
3. Sokol RJ, Devereaux M, Khandwala RA. Effect of dietary lipid and vitamin E on mitochondrial lipid peroxidation and hepatic injury in the bile duct ligated rat. J Lipid Res. 1991;32:1349–57.
4. Sokol RJ, Heubi JE, Balistreri WF. Improved hepatic function following vitamin E repletion during childhood cholestasis. Hepatology. 1983;3:848 (abstr.).
5. Vuilleumier J-P, Keller HE, Gysel D, Hunziker F. Clinical chemical methods for the routine assessment of the vitamin status in human populations. Part I: The fat-soluble vitamin A and E, and β-carotene. Int J Vitam Nutr Res. 1983;53:265–72.
6. Celenk A, Tuchschmid P, Rieser F, Duc G. Effect of vitamin E substitution in very low birth weight infants. Biol Neonat. 1987;52(suppl. 1):131–40.
7. Paglia DE, Valentine WN. Studies on the quantitative and qualitative characterization of erythrocyte glutathione peroxidase. J Lab Clin Med. 1967;70:158–69.

9
Mechanisms of bile salt toxicity

J. SCHÖLMERICH and R. STRAUB

INTRODUCTION

Bile acids are amphiphilic compounds with a steroid nucleus and differ with regard to their physicochemical properties due to hydroxylation and conjugation. They are produced by the liver from endogenous or exogenous cholesterol by different metabolic pathways[1]. Several physiological functions of bile salts are known, i.e. micelle formation in order to absorb fat and related substances such as fat-soluble vitamins, solubilization of lipids in bile and induction of bile acid-dependent bile flow[2]. It is not known if they have additional roles in the liver cell; however, it has been found that they may act as antioxidants[3]. They are reabsorbed during enterohepatic circulation in the small bowel and in particular in the terminal ileum by an active transport[4], taken up by the liver, and resecreted into bile. Inside the hepatocyte they are bound to 'bile acid binders', a major one in the rat being 3α-hydroxy steroid dehydrogenase (3α-HSD), an enzyme capable of oxidizing and reducing 3α-hydroxy bile salts[5]. Other bile acid binders have been identified, such as glutathione transferase and ligandin[6]. In humans the major binding protein in cytosol is another oxidoreductase, different from 3α-HSD[7]. Depending on their structure, bile acids may be found in different compartments of the cell[8].

There are species differences with respect to the major bile acids[9]; however, it is common that tri- and dihydroxylated bile acids are primarily synthesized in the liver (= primary bile acids), which are then transformed mostly by bacterial dehydroxylation into mono- and dihydroxy bile acids in the bowel lumen (= secondary bile acids). Isomerization, for example, β-hydroxylation in the 7-position of the steroid nucleus, may occur (= tertiary bile acids)[4]. Bile acids are conjugated by the liver, mostly with amino acids into taurine or glycine conjugates. The relation of conjugates depends upon the species; furthermore, sulphation, glucuronidation and glucosidation occur[10]. Therefore in bile mostly primary or tertiary bile salts in amidated form are found in most species. In the rat taurine conjugation is predominant, while in humans glycine is the major conjugate[4].

It has been found in several disease states and experimental models that

Table 1   Questions related to the mechanisms of bile acid toxicity

---

1. Is toxicity a consequence of cholestasis or vice-versa, or is there no correlation?
2. What signs of toxicity are found?
3. What organelles are involved?
4. What mediators are involved?
5. What studies have to be done?

---

bile acids can have cholestatic and toxic effects on the liver. This is particularly so in cholestatic liver disorders[11], but occurs also when the dihydroxylated bile salt chenodeoxycholic acid (CDCA) is used for gallstone dissolution[12]. In this context morphological and biochemical abnormalities have been observed. The former manifest themselves in mitochondrial changes[13], signs of liver cell necrosis[14], and expansion of the endoplasmic reticulum[15]; the latter appear as an increase of serum transaminases[16].

Interestingly, the hydrophilic bile salt ursodeoxycholic acid (UDCA) does not produce, or at least to a lesser extent produces signs of liver abnormalities in several species[17], and this bile salt even improves liver function tests in several liver disorders[18–20]. Thus, it seems to be of interest to study the mechanism of bile salt toxicity in the liver. This review will deal with five questions related to this problem (Table 1).

CHOLESTASIS AND TOXICITY

Bile acid transport by the hepatocyte is different for each bile acid depending on its conjugation and the position of the hydroxyl groups[21]. It was thought that this difference was due to differences in uptake[21]; however, it was later found that secretion at the canalicular pole was the limiting step leading to the definition of the secretory rate maximum (SRm)[22]. Furthermore, it was suggested that the SRm was a function of the toxicity of the bile acid in question when a correlation between morphological signs of bile salt toxicity and the decrease in bile flow was found. Each bile salt has its own SRm (Table 2)[23], and the fall in bile salt secretion is accompanied or even preceded by a fall in cholesterol or phospholipid secretion. In addition it was found that SRm is inversely proportional to the ability of a bile salt to induce phospholipid secretion and non-linearly correlated to the critical micellar concentration (CMC) (Fig. 1). It has been speculated that depletion of the intracellular pool of phospholipids may be a cause of bile salt-induced cholestasis[24]. Finally, a change of the cholesterol/phospholipid ratio in the canalicular membrane has been found to be associated with taurolithocholate (TLCA)-induced cholestasis (Table 3)[25]. Interestingly, again the addition of the taurine conjugate of UDCA (TUDCA) is able to eliminate or at least attenuate the cholestatic effect of other bile salts, and in fact to increase the SRm (Fig. 2)[26–30]. The 7β-hydroxylated bile salt β-muricholic acid has similar protective properties[31]; sulphation is also a protective mechanism[32].

Interestingly, however, the cholestasis induced by increasing bile salt load above the SRm is reversible when bile salt supply is stopped[33]; this seems to be an argument against toxicity as a cause of cholestasis. In addition, it

Table 2 Critical micellar concentration (CMC), secretory rate maximum (SRm), and ability to induce phospholipid secretion (ΔPL) in relation to bile salt secretion (ΔBSS) of different taurine-conjugated bile salts

Bile salt	CMC (mmol/l)	SRm (nmol/g per min)	$\Delta PL/\Delta BSS$ (nmol/μmol)
TUCA	52	193 $\pm$ 32	13 $\pm$ 4
THCA	14	541	26
TCA	10	136 $\pm$ 35	66 $\pm$ 9
THDCA	11	391 $\pm$ 4	23 $\pm$ 2
TUDCA	8	390 $\pm$ 25	22 $\pm$ 4
TCDCA	7	32 $\pm$ 8	200 $\pm$ 78
TDHCA	250	269 $\pm$ 27	2 $\pm$ 2
T-3α7α 12 = 0	70	162 $\pm$ 11	65 $\pm$ 1
T-3α 7 = 0	35	95 $\pm$ 29	73 $\pm$ 12

Table 3 Effect of LCA and TLCA infusion on composition of liver cell plasma membrane fractions[25]

	LCA (30 min)	TLCA (30 min)	Control (30 min)
Protein[a]	0.18 $\pm$ 0.01	0.21 $\pm$ 0.03	0.25 $\pm$ 0.01
Cholesterol[b]	1433.14 $\pm$ 186.31	545.17 $\pm$ 43.24	226.17 $\pm$ 6.27
Phospholipids[b]	735.86 $\pm$ 20.14	875.17 $\pm$ 174.63	739.17 $\pm$ 17.71
LCA[b]	425.00 $\pm$ 42.00	n.d.	n.d.

[a]In mg/g liver. [b]In nmol/mg protein.

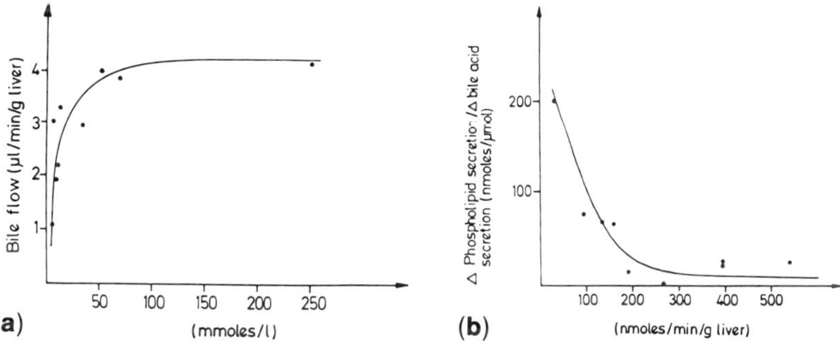

Fig. 1 Correlation between critical micellar concentrations (CMC) of, and bile flow induced by, different bile salts in the isolated perfused rat liver (**a**). Relation between secretory rate maximum (SRm) and the ability to induce phospholipid secretion of different bile salts (**b**)

has been found that there are species differences in the cholestatic effects of bile salts while toxicity seems to be more or less identical[34]; these differences are also present with respect to uptake[35]. Furthermore, it was shown that in the rat the order of cell toxicity is inversely proportional to the SRm, while this is not entirely so in the hamster (Table 4)[36].

Finally, there is a strong argument against a direct relation between

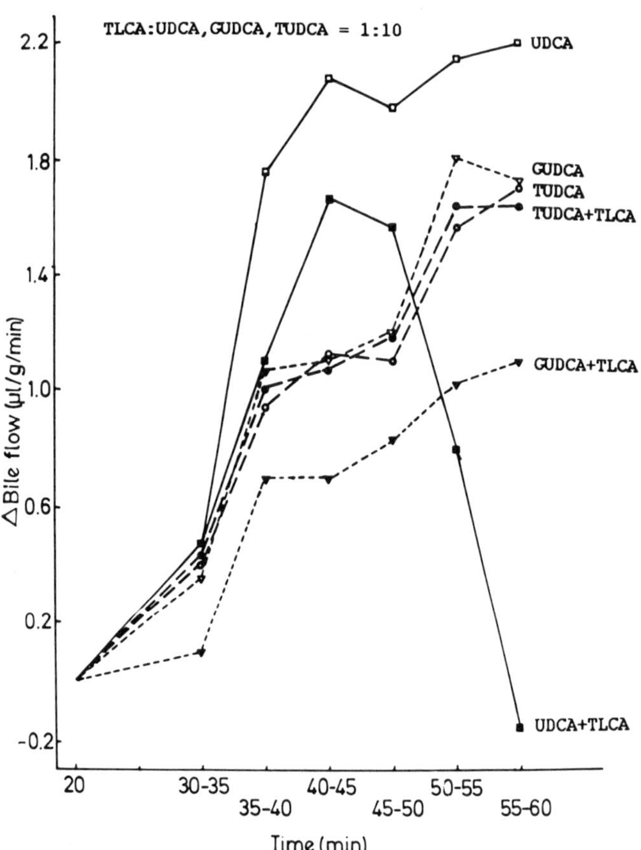

Fig. 2 Protective effects of ursodeoxycholate and its conjugates against taurolithocholate-induced cholestasis

Table 4 Species differences in SRm and cytotoxicity of bile salts[36]

	Rat	Hamster
SRm (order)	TUDCA > TCA > TCDCA	TCA > TCDCA > TUDCA
Cytotoxicity (order)	TCDCA > TCA > TUDCA	TCDCA > TCA > TUDCA

cholestasis and toxicity: while taurolithocholate induces cholestasis in the rat liver when perfused in orthograde fashion it does not when perfused in retrograde direction (Fig. 3). Accordingly, canalicular changes associated with cholestasis (Fig. 4) occur more frequently with orthograde as compared to retrograde perfusion; however, the number of necrotic cells as a sign of toxicity is 10-fold higher in retrograde perfused livers (Table 5)[37]. Taking these findings together it seems that there is no clear correlation between cholestasis and toxicity and vice-versa. Both seem, at least to some extent, to be independent from each other. Therefore, toxicity must not necessarily

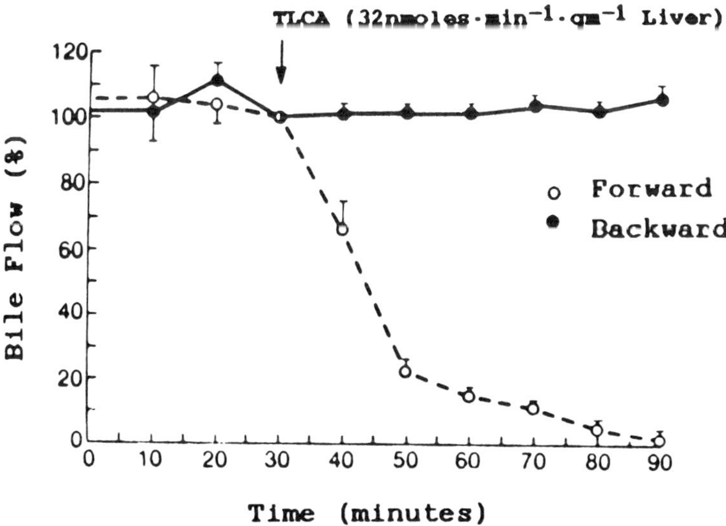

Fig. 3 Effect of antegrade and retrograde liver perfusion with taurolithocholate on bile flow[37]

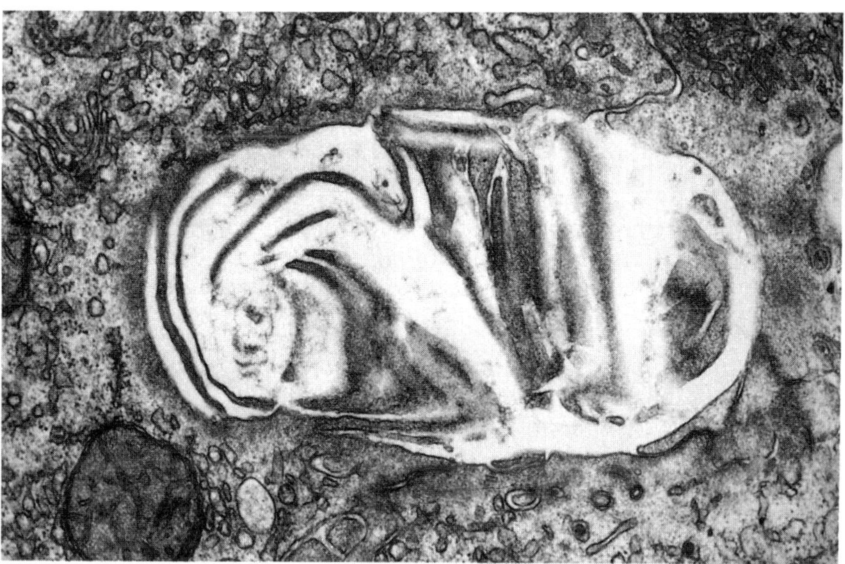

Fig. 4 Typical appearance of a canaliculus in taurolithocholate-induced cholestasis[37]

be correlated to the physicochemical properties of bile salts, in contrast to cholestasis, where such a correlation has been proven.

SIGNS OF TOXICITY

A number of signs of toxicity have been described. Liver cell hydropic swelling and necrosis can be seen. Furthermore, proteins are released into

Table 5 Effects of TLCA on tissue injury in the perfused rat liver[37]

	Focal cell necrosis (%)		Canalicular changes (%)	
	PP	*PV*	*PP*	*PV*
Forward perfusion (8 μmol/l)	0.96–1.28	0	89–93	4–7
Backward perfusion (8 μmol/l)	0	9.3–10.1	0	20–23

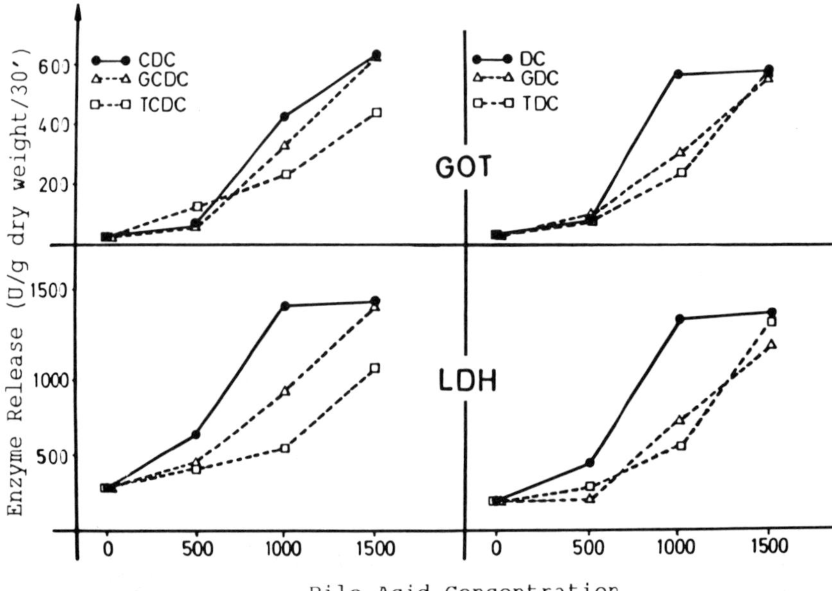

Fig. 5 Enzyme release from isolated hepatocytes with CDCA and DCA and their conjugates at different concentrations

bile and into the circulation[38]. Isolated hepatocytes have been used to study the toxic effects of bile salts, and it was found that mono- and dihydroxylated bile salts induced enzyme leakage (Fig. 5) in a dose- and time-dependent fashion, while conjugation and hydroxylation of the bile salts were correlated with the effects only to some extent[39]. Furthermore, the time course was different for TLCA and CDCA (Fig. 6). In addition, it was found that urea synthesis of these hepatocytes decreased, and that the hormone control of urea synthesis was lost (Fig. 7)[39].

A similar phenomenon was seen in cells isolated from cholestatic rat livers[40]. The toxic effects on cells were enhanced by cyclosporin A[41] and decreased by sulphation[42]. Similar findings were found in erythrocytes[43]. In some studies it was reported that TUDCA ameliorated or eliminated these effects of toxic bile salts in hepatocyte cultures[44]; however, on freshly isolated hepatocytes we could not demonstrate this effect[45]. Thus, in isolated

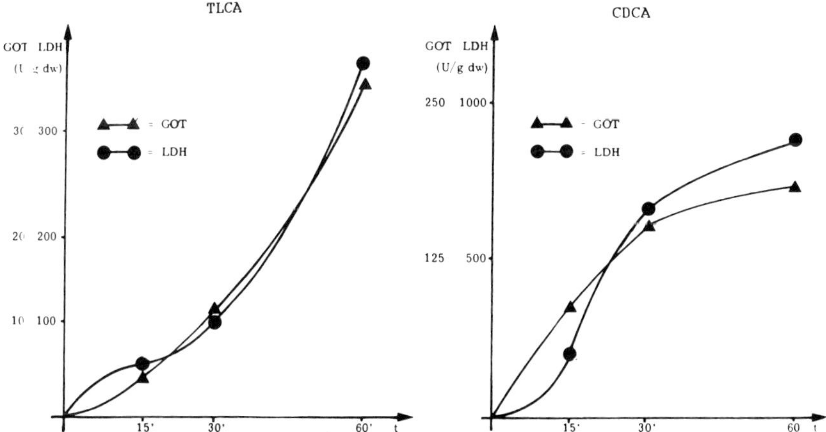

Fig. 6 Time-dependency of enzyme release in TLCA and TDCA incubation of isolated rat liver cells

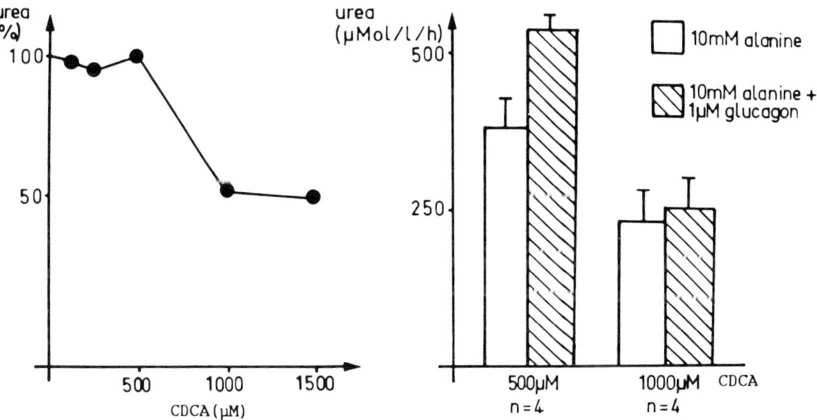

Fig. 7 Dose-dependent effect of CDCA on urea synthesis of isolated hepatocytes (left part) and loss of glucagon control of urea synthesis from alanine at 1000 µmol/l CDCA (right part)

hepatocytes enzyme leakage, decreased function, and morphological changes were found, indicating slightly different effects of different bile salts whereby the dihydroxylated bile salts CDCA and deoxycholic acid (DCA) seemed to have more detergent-like effects while TLCA was acting probably intracellularly. In the perfused liver enzyme release and morphological changes have been found, as well as in the whole animal. Some species differences seem to exist.

ORGANELLE INVOLVEMENT

The findings discussed so far do not give very specific hints with regard to the intracellular localization of the damage induced by bile salts; however,

Table 6 Distribution of bile salts in rat liver (%)[8]

	CA (*conj.*)	CDCA (*conj.*)	LCA
Nuclei	41	29	17
Microsomes	17	19	11
Mitochondria	9	15	3
Cytosol (bound)	22	33	68
Cytosol (free)	11	4	1

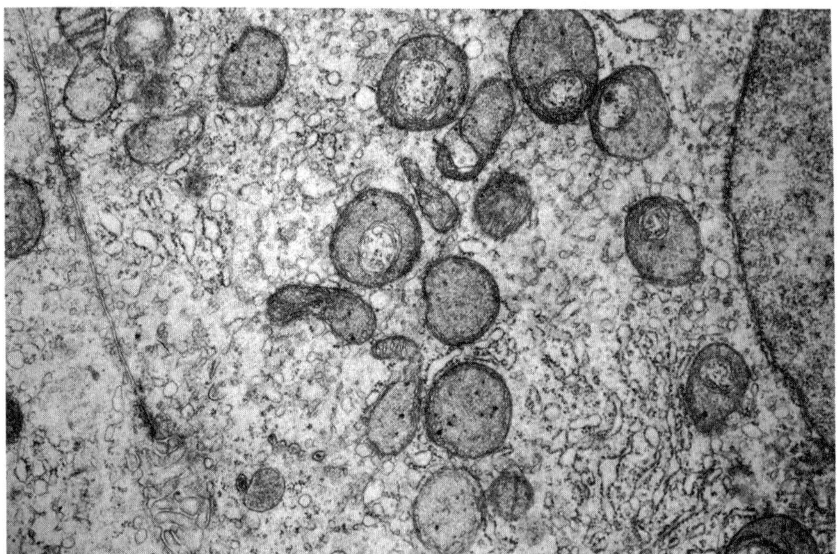

Fig. 8 Whorling of mitochondria in rats treated with CDCA[13]

disturbed urea synthesis and GOT release occurring before cell lysis point to a possible involvement of mitochondria. In order to analyse organelle involvement further, it is of interest to study the intracellular distribution of bile salts.

Surprisingly little is known on this aspect. Data are conflicting[8,46], and this might be due to technical problems with organelle fractionation. It seems obvious, however, that in addition to bound and free fractions in the cytosol, nuclei, microsomes, and mitochondria are involved (Table 6). It is of interest that the amount being free or bound in the cytosol varies widely depending on the hydrophobic properties of the bile salt. Binding is not irreversible[47]. Obstructive jaundice, however, is not associated with increased tissue binding in men[48]. Finally, mitochondria seem to be involved in bile acid metabolism. The formation of LCA, CDCA and α- and β-muricholic acid has been described[49]. In contrast, conjugating enzymes are probably not associated with mitochondria[50]. Interestingly, several groups have found morphological abnormalities of mitochondria in men under treatment with CDCA[51] and in rats given CDCA (Fig. 8)[13]. In addition, effects on mitochondrial functions

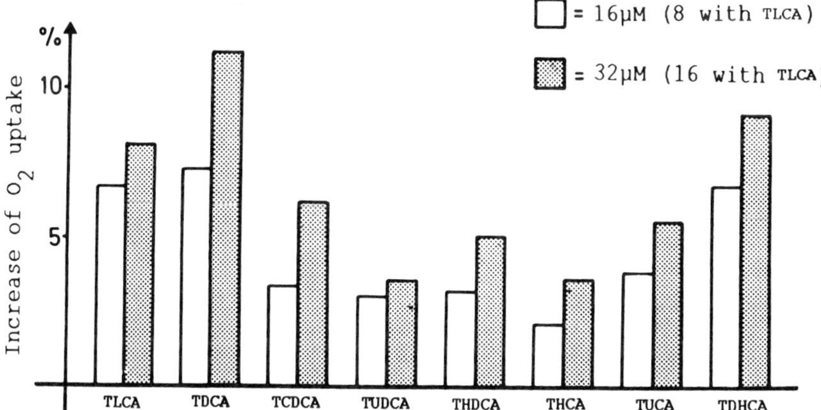

Fig. 9 Maximal increase of oxygen uptake by the isolated perfused rat liver under the influence of different bile salts at different concentrations

have been described. An uncoupling of oxidative phosphorylation[52], and an enhancement of state 4 mitochondrial respiration[53] have been observed. There have, however, been conflicting reports in rats with biliary obstruction[54].

Only a few other morphological abnormalities, including increased smooth endoplasmic reticulum[13,51,55], distension of the Golgi vesicles[13], and changes of ITO cells[51] have been found. Thus, at the present time little is known about organelle involvement, and even less about the functional consequences; however, some lines of evidence indicate that mitochondria might be of interest.

MEDIATORS

Considering mitochondrial involvement it is an obvious idea to look for abnormal oxygen metabolism. Van Dyke *et al.* (1983) found that the transcellular transport of taurocholic acid (TCA) does not increase oxygen consumption by rat liver[56]. When the findings of these authors are carefully studied, however, there seems to be an increase of O_2 uptake with a rapid loading of the liver with TCA as a bolus. When we studied the oxygen uptake of the isolated perfused rat liver with constant perfusate concentrations of different bile salts[57], it was found that the more toxic bile salts TLCA, TDCA and TCDCA, as well as the 3-keto bile salt TDHCA, led to a more pronounced increase of oxygen uptake as compared to other bile salts, while TCA and β-tauromuricholate did not result in any relevant increase (Fig. 9). It was furthermore found that those bile acids protecting the liver against TLCA induced cholestasis[30] also prevented the increase of O_2 uptake, at least to some extent. In particular TDHCA and taurourocholate (TUC) did not lead to significant protection. Furthermore, when cell toxicity was studied it became obvious that 'non-protective' bile salts with respect to O_2 uptake did even enhance morphological changes induced by TLCA (Table 7). Finally,

Table 7 Cell necrosis with TLCA – protection by other bile salts

	Number/625 cells
TLCA (8 μmol/l)	7.2 ± 1.0
+ TCA (16 μmol/l)	0
+ THCA (16 μmol/l)	1.7 ± 1.5
+ TUDCA (16 μmol/l)	2.7 ± 0.6
+ TUCA (16 μmol/l)	10.0 ± 4.0
+ TDHCA (16 μmol/l)	22.7 ± 4.5

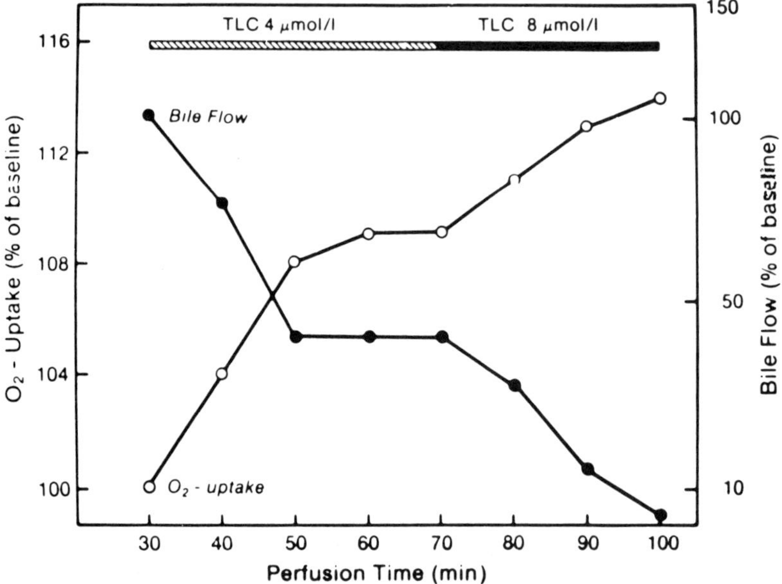

Fig. 10 Effect of antegrade perfusion with TLCA in the isolated perfused rat liver on bile flow and oxygen uptake

the model of orthograde and retrograde perfusion gives some hints to a correlation between O_2 uptake and toxicity but not cholestasis[37]. It is found that in the orthograde perfused rat liver bile flow fell rapidly while O_2 uptake increased[57]. In contrast, in the retrograde perfused rat liver bile flow increased and O_2 uptake also increased. In the latter group, however, toxicity was found (Figs 10 and 11). Thus it seems that bile salts do induce changes in oxygen metabolism, and that there is a relation to toxicity.

There are several possible ways by which hepatotoxicity can be oxygen-dependent[58]. The most general principle is that of oxygen radicals and peroxidation[59,60]. Interestingly, it has been found that bile salts act as antioxidants by inhibiting peroxidation. This results from scavenging of peroxy radicals by direct oxidation of the bile salt. In particular, 7-keto bile salts were found to be the most abundant products. However, at higher concentrations of lipids bile salts were found by the same authors to enhance

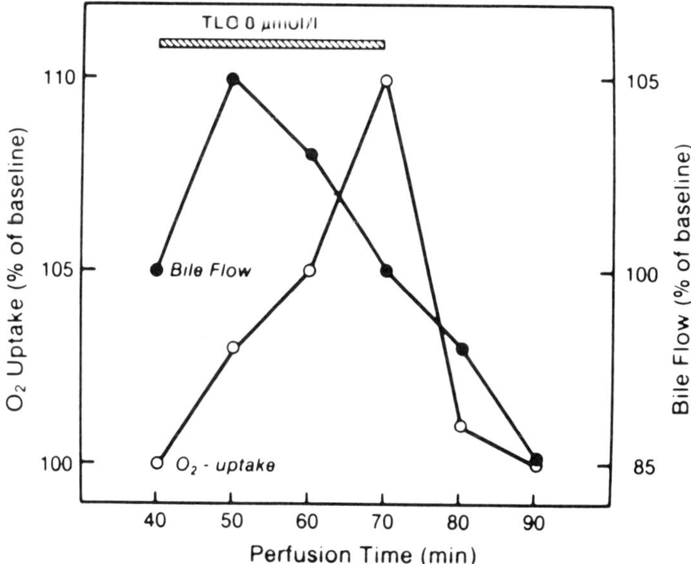

Fig. 11 Effect of retrograde perfusion with TLCA in the isolated perfused rat liver on bile flow and oxygen uptake

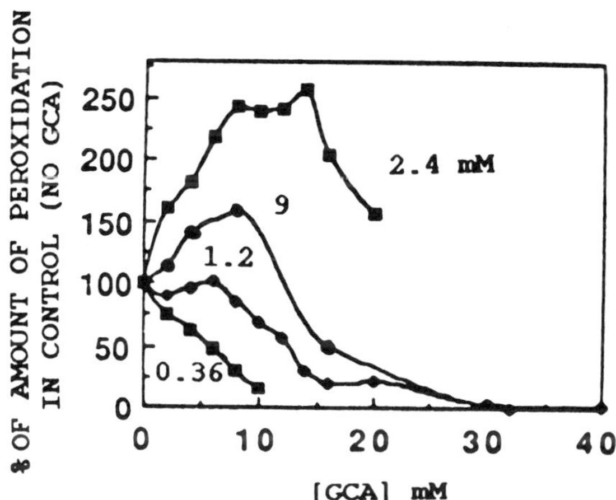

Fig. 12 Effect of glycocholate on lineolate peroxidation at different concentrations of lineolate and glycocholate[3]

lipid peroxidation (Fig. 12)[3]. In microsomal membranes a slight increase of lipid peroxidation products (LPO) was found, while in cholestasis the effect was less pronounced[61]. In isolated hepatocytes LCA, DCA and CDCA at concentrations of 10–100 µmol/l enhanced LPO formation and ornithine decarboxylase activity, and this was suppressed by superoxide dismutase or α-tocopherol. In accordance, loss of cell viability induced by 100 µmol/l of

Table 8 Effect of DCA on chemiluminescence of colonic mucosa[63]

	Chemiluminescence (cpm)
Basal	4963 ± 694
DOC (5 mmol/l)	52060 ± 6971
Xanthine/xanthine-oxidase	48722 ± 5197

these bile salts was prevented by the antioxidants[62]. Furthermore, DCA increased the chemiluminescence and ornithine decarboxylase of ODC activity in colonic epithelial cells to a similar extent as xanthine–xanthine oxidase, and these actions were blocked by radical scavengers (Table 8)[63].

Here the question arises how bile salts can induce the generation of oxygen radicals which then may lead to LPO formation. Taking into account observations that bile salts are transformed at least transiently to keto-forms during intracellular passage and/or metabolism[64] whereby in particular 7-keto forms occur[3,64], and that in addition one of the major binding proteins also acts on 3-keto bile salts[65], it might be helpful to look at other compounds having ring structures and keto-groups which induce oxidative stress via 'redox cycling'[66–68].

This phenomenon is well studied, i.e. for nitrofurantoin[66], and it has been shown that this compound induces a striking increase of excretion of reduced glutathione (GSSG) into bile with a concomitant increase in bile flow in a dose-dependent fashion (Fig. 13). These findings fit to some extent to the action of 'toxic' bile salts where bile flow is less affected than bile salt secretion since the 'independent fraction' may be increased due to increased GSSG excretion. This has been shown in experiments where hydrogen peroxide, diamide, and other thiol oxidizing agents were used[69,70]. Redox cycling acts as shown in Fig. 14, ultimately leading to the formation of toxic oxygen radicals from the superoxide anion and to the depletion of scavenger systems such as glutathione. The fact that bile salts inhibit enzymes necessary for detoxication[71] such as glutathione S-transferase – also a bile salt binder[6] – might further enhance this problem.

It is therefore very interesting that it was recently found that the major bile salt binder of rat liver, namely 3α-HSD[5,7] catalyses a cyclical oxidation–reduction of the C_3 position of different bile salts, which was shown by the constant decrease of the $^3H/^{14}C$ ratio of double-labelled bile salts (Table 9). The fact that ^3H loss from LCA ceased rapidly over time is probably due to its compartmentation in intact hepatocytes[72]. The same group later showed that this redox cycling also occurs in the isolated perfused rat liver[73] and also involves bile salt precursors[74].

A final argument in favour of redox cycling induced by bile salts is a preliminary experiment showing that cyanide could not suppress oxygen uptake completely when TDCA was present (Fig. 15) – this is a typical effect of other redox cyclers.

Reactive oxygen intermediates have been suggested to play a role in several models of liver tissue injury[60]. It is of particular importance that substances

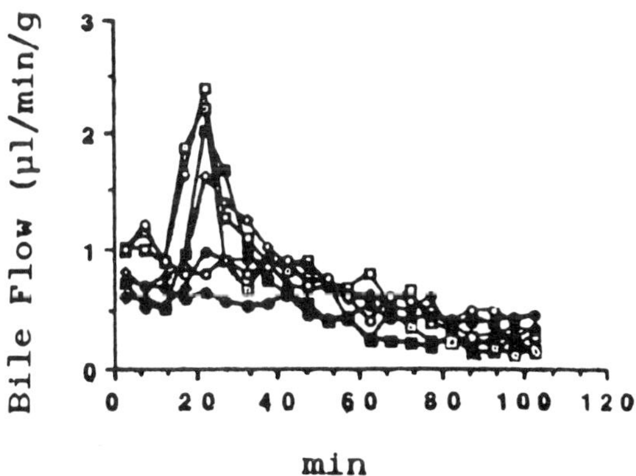

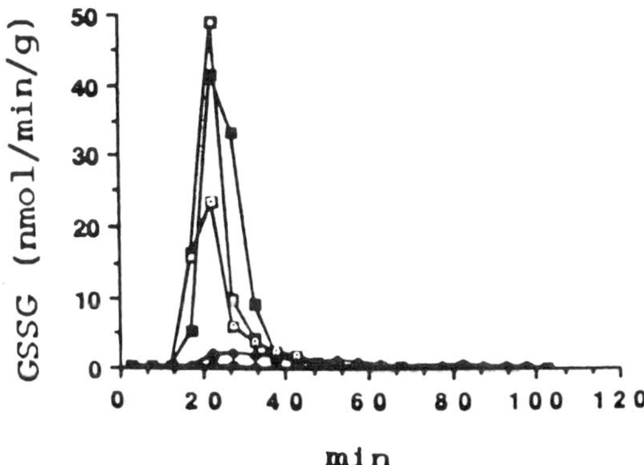

Fig. 13 Effect of nitrofurantoin on bile flow and GSSG release into bile at different concentrations[66]

which can inhibit enzymes necessary to regenerate the endogenous anti-oxidant potential of the cell, such as glutathione reductase, can aggravate the damage induced by the primary noxious agent.

It has recently been suggested that intracellular free calcium plays an important role in liver cell injury and death[75,76]. It was found that the activation of calcium-dependent proteases and protein kinase C may be a secondary messenger for cell death. It was further shown that free calcium increased the toxic effects of bile salts[77]. Interestingly, cell blebbing, typical for calcium-mediated processes, was found in our early studies on isolated hepatocytes (Fig. 16)[37]. Bile salts were found to increase cellular free calcium in cultured kidney cells[78]. It was furthermore shown[79] that the increase of intracellular calcium induced by hepatotoxic bile salts occurred at the concentrations found to be the 'thresholds' for cell damage as measured by enzyme release (Fig. 17)[37]. These authors thought the calcium to come from the extracellular compartment. Others, in contrast, have shown that calcium

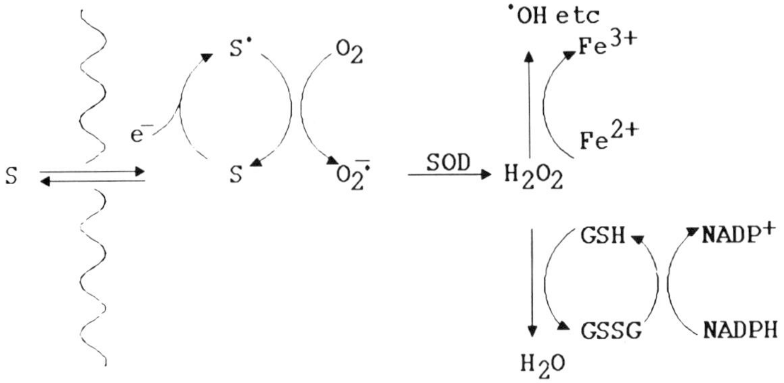

S
e^-
S·
O_2
S
$O_2^{-\cdot}$
SOD
H_2O_2
·OH etc
Fe^{3+}
Fe^{2+}
GSH
GSSG
H_2O
$NADP^+$
NADPH

S = Nitrofurantoin
  = Diquat
  = BS (i.e. mono- dihydroxy- and ketobile-salts)?

Fig. 14 Schematic representation of 'redox cycling'

Table 9 Redox cycling of bile salts by 3α-HSD (rat liver)[72]

| | Percentage initial $^3H/^{14}C$ ratio | | | |
| | LCA | | CDCA | |
Time (min)	Cells	Medium	Cells	Medium
5	69	88	40	74
10	58	79	31	48
20	48	65	22	30
30	40	53	17	20

is released from the endoplasmic reticulum under the influence of bile salts, in particular TLCA[80-83]. This also occurs in other cell types; however, the latest study, although using the intact rat liver instead of isolated cells, did not find a change of calcium fluxes after 10–30 min perfusion with the same bile salts (5 and 25 μmol/l)[84]. It is of interest, in addition, that taurine is protective against oxygen- and calcium-induced damage on isolated liver cells[85]. It is therefore possible that the unexplained difference between TUDCA and (G)UDCA in protection[86] may be due to the taurine itself, thus explaining why TUDCA is indeed protective against TLCA-induced liver damage. However, this has to be studied further since taurine only is not as protective as TUDCA.

NON-PARENCHYMAL CELLS

Finally, it has to be discussed that bile salts affect not only hepatocytes but also a variety of other cell types[78,82]. Since some cells may release substances which in turn might affect hepatocytes such as oxygen radicals, leukotrienes, cytokines, and other mediators, such effects might be of importance for bile

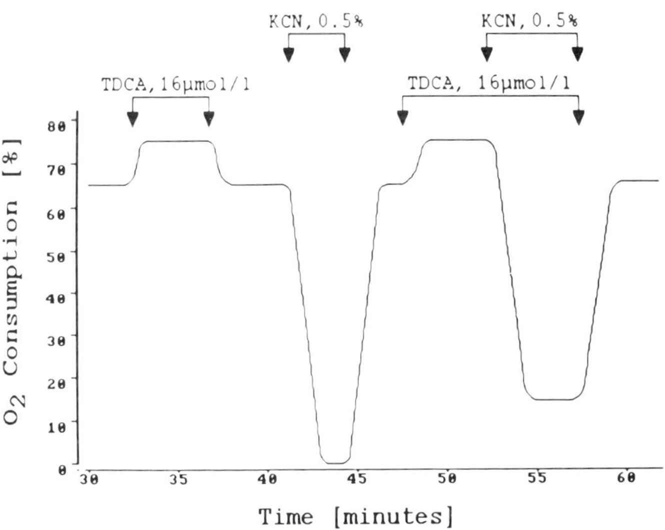

Fig. 15   Effect of the presence of TDCA on the suppression of oxygen uptake by cyanide in the isolated perfused rat liver

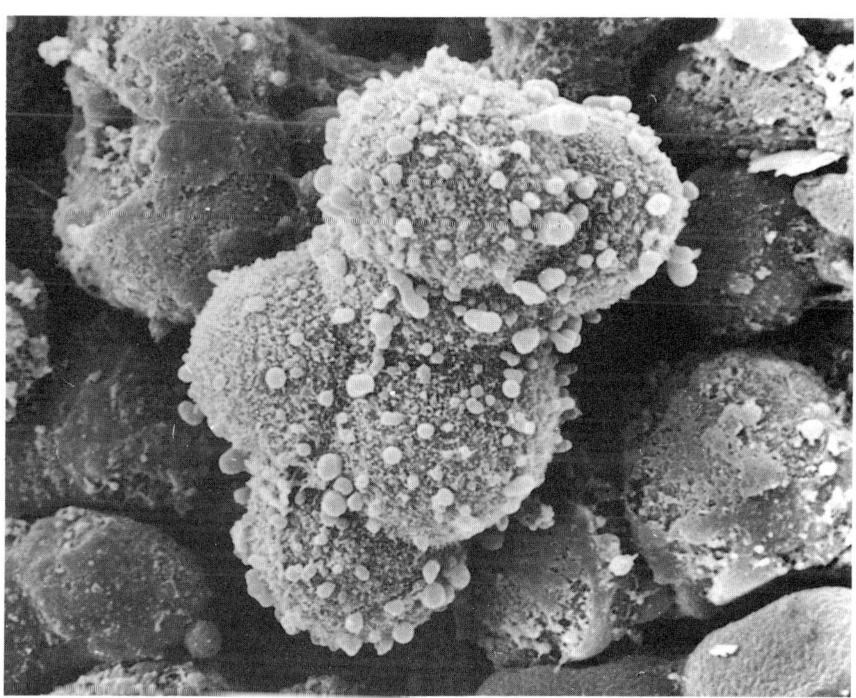

Fig. 16   Blebbing of isolated rat liver cells under the influence of DCA (1000 μmol/l)

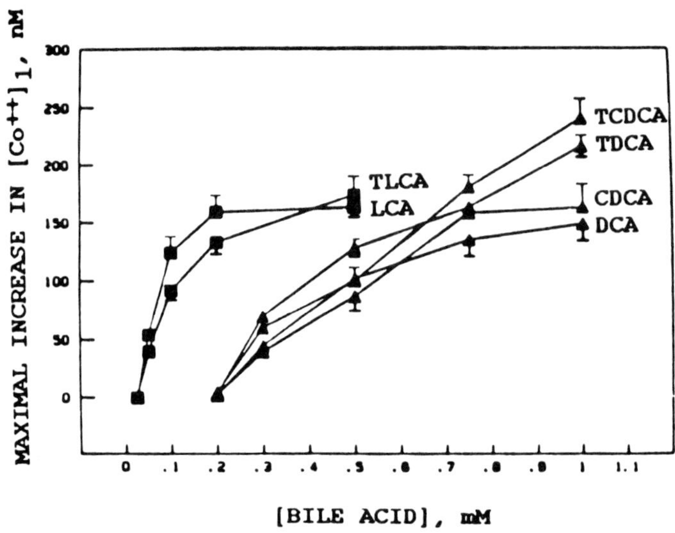

Fig. 17 Maximal increase of intracellular calcium induced by different bile salts at different concentrations[79]

Table 10 Effect of LCA on O_2 release from PMNs[87]

	DMF	*LCA*
Hanks solution	0.8 ± 0.5	0.5 ± 0.2
Phorbolacetate (2 ng/ml)	3.6 ± 1.1	29.6 ± 3.2
		$p < 0.01$

Table 11 Bile salts and leukotrienes[88]

	TCA Bolus	
	3 μmol, n = 8	*12 μmol*, n = 6
ΔBSS	$+ 60 \pm 4\%$	$+ 192 \pm 12\%$
ΔBLT	$+ 30 \pm 4\%$	$+ 80 \pm 9\%$

Vice-versa high $LTC_4 \Rightarrow$ BSS ↓

salt toxicity. For example, it was found that LCA (32 μmol/l) stimulated the release of superoxide anion from activated neutrophils (Table 10)[87]. An increased release of leukotriene C_4 from the perfused rat liver was found with TCA, and LTC_4 in turn induced cholestasis (Table 11)[88]. Tumour necrosis factor and interleukin-6 are cholestatic, and this explains the mechanism of endotoxin-induced liver damage at least to some extent[89].

STUDIES TO BE DONE

In summary, a number of possible mechanisms of bile salt toxicity are suggested from the literature and from a few experiments of our group

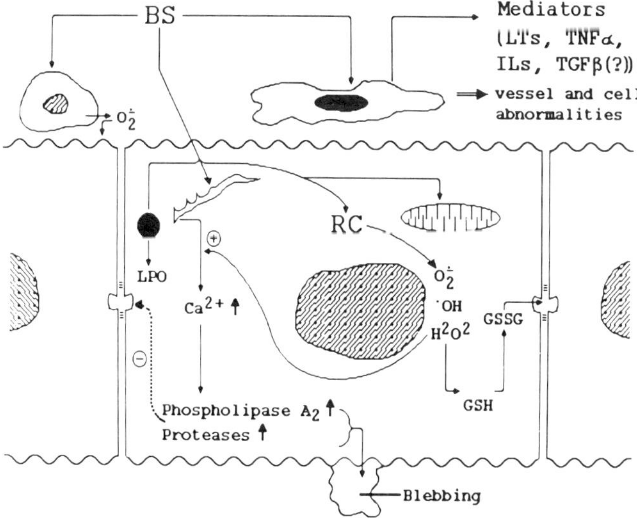

Fig. 18   Possible mechanisms of bile salt toxicity in the liver

(Fig. 18). It could well be that several of these mechanisms act together. Studies should be done to analyse the role of these mechanisms. In particular, reactive oxygen products, a possible redox cycling and the role of calcium should be studied in concert. Mitochondrial functions need to be analysed, and in particular the role of cell–cell interactions in bile acid-related toxicity remains to be studied. Here, cytokines and other mediators may have a leading role.

In conclusion, several hints with respect to possible mechanisms of toxicity are available. None of these have been proven and probably no single mechanism exists; however, it is surprising how little has been done. This might be due to the prevailing interest in bile salt transport secretion which also is the cause of the sole focus on hepatocytes neglecting the other cellular compounds of the liver. A number of ways forward have been suggested in this chapter, and the results are awaited.

References

1. Lester R, Pyrer JS, Little JM, Adcock EW. What is meant by the term 'bile acid'? Am J Physiol. 1983;244:G107–10.
2. Hofmann AF, Roda A. Physicochemical properties of bile acids and their relationship to biological properties: an overview of the problem. J Lipid Res. 1984;25:1477–89.
3. DeLange RJ, Glazer AN. Bile acids: antioxidants or enhancers of peroxidation depending on lipid concentration. Arch Biochem Biophys. 1990;276:19–25.
4. Hofmann AF. Chemistry and enterohepatic circulation of bile acids. Hepatology (suppl.) 1984;4:4S–14S.
5. Stolz A, Takikawa H, Sugiyama Y, Kuhlenkamp J, Kaplowitz N. 3α-Hydroxysteroid dehydrogenase activity of the Y'bile acid binders in rat liver cytosol. Identification, kinetics, and physiological significance. J Clin Invest. 1987;79:427–34.

6. Takikawa H, Sugiyama Y, Kaplowitz N. Binding of bile acids by glutathione S-transferase from rat liver. J Lipid Res. 1986;27:955–66.

7. Takikawa H, Stolz A, Sugiyama Y, Yoshida H, Yamanaka M, Kaplowitz N. Relationship between the newly identified bile acid binder and bile acid oxidoreductases in human liver. J Biol Chem. 1990;265:2132–6.

8. Strange RC, Chapman BT, Johnston JD, Nimmo IA, Percy-Robb IW. Partitioning of bile acids into subcellular organelles and the *in vivo* distribution of bile acids in rat liver. Biochim Biophys Acta. 1979;573:535–45.

9. Haslewood GAD. The biological significance of chemical differences in bile salts. Biol Rev. 1964;39:537–74.

10. Wietholtz H, Marschall H-U, Reuschenbach R, Matern H, Matern S. Urinary excretion of bile acid glucosides and glucuronides in extraheptic cholestasis. Hepatology. 1991;13:656–62.

11. Raedsch R, Lauterburg B, Hofmann AF. Altered bile acid metabolism in primary biliary cirrhosis. Dig Dis Sci. 1981;26:394–401.

12. Leuschner U, Schneider M, Korte L. Der Einfluß von Chenodesoxycholsäure und Ursodesoxycholsäure auf die Leberstruktur der Ratte. Z Gastroenterol. 1979;17:244–56.

13. Shefer S, Zaki FG, Salen G. Early morphologic and enzymatic changes in livers of rats treated with chenodeoxycholic and ursodeoxycholic acids. Hepatology. 1983;3:201–8.

14. Koch MM, Giampieri MP, Lorenzini I, Iezequel AM, Orlandi F. Effect of chenodeoxycholic acid on liver structure and function in man: a stereological and biochemical study. Digest. 1980;20:8–21.

15. Leuschner VU, Czygan P, Liersch M, Fröhling W, Stiehl A. Morphologische Untersuchungen zur Toxizität sulfatierter und nichtsulfatierter Lithocholsäure an der perfundierten Rattenleber. Gastroenterologie. 1977;15:246–53.

16. Marks JW, Sue SO, Peralman BJ, Bonorris GG, Varady P, Lachin JM, Schoenfield LJ. Sulfation of lithocholate as a possible modifier of chenodeoxycholic acid-induced elevations of serum transaminase in patients with gallstones. J Clin Invest. 1981;68:1190–6.

17. Miyai K, Javitt NB, Gochman N, Jones M, Baker D. Hepatotoxicity of bile acids in rabbits. Ursodeoxycholic acid is less toxic than chenodeoxycholic acid. Lab Invest. 1982;46:428–37.

18. Poupon R, Chretien Y, Poupon RE, Ballet F, Calmus Y, Darnis F. Is ursodeoxycholic acid an effective treatment for primary biliary cirrhosis? Lancet. 1987;1:834–6.

19. Leuschner U, Leuschner M, Sieratzki J, Kurtz W, Hubner K. Gallstone dissolution with ursodeoxycholic acid in patients with chronic active hepatitis and two years follow-up. A pilot study. Dig Dis Sci. 1985;30:642–9.

20. Podda M, Ghezzi C, Battezzati PM, Crosignani A, Zuin M, Roda A. Effects of ursodeoxycholic acid and taurine on serum liver enzymes and bile acids in chronic hepatitis. Gastroenterology. 1990;98:1044–50.

21. Hoffman NE, Iser JH, Smallwood RA. Hepatic bile acid transport: effect of conjugation and position of hydroxyl groups. Am J Physiol. 1975;229:298–302.

22. Hardison WGM, Hatoff DE, Miyai K, Weiner RG. Nature of bile acid maximum secretory rate in the rat. Am J Physiol. 1981;241:G337–43.

23. Baumgartner U, Schölmerich J, Leible P, Farthmann EH, Gerok W. Cholestatic and choleretic potency of differently hydroxylated bile salts. Biochem Biophys Acta. (In press).

24. Bernwell S, Yousef IM, Tuchweber B, Weber A, Roy CC. Pathogenesis of bile acid induced cholestasis. Hepatology. 1986;6:772 (abstr.).

25. Kakis G, Yousef IM. Mechanism of cholic acid protection in lithocholate-induced intrahepatic cholestasis in rats. Gastroenterology. 1980;78:1402–11.

26. Kitani K, Ohta M, Kanai S. Tauroursodeoxycholate prevents biliary protein excretion induced by other bile salts in rat. Am J Physiol. 1985;248:G407–17.

27. Kanai S, Kitani K. Glycoursodeoxycholate is as effective as tauroursodeoxycholate in preventing the taurocholate-induced cholestasis in the rat. Res Commun Chem Pathol Pharmacol. 1983;42:423–30.

28. Heuman DM, Mills AS, McCall J, Hylemon PB, Pandak WM, Vlahcevic ZR. Conjugates or ursodeoxycholate protect against cholestasis and hepatocellular necrosis caused by more hydrophobic bile salts. *In vivo* studies in the rat. Gastroenterology. 1991;100:203–11.

29. Schölmerich J, Baumgartner U, Miyai K, Gerok W. Tauroursodeoxycholate prevents taurolithocholate-induced cholestasis and toxicity in rat liver. J Hepatol. 1990;10:280–3.

30. Schölmerich J, Kitamura S, Baumgartner U, Miyai K, Gerok W. Taurohyocholate,

taurocholate, and tauroursodeoxycholate but not tauroursocholate and taurodehydro-cholate counteract effects of taurolithocholate in rat liver. Res Exp Med. 1990;190:121–9.
31. Zhao XM, Montet JC. Anticholestatic properties of β-muricholate acid. Gastroenterology. 1991;100:A816 (abstr.).
32. Yousef IM, Mignault D, Tuchweber B. High choleretic activity and reduced detergent properties of sulfated bile acids prevent bile acid induced cholestasis in rats. Hepatology. 1990;12:A1003 (abstr.).
33. Herz R, Paumgartner G, Preisig R. Inhibition of bile formation by high doses of taurocholate in the perfused rat liver. Scand J Gastroenterol. 1976;11:741–6.
34. Rutishauser SCB, Stone SL. Comparative effects of sodium taurodeoxycholate and sodium taurocholate on bile secretion in the rat, dog and rabbit. J Physiol. 1975;245:583–98.
35. Aldini R, Roda A, Grigolo B, Paselli L, Morselli AM, Roda E, Barbara L. Species differences in the hepatic uptake of bile acids. Hepatology. 1983;3:820 (abstr.).
36. Kitani K, Kanai S, Ohta M, Sato Y. Differing transport maxima values for taurine-conjugated bile salts in rats and hamsters. Am J Physiol. 1986;251:G852–8.
37. Baumgartner U, Hardison WGM, Miyai K. Reduced cholestatic potency of taurolitho-cholate during backward perfusion of the rat liver. Lab Invest. 1987;56:576–82.
38. Schmucker DL, Ohta M, Kanai S, Sato Y, Kitani K. Hepatic injury induced by bile salts: correlation between biochemical and morphological events. Hepatology. 1990;12:1216–21.
39. Schölmerich J, Becher M-S, Schmidt K, Schubert R, Kremer B, Feldhaus S, Gerok W. Influence of hydroxylation and conjugation of bile salts on their membrane-damaging properties – studies on isolated hepatocytes and lipid membrane vesicles. Hepatology. 1984;4:661–6.
40. Schölmerich J, Becher M-S, Baumgartner U, Gerok W. Loss of glucagon control of gluconeogenesis in liver cells from rats with bile duct obstruction. Biochem Biophys Res Commun. 1985;126:1146–53.
41. Lee WM, Hatley WL, Kennedy JW. Cyclosporin enhances the hepatotoxicity of conjugated bile acids. Hepatology. 1989;10:613 (abstr.).
42. Ammon HV, Loefler RF, Tapper EJ, Lewand D, Komorowski RH. Sulfation abolishes the toxic effects of deoxycholate. Gastroenterology. 1982;82:1007 (abstr.).
43. Coleman R, Lowe PJ, Billington D. Membrane lipid composition and susceptibility to bile salt damage. Biochim Biophys Acta. 1980;599:294–300.
44. Galle PR, Theilmann L, Raedsch R, Otto G, Stiehl A. Ursodeoxycholate reduces hepatotox-icity of bile salts in primary human hepatocytes. Hepatology. 1990;3(1):486–91.
45. Baumgartner U, Schölmerich J. Ursodeoxycholate does not prevent bile acid toxicity on freshly isolated rat hepatocytes. J Hepatol. 1991;13(suppl.1):95.
46. Lamri Y, Roda A, Dumont M, Feldmann G, Erlinger S. Immunoperoxidase localization of bile salts in rat liver cells. Evidence for a role of the Golgi apparatus in bile salt transport. J Clin Invest. 1988;82:1173–82.
47. Miskovitz PF, Javitt JB. Lithocholic acid metabolism: tissue-bound lithocholic acid and hepatotoxicity. Hepatology. 1980;1:1039 (abstr.).
48. Yanagisawa J, Nagai M, Hirano Y, Fujii T, Nakayama F. Lithocholate in liver tissue with obstructive jaundice. Gastroenterol Jpn. 1989;24:156–8.
49. Mitropoulos KA, Myant NB. The formation of lithocholic acid, chenodeoxycholic acid and α- and β-muricholic acids from cholesterol incubated with rat liver mitochondria. Biochem J. 1967;103:472–9.
50. Lim WC, Jordan TW. Subcellular distribution of hepatic bile acid-conjugating enzymes. Biochem J. 1981;197:611–18.
51. Chiarantini E, Arcangeli A, Romagnoli P, Buzzelli G, Salvadori G, Gentilini P. Functional and ultrastructural changes in the liver during CDCA treatment. Ital J Gastroenterol. 1980;12:224–7.
52. Lee MJ, Whitehouse MW. Inhibition of electron transport and coupled phosphorylation in liver mitochondria by cholanic (bile) acids and their conjugates. Biochem Biophys Acta. 1965;100:317–28.
53. Gregus Z, Varga F, Fischer E. Effect of bile acids on the biliary excretion of amaranth and the respiration of liver mitochondria. Acta Physiol Acad Sci Hung. 1982;59:89–97.
54. Koyama K, Ito K, Ouchi K, Sato T. Mitochondrial function in rat liver in biliary obstruction. Tohoku J Exp Med. 1980;131:59–69.

55. Kolde G, Herwig J, Themann H. Normoactive hypertrophic endoplasmic reticulum in taurolithocholate-induced cholestasis in rats. Virchows Arch. 1981;37:103–8.
56. van Dyke RW, Bollan JL, Scharschmidt BF. Oxygen consumption by rat liver: effects of taurocholate and sulfobromophthalein transport, glucagon and cation substitution. Am J Physiol. 1983;244:G523–31.
57. Schölmerich J, Baumgartner U, Miyai K, Gerok W. Hepatic passage of bile acids increases oxygen uptake by the perfused rat liver. Res Exp Med. 1990;190:69–75.
58. Keller BJ, Yamanaka H, Liang D, Kauffman FC, Thurman RG. O_2-dependent hepatotoxicity due to ethylhexanol in the perfused rat liver: mitochondria as a site of action. J Pharmacol Exp Ther. 1990;252:1355–60.
59. McCord JM. Radical explanations for old observations. Gastroenterology. 1987;92:2026–8.
60. Arthur MJP. Reactive oxygen intermediates and liver injury. J Hepatol. 1988;6:125–31.
61. Malik R, Zanninelli G, Gollan J. Is lipid peroxidation a mediator of cholestatic liver injury? Effects of cholestasis and bile salts on the peroxidation of hepatic microsomes. Gastroenterology. 1991;100:A770 (abstr.).
62. Seto Y, Nakashima T, Nakajima T, Shima T, Sakamoto Y, Okuno T, Takino T. Involvement of oxygen radicals in bile acid induced hepatocytes injury. Hepatology. 1988;8:1452 (abstr.).
63. Craven PA, Pfanstiel J, Saito R, DeRubertis FR. Actions of sulfasalazine and 5-aminosalicylic acid as reactive oxygen scavengers in the suppression of bile acid-induced increases in colonic epithelial cell loss and proliferative activity. Gastroenterology. 1987;92:1998–2006.
64. Zimniak P, Holsztynska EJ, Lester R, Waxman DJ, Radominska A. Detoxification of lithocholic acid. Elucidation of the pathways of oxidative metabolism in rat liver microsomes. J Lipid Res. 1989;30:907–18.
65. Kudo K, Amuro Y, Hada T, Higashino K. Purification and properties of 3α-hydroxysteroid dehydrogenase as a 3-keto bile acid reductase from human liver cytosol. Biochim Biophys Acta. 1990;1046:12–18.
66. Hoener B, Noach A, Andrup M, Yen T-SB. Nitrofurantoin produces oxidative stress and loss of glutathione and protein thiols in the isolated perfused rat liver. Pharmacology. 1989;38:363–73.
67. Sandy MS, Moldeus P, Ross D, Smith MT. Cytotoxicity of the redox cycling compound diquat in isolated hepatocytes: involvement of hydrogen peroxide and transition metals. Arch Biochem Biophys. 1987;259:29–37.
68. Kass GEN, Duddy SK, Orrenius S. Activation of hepatocyte protein kinase C by redox-cycling quinones. Biochem J. 1989;260:499–507.
69. Akerboom TPM, Bilzer M, Sies H. Relation between glutathione redox changes and biliary excretion of taurocholate in perfused rat liver. J Biol Chem. 1984;259:5838–43.
70. Ballatori N, Truong AT. Altered hepatic junctional permeability, bile acid excretion and glutathione efflux during oxidant challenge. J Pharmacol Exp Ther. 1989;251:1069–75.
71. Singh SV, Leal T, Awasthi YC. Inhibition of human glutathione S-transferases by bile acids. Toxicol Appl Pharmacol. 1988;95:248–54.
72. Takikawa H, Stolz A, Kaplowitz N. Cyclical oxidation–reduction of the C_3 position on bile acids catalyzed by rat hepatic 3α-hydroxysteroid dehydrogenase. I. Studies with the purified enzyme, isolated rat hepatocytes, and inhibition by indomethacin. J Clin Invest. 1987;80:852–60.
73. Takikawa H, Ookhtens M, Stolz A, Kaplowitz N. Cyclical oxidation–reduction of the C_3 position on bile acids catalyzed by 3α-hydroxysteroid dehydrogenase. II. Studies in the prograde and retrograde single-pass, perfused rat liver and inhibition by indomethacin. J Clin Invest. 1987;80:861–6.
74. Takikawa H, Stolz A, Kuroki S, Kaplowitz N. Oxidation and reduction of bile acid precursors by rat hepatic 3α-hydroxysteroid dehydrogenase and inhibition by bile acids and indomethacin. Biochim Biophys Acta. 1990;1043:153–6.
75. Lemasters JJ, DeGuiseppi J, Nieminen A-L, Herman B. Blebbing, free Ca^{2+} and mitochondrial membrane potential preceding cell death in hepatocytes. Nature. 1987;325:78–81.
76. Orrenius S, Nicotera P. Studies of Ca^{2+}-mediated toxicity in hepatocytes. Klin Wochenschr. 1986;64(suppl.VII):138–41.
77. van der Meer R, Termont DSML, de Vries HT. Differential effects of calcium ions and calcium phosphate on cytotoxicity of bile acids. Am J Physiol. 1991;260:G142–7.
78. Montrose MH, Lester R, Zimniak P, Anwer MS, Murer H. Bile acids increase cellular free

calcium in cultured kidney cells (LLC-PK$_1$). Pflügers Arch. 1988;412:164–71.

79. Anwer MS, Engelking LR, Nolan K, Sullivan D, Zimniak P, Lester R. Hepatotoxic bile acids increase cytosolic Ca^{++} activity of isolated rat hepatocytes. Hepatology. 1988;8:887–91.

80. Combettes L, Dumont M, Berthon B, Erlinger S, Claret M. Release of calcium from the endoplasmic reticulum by bile acids in rat liver cells. J Biol Chem. 1988;263:2299–303.

81. Combettes L, Dumont M, Berthon B, Erlinger S, Claret M. Effect of the bile acid taurolithocholate on cell calcium in saponin-treated rat hepatocytes. FEBS Lett. 1988;227:161–6.

82. Coquil J-F, Berthon B, Chomiki N, Combettes L, Jourdon P, Schteingart C, Erlinger S, Claret M. Effects of taurolithocholate, a Ca^{2+}-mobilizing agent, on cell Ca^{2+} in rat hepatocytes, human platelets and neuroblastoma NG108-15 cell line. Biochem J. 1991;273:153–60.

83. Combettes L, Berthon B, Doucet E, Erlinger S, Claret M. Taurolithocholate permeabilizes the hormone-sensitive intracellular calcium pool independently of extracellular calcium in rat hepatocytes. Hepatology. 1989;10:595.

84. Farrell GC, Duddy SK, Kass GEN, Llopis J, Gahm A. Orrenius S. Release of Ca^{2+} from the endoplasmic reticulum is not the mechanism for bile acid-induced cholestasis and hepatotoxicity in the intact rat liver. J Clin Invest. 1990;85:1255–9.

85. Nakashima T, Seto Y, Nakajima T, Shima T, Sakamoto Y, Cho N, Sano A, Iwai M, Kagawa K, Okanoue T, Kashima K. Calcium-associated cytoprotective effect of taurine on the calcium and oxygen paradoxes in isolated rat hepatocytes. Liver. 1990;10:167–72.

86. Schölmerich J, Baumgartner U, Farthmann EH, Gerok W. Taurine conjugation is necessary for the protective effect of ursodeoxycholate in taurolithocholate induced cholestasis. J Hepatol. 1989;9(suppl.1):82.

87. Dahm LJ, Hewett JA, Roth RA. Bile and bile salts potentiate superoxide anion release from activated, rat peritoneal neutrophils. Toxicol Appl Pharmacol. 1988;95:82–92.

88. Rodriguez CM, Quiroga J, Prieto J. Physiological role of peptidoleukotrienes (LT) in bile salt (BS) transport. J Hepatol. 1990;11:S53 (abstr.).

89. Whiting JF, Rosenbluth AB, Narciso JP, Gollan JL. Tumor necrosis factor-α inhibits taurocholate uptake by hepatocytes: implications for the pathogenesis of endotoxin-induced cholestasis. Gastroenterology. 1991;100:A811 (abstr.).

10
The enterohepatic circulation of bile acids in cholestasis

A. F. HOFMANN

INTRODUCTION

Vectorial transport into bile of bile acids, bilirubin, biliary lipids, oxidized glutathione and polar biotransformation products of sex hormones and drugs is a major hepatocyte function[1]. In cholestasis this vectorial transport is impaired and in principle could even cease completely. This chapter will consider the enterohepatic circulation from two aspects: the first is the disturbance in bile acid metabolism *per se* caused by cholestasis; the second is the consequence(s) of these disturbances in bile acid metabolism. The second point must be divided into two topics: (a) the effect of partial or complete loss of vectorial secretion of bile acids on biliary and intestinal function, that is, the effect of bile acid deficiency on these tissues; and (b) the effect of bile acid retention on hepatocyte function as well as the function of other tissues, that is the effect of bile acid retention on hepatic and extrahepatic metabolism. Finally, approaches to therapy will be discussed briefly.

DISTURBANCES IN BILE ACID METABOLISM IN CHOLESTASIS

Bile acid biosynthesis of primary bile acids in health

In the healthy adult, bile acid biosynthesis from cholesterol averages 500–1500 µmol/day, the amount depending on genetic factors as well as dietary composition[2]. The two bile acids biosynthesized in humans are named chenodeoxycholic acid (3,7-dihydroxy-5-cholan-24-oic acid) and cholic acid (3,7,12-trihydroxy-5-cholan-24-oic acid), these bile acids being denoted primary bile acids. The term primary is used to distinguish those bile acids formed in the liver from cholesterol from those bile acids resulting from dehydroxylation or dehydrogenation of primary bile acids; such bile acids produced by bacterial enzymes are termed secondary bile acids[2]. About twice as much cholic acid as chenodeoxycholic acid (CDCA) is synthesized[3]. With increased caloric intake or increased fibre intake, bile acid biosynthesis

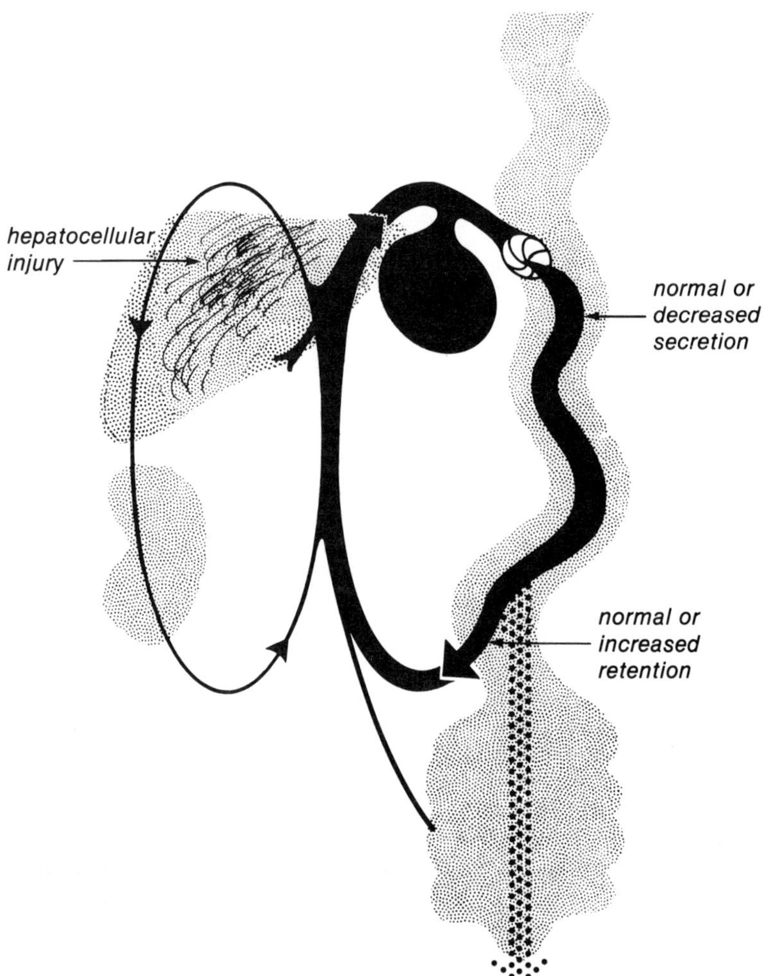

Fig. 1 Schematic depiction of the proposed abnormality in the enterohepatic circulation of bile acids in incomplete cholestasis. Up-regulation of active ileal transport of bile acids causes inappropriate conservation of endogenous, hepatotoxic bile acids contributing to liver injury. The figure has been published previously[60]

increases, presumably because of increased faecal loss. Bile acid biosynthesis decreases in old age, extrapolating to no synthesis at 100 years[4].

In the steady state, bile acid biosynthesis is equal to faecal loss, since normal urinary bile acid excretion is less than $10\,\mu$mol/day[5]. The efficient conservation of bile acids by active ileal transport, as well as passive absorption in the small and large intestine, results in the accumulation of a large bile acid pool 5000–10000 μmol in size, which cycles six to ten times daily (for a summary of pool size measurements, see ref. 3). The larger the pool, the smaller the cycling frequency; the product, bile acid secretion, is thus independent of either pool size or recycling frequency, at least in most adults[6]. The constancy of bile acid secretion results from two homeostatic mechanisms: (1) negative feedback of bile acid biosynthesis[7] and (2) negative feedback inhibition of active ileal transport[8]. The latter homeostatic mechanism has only recently been recognized.

Bile acid biosynthesis in cholestasis

Bile acid biosynthesis from cholesterol

In complete cholestasis, faecal elimination falls to very low levels. Urinary excretion increases many-fold, but the highest values that have been reported are about $200\,\mu mol/day$[5]. This means that bile acid biosynthesis must decrease by a factor of two to seven. It is most reasonable to propose that bile acid biosynthesis decreases at intermediate levels of cholestasis, at least in humans.

In the steady state, in health, cholesterol biosynthesis is considerably greater than bile acid biosynthesis. Cholesterol balance is maintained by a high rate of biliary excretion of cholesterol ($2000–3000\,\mu mol/day$) (cf. refs 9 and 10). There is a variable, but generally small, input of cholesterol into the exchangeable cholesterol pool from the intestinal absorption of dietary cholesterol; intestinal absorption of dietary cholesterol is generally relatively unimportant in cholesterol balance in humans[11]. The majority of the cholesterol molecules absorbed from the intestine originate in biliary cholesterol excretion. Biliary lipid secretion in humans is characterized by a higher cholesterol/phospholipid ratio than any other vertebrate identified to date, indicating that the vesicles formed in the human hepatocyte are extremely cholesterol-rich[12].

In complete cholestasis, biliary excretion of cholesterol should approach zero. Absorption of dietary cholesterol should also cease, since bile acids are required for cholesterol absorption. Cholesterol cannot be excreted in urine because of its insolubility in water. Therefore, in complete cholestasis, in the steady state, cholesterol biosynthesis should become equivalent to bile acid biosynthesis, both being extremely suppressed. Cholesterol balance is maintained entirely by urinary excretion of bile acids. This reasoning, for which there is good experimental support, indicates that in cholestasis, cholesterol biosynthesis must decrease to a greater extent than bile acid biosynthesis. Of course, blood levels of cholesterol become markedly elevated, presumably because of reflux of cholesterol-rich vesicles from the hepatocyte into plasma[13]. In incomplete cholestasis there is also likely to be regurgitation of cholesterol-rich vesicles into plasma. In this situation the intestinal absorption of dietary and biliary cholesterol contributes to the cholesterol input into the cholesterol metabolic pool. Ursodeoxycholic acid (UDCA) improves cholesterol balance by inhibiting intestinal cholesterol absorption[14,15].

Additional hydroxylation of primary bile acids

Since cholesterol has a 3-hydroxy group, and since the rate-limiting enzyme in bile acid biosynthesis is considered to be cholesterol 7-hydroxylase, all primary bile acids must have a 3- and a 7-hydroxy group. CDCA is therefore the most primitive bile acid from the point of view of nuclear hydroxylation. CA is not formed by 12-hydroxylation of CDCA, but by 12-hydroxylation of a 3-oxo, 7-hydroxy-intermediate in CDCA biosynthesis, at least in mammals. As noted above, two-thirds of the precursor molecules are hydroxylated resulting in CA biosynthesis being about twice as great as CDCA biosynthesis. In some cholestatic conditions it is likely that the 3-oxo precursor will undergo more complete hydroxylation, resulting in CA constituting a higher proportion of bile acid biosynthesis than the usual 66%.

In other vertebrates an additional hydroxy group may be added at the level of the intermediate or directly to CDCA during normal bile acid biosynthesis. This additional hydroxy group may be present at a variety of carbon atoms on the steroid nucleus, and a few examples can be cited: 1 (carbon), Australian opossum[16]; 6, pigs, many rodents; 12, most mammals; and 16, the stork[17]. Additional hydroxylations occur in fetal development in humans (at the 1, 2, or 4 positions), and such atypical hydroxylated bile acids are present in meconium[18].

In cholestasis, bile acids accumulate in the hepatocyte and additional hydroxylation occurs – mostly at the 1 or 6 positions[5,19]. The amount of such atypical hydroxylation as a proportion of total bile acid biosythesis is small. Ostrow has recently tabulated the changes in bile acid metabolism occurring in cholestasis[5].

In bile acid biosynthesis, nuclear changes are generally considered to precede side-chain changes, at least for the majority of bile acids. In cholestasis a small fraction of bile acids are formed in which the normal side-chain oxidative cleavage occurs, but the nucleus remains unchanged. The resulting molecule (3β-hydroxy-5-chol-24-enic acid or 3β-hydroxy-5-cholenic acid) has the nucleus of cholesterol, yet the C5 side-chain of the common natural bile acids[20,21]. It is not impossible that intermediates occurring in bile acid biosynthesis after 7-hydroxy cholesterol, for example the 3-oxo-Δ^4-7-hydroxy derivative of cholesterol, might undergo cleavage of the side-chain with the result that an atypical bile acid is formed having a nuclear structure between cholesterol and bile acids, and the normal side-chain of the 'mature' bile acid. This point is mentioned only because the presence of such atypical bile acids in small proportions does not necessarily indicate an inborn error in bile acid biosynthesis[22].

One other change occurs in cholestasis – the disappearance of deoxycholic acid from biliary bile acids[23]. The reasons for this occurrence are not well understood. Obviously, in cholestasis, deoxycholic acid is not formed because bile acids do not enter the small intestine. In incomplete cholestasis there are two possible explanations. One possibility is that ileal absorption is so efficient that only greatly decreased amounts of bile acids enter the caecum (where deoxycholic acid formation occurs, mediated by anaerobic bacteria). The second possibility is that for some reason in cholestasis, 7-dehydroxylation does not occur. The first possibility is more likely, in my judgement, since ileal transport of bile acids is now known, at least in rodents, to be regulated by feedback inhibition[8]. In cholestasis, upregulation should occur, leading to more efficient ileal absorption and, in turn, to a smaller fraction of bile acids entering the colon.

Conjugation of bile acids

In the healthy adult, CDCA and CA are virtually completely conjugated with glycine or taurine before secretion into bile[24]. Such a mode of conjugation is now termed aminoacyl amidation (or *N*-acylation). Extensive sulphation or glucuronidation (in 'ethereal linkage') of the nuclear hydroxy groups does not occur to any appreciable extent for these two primary bile acids. In humans a fraction of lithocholic acid (LBA) (formed in the colon by bacterial 7-dehydroxylation of CDCA) is absorbed and returns to the liver. Here it is fully amidated and in part 3-sulphated[25]. The rate of such sulphation can be estimated as follows. About 250–500 μmol/day of CDCA is synthesized. Absorption of lithocholic acid (LCA) from the colon is about 50–150 μmol/day, of which 50–80% is sulphated[26]. This reckoning gives a daily LCA sulphation rate of 25–120 μmol/day.

In contrast to sulphation, amidation is required not only for newly synthesized bile acids, but also for unconjugated bile acids formed in the small intestine by bacterial deconjugation and subsequently absorbed. The amount of such amidation used in 'reconjugation' of previously conjugated bile acids exceeds that required for amidation of newly biosynthesized bile acids[26,27]. The amount of bile acid amidation is in the range of 1500–3000 μmol/day. Thus the daily rate of bile acid amidation greatly exceeds the daily rate of bile acid sulphation. Ester glucuronidation of the carboxyl group (on the side-chain) cannot occur once the carboxyl group is amidated with glycine or taurine.

In complete cholestasis, CDCA is sulphated (mostly, but not entirely at the 3-position) and the sulphates are rapidly excreted in urine[28–30]. Indeed, renal clearance is so high that plasma levels of sulphated CDCA remain low, even though urinary excretion of sulphated CDCA increases greatly[29]. LCA is not present in the circulating bile acids; thus, CDCA is the only bile acid that undergoes considerable sulphation. CA is also sulphated, but to a much lesser extent so that urinary bile acids contain mostly unsulphated amidates of CA and both sulphated and unsulphated amidates of CDCA. Glucuronidation[31] and glycosylation[32] (both mostly on the 3-hydroxy group) also occur at increased rates, but the magnitude of such uncommon conjugation steps remains quite low. The novel conjugates – sulphates, glucuronides, and glycosides – are excreted predominantly in urine; there is little increase in their biliary excretion.

In health about 75% of bile acids are amidated with glycine. This percentage is a resultant of the proportion (of glycine versus taurine) used for conjugation and the proportion of their corresponding amidates undergoing deconjugation[33] It is likely that the proportion of bile acids conjugated with glycine in the hepatocyte is > 75%, and that the steady state proportion of 75% is the result of taurine-amidated bile acids being more resistant to bacterial conjugation than glycine-amidated bile acids.

In cholestasis a greater proportion of bile acids becomes amidated with taurine[5]. The simplest explanation for this change in the proportion of amidates in the steady state is that the overall rate of bile acid amidation decreases in cholestasis. This decrease occurs for two reasons. The first is that there is decreased demand for the conjugation of newly formed bile acids, since biosynthesis decreases. The second is that there is a decreased return of unconjugated bile acids to the liver, because the secretion of conjugated bile acids into the intestine is less.

There is considerable evidence that the cholyl N-amino acid transferase prefers to conjugate bile acids with taurine (rather than glycine)[34]. There is also considerable evidence in both animals and humans that the supply of taurine in the hepatocyte is rate-limiting for taurine conjugation[35]. Accordingly, the most reasonable hypothesis for the increased conjugation with taurine in cholestasis is that hepatocyte taurine increases because of a decreased demand for conjugation.

PHYSIOLOGY OF BILE ACIDS IN CHOLESTASIS

Macro events

In total cholestasis, bile acid secretion, that is secretion into the duodenum is likely to cease. In incomplete cholestasis, biliary bile acid secretion is maintained at near normal levels, at least in early cholestasis (cf. ref. 36). Presumably, as cholestasis increases, there is a progressive decrease in secretion of bile acids into the duodenum, and a decreased load of bile acids to the ileum. In the healthy adult, ileal absorption provides most of the bile acid load for the liver to secrete[37]. As noted, recent work in animals has shown that ileal transport of bile acids is regulated by negative feedback inhibition[8]. If these data can be extrapolated to humans, in cholestasis, as bile acid secretion into the intestine decreases there should be progressive upregulation of ileal transport. As a consequence, the efficiency of bile acid transport should increase, and the fractional turnover of bile acids, especially that of conjugates of CA, should be prolonged.

Micro events

Two limiting situations can be envisioned. If there is true loss of canalicular transport of bile acids, then bile formation will decrease greatly. Presumably, until total cholestasis obtains, there are always some bile acid molecules for each hepatocyte to deal with. These arise from biosynthesis within the hepatocyte, or are present in sinusoidal plasma, where they originate from biliary secretion by other (non-cholestatic) hepatocytes. In the first situation, such bile acids can only exit the hepatocyte by a sinusoidal (basolateral) membrane transport system. In experimental cholestasis bile acid transporters that are usually in the canalicular domain become present in the basolateral domain[38]. In the second situation, bile acids are secreted into the canaliculus and are reabsorbed either actively or passively by the biliary ductular epithelial cells. Paracellular transport might also contribute. In this scenario there is continuous cholehepatic shunting of conjugated bile acids (cf. ref. 39). Preliminary evidence consistent with this possibility has also been presented[40]. Obviously a combination of the two limiting cases could occur. In the second case which involves cholehepatic shunting, a non-absorbable residue of molecules such as phospholipid, cholesterol, and bilirubin diglucuronide might remain in the ductular lumen. Were the viscosity of this residuum to become high, conceivably 'plugs' might occur, in which case distal obstruction of the biliary tree would now become proximal obstruction of the biliary tree. It may be useful to examine these possibilities experimentally.

PATHOLOGICAL CONSEQUENCES OF CHOLESTASIS

Deficiency of bile acids in the biliary tract and small intestine

The absence of bile acids in the small intestine is well tolerated in the adult animal, provided nutrition is maintained and fat-soluble vitamin deficiency supplementation is administered. This pathological condition is conveniently created in the dog by constructing a cholecysto-pyelostomy after ligation of the common bile duct[41]. Other groups have prepared rats with chronic external biliary fistula (cf. ref. 42).

The major physiological role of bile acids in the small intestine is to promote lipid absorption. Bile acid deficiency in the small intestine results in defective lipid digestion. Hydrolysis of dietary triglyceride (lipolysis) proceeds to completion, but vesicles composed mostly of lipolytic products (fatty acids and monoglycerides) are not converted into mixed micelles. These lipids are absorbed more slowly, since presumably uptake is from monomers. It is likely that movement of molecules from vesicles to the monomeric phase is slower than movement of molecules from micelles to the monomeric phase. For a given chain length the absorption efficiency of long-chain fatty acids is considerably less than that of unsaturated fatty acids[43], presumably because saturated fatty acids have a lower aqueous solubility. Absorption of fat-soluble vitamins is greatly impaired because of their extremely low aqueous solubility.

Detailed physiological studies of the absorption of non-lipids in the absence of bile acids in the intestinal lumen have not been reported. Bile acids are now recognized to associate with divalent cations at a concentration well below their critical micellization concentration (CMC)[44]. Accordingly, it is likely that the efficiency of iron and calcium absorption decreases in cholestatic conditions, at least for a given intraluminal concentration (cf. ref. 45).

Bile acid retention

Bile duct ligation, in contrast to bile duct exteriorization, leads to secondary biliary cirrhosis and death in most animals. It is the current view that hepatocyte death is caused by increased bile acid retention in the hepatocyte.

The only reasonable candidates for cytotoxic bile acids are the conjugates of CDCA, a primary bile acid, and DCA, a secondary bile acid. In complete cholestasis, DCA conjugates are not present, so that cytotoxicity must be caused by CDCA conjugates. The administration of CDCA to gallstone patients may convert the circulating bile acids to > 90% CDCA, and hepatotoxicity may not occur[46]. Such observations indicate that CDCA conjugates are not usually cytotoxic in humans, provided their concentration in the hepatocyte is kept low by efficient canalicular secretion.

With isolated hepatocytes[47,48], mast cells[49], in the perfused large intestine[50], or in the isolated perfused liver[51,52], CDCA and/or its conjugates are clearly cytotoxic in a dose-dependent manner. CA and its conjugates are also cytotoxic, but at considerably higher concentrations. In contrast, UDCA and its conjugates are not cytotoxic[49-54].

The mechanism of bile acid cytotoxicity has not been elucidated. The bile acid molecule is sufficiently small that molecules not bound to cytosolic proteins will enter organelles such as mitochondria and nuclei. Mechanistic studies of bile acid cytotoxicity will be of interest.

The above discussion has considered only the hepatocyte. In cholestasis, there is also increased exposure of the renal tubular epithelium to bile acids. In incomplete cholestasis, if there were a great increase in the concentration of unconjugated bile acids in plasma, it is possible that bile acid concentrations in peripheral tissues might increase considerably, since unconjugated dihydroxy bile acids readily cross endothelial and epithelial cell membranes rapidly by passive mechanisms.

THERAPEUTIC IMPLICATIONS

Overview

If CDCA amidates are truly 'killer molecules' in cholestasis, then four therapeutic approaches can be considered, namely (1) decrease their biosynthesis, (2) decrease their proportion in circulating bile acids so as to diminish the mean cytotoxicity of the circulating bile acids, (3) increase their detoxification by additional hydroxylation or additional sulphation, or (4) decrease their inappropriate intestinal conservation.

Specific therapeutic approaches

Suppression of synthesis of CDCA

Since biosynthesis of primary bile acids is already greatly suppressed in cholestasis, it is difficult to suppose that it could be suppressed to any greater extent.

Decreasing the proportion of CDCA in circulating bile acids

Administration of CA, DCA, or UDCA decreases the proportion of CDCA in circulating bile acids. Administration of CA or DCA causes enrichment in DCA amidates, which possess similar cytotoxicity to CDCA amidates. The only bile acid whose administration markedly decreases the cytotoxicity of the bile acid pool is UDCA, and that is in part the rationale of UDCA therapy for chronic cholestatic liver disease. UDCA administration decreases cholesterol absorption, suppresses the normal compensatory increase in cholesterol biosynthesis that is associated with decreased cholesterol absorption, induces increased turnover of primary bile acid amidates by competition for ileal transport, and suppresses the usual hepatic compensatory response to increased bile acid loss (cf. refs 55 and 56).

Increasing the detoxification of CDCA amidates

In mammals, 12-hydroxylation of bile acids does not occur. Increased glucuronidation of bile acids can be achieved by phenobarbital administration, but the effect is modest and is not clinically useful[57]. It is not known whether sulphate administration, either orally or parenterally, could induce increased bile acid sulphation.

Preventing inappropriate ileal conservation

In incomplete cholestasis it would appear useful to decrease inappropriate ileal conservation. Four approaches are possible.

The first approach is to decrease the flux to the ileum. This can be done by biliary drainage. Historically, this was done by duodenal intubation and aspiration of bile[58]. More recently a partial biliary diversion has been performed surgically, and has been reported to be useful clinically[59].

The second approach is to decrease the intraluminal concentration of bile acids. This is commonly done by the administration of bile acid sequestrants such as cholestyramine or colestipol. The binding of these agents is inefficient, as less than 10% of the sites are occupied by bile acids. Presumably, this is because of successful competition by other ions such as carbonate[60].

The third approach is to inhibit the ileal transport system either competitively or non-competitively. This is presently being achieved by UDCA administration, but the competitive inhibition is rather weak. It should be possible to develop much more potent inhibitors of ileal transport.

The final approach is to remove or bypass the ileum surgically. This has been shown to be effective in improving the pruritus of chronic cholestatic disease in two patients who did not respond to UDCA. More details are given in the report of Whitington *et al.* in Chapter 17 in this volume.

EPILOGUE

The experimental evidence that CDCA and DCA are cytotoxic is convincing. It is a reasonable working hypothesis that retention of cytotoxic bile acids is the key pathochemical defect responsible for secondary biliary cirrhosis. This is not a new idea and was articulated clearly by the late James Carey[61], as well as the late Hans Popper[62]. With the availability of UDCA, a non-cytotoxic analogue of CDCA, it has proved possible to decrease the cytotoxicity of the circulating bile acid pool and decrease cytotoxic injury.

The development of UDCA as therapy for chronic cholestatic liver disease is a useful advance, but it should be remembered that therapy of obstruction of the large bile ducts has also improved greatly because of the ability of the interventional radiologist to drain the obstructed biliary tree. For chronic cholestatic liver disease it seems most important to attack the fundamental disturbance in the disease process which is likely to be immunological. What can now be done – either medically or surgically – is to decrease the consequences of bile acid retention. Thus, some progress has been made.

Acknowledgements

The author's work is supported by NIH Grants DK 21506 and DK 32130, as well as grants-in-aid from the Falk Foundation e.v., Freiburg, Germany. This chapter was prepared during the tenure of a fellowship from the Alexander von Humboldt Foundation, Bonn, Germany.

References

1. Hofmann, AF. Overview of bile secretion. In: Schultz SG, editor. Handbook of physiology: section on the gastrointestinal system. Bethesda: American Physiological Society; 1989: 549–66.
2. Hofmann AF. Enterohepatic circulation of bile acids. In: Schultz SG, editor. Handbook of physiology: section on the gastrointestinal system. Bethesda: American Physiological Society; 1989:567–96.
3. Hofmann AF, Cummings SA. Measurement of bile acid and cholesterol kinetics in man by isotope dilution: principles and applications. In: Barbara L, Dowling RH, Hofmann AF, Roda E, editors. Bile acids in gastroenterology. Lancaster: MTP Press; 1983:75–117
4. Einarsson K, Nilsell K, Leijd B, Angelin B. Influence of age on secretion of cholesterol and synthesis of bile acids by the liver. N Engl J Med. 1985;313:277–82.
5. Ostrow JD. Metabolism of bile salts in cholestasis in humans. In: Tavoloni N, Berk PD, editors. Hepatic anion transport and bile secretion. New York: M Dekker; 1992:(in press).
6. LaRusso NF, Szczepanik PA, Hofmann AF, Coffin SB. Effect of deoxycholic acid ingestion on bile acid metabolism and biliary lipid secretion in normal subjects. Gastroenterology. 1977;72:132–40.
7. Vlahcevic ZR, Heuman DM, Hylemon PB. Regulation of bile acid biosynthesis. Hepatology. 1991;13:590–600.
8. Lillienau J, Munoz J, Longmire-Cook SJ, Hagey LR, Crombie DL, Hofmann AF. Negative feedback regulation of the ileal bile acid transport system: the second site of regulation of the enterohepatic circulation (submitted).
9. Northfield TC, Hofmann AF. Biliary lipid output during three meals and an overnight fast. I. Relationship to bile acid pool size and cholesterol saturation of bile in gallstone and control subjects. Gut. 1975;16:1–11.
10. LaRusso NF, Hoffman NE, Hofmann AF, Northfield TC, Thistle JL. Effect of primary bile acid ingestion on bile acid metabolism and biliary lipid secretion in gallstones patients. Gastroenterology. 1975;69:1301–14.
11. Turley SD, Dietschy JM. The metabolism and excretion of cholesterol by the liver. In: Arias IM, Jakoby WB, Popper H, Schachter D, Shafritz DA, editors. The liver: biology and pathobiology, 2nd edn. New York: Raven Press; 1988:617–41.
12. Small DM. The formation of gallstones. Adv Intern Med. 1970;16:243–64.
13. Seidel D. Lipoproteins in liver disease. J Clin Chem Biochem. 1987;9:541–51.
14. Ponz de Leon M, Carulli N, Loria P, Iori R, Zironi F. Cholesterol absorption during bile

acid feeding. Effect of ursodeoxycholic acid (UDCA) administration. Gastroenterology. 1980;78:214–19.

15. Hardison WGM, Grundy SM. Effect of ursodeoxycholate and its taurine conjugate on bile acid synthesis and cholesterol absorption. Gastroenterology. 1984;87:130–5.

16. Lee SP, Lester R, J. St Pyrek. Vulpecholic acid (1α,3α,7α-trihydroxy-5β-cholan-24-oic acid): a novel bile acid of a marsupial, *Trichosurus vulpecula* (Lesson). J Lipid Res. 1987;28: 19–31.

17. Haslewood GAD. The biological importance of bile salts. Amsterdam: North-Holland, 1978.

18. Bact P, Walker K. Developmental pattern of bile acid metabolism as revealed by bile acid analysis of meconium. Gastroenterology. 1980;78:671–6.

19. Bremmelgaard A, Sjövall J. Hydroxylation of cholic, chenodeoxycholic, and deoxycholic acid in patients with intrahepatic cholestasis. J Lipid Res. 1980;21:1072–81.

20. Takikawa H, Otsuka H, Beppu T, Seyama Y. Determination of 3-hydroxy-5-cholenoic acid in serum of hepatobiliary diseases – its glucuronidated and sulfated conjugates. Biochem Med. 1985;33:393–400.

21. Sugiyama K, Okuyama S, Imoto M, Okomura K, Takagi K, Satake T. Clinical evaluation of serum 3β-hydroxy-5-chenoic acid in hepatobiliary diseases. Gastroenterol Jpn. 1986;21:608–16.

22. Ichimiya H, Egestad B, Nazer H, Baginski ES, Clayton PT, Sjövall J. Bile acids and bile alcohols in a child with hepatic 3β-hydroxy-Δ^5-C27-steroid dehydrogenase deficiency: effects of chenodeoxycholic acid treatment. J Lipid Res. 1991;32:829–41.

23. Rossi SS, Crombie D, Steinbach JH, Lindor K, Dickson ER, Hofmann AF. Biliary bile acid composition in untreated primary biliary cirrhosis and sclerosing cholangitis: neither disease-specific nor of prognostic value. Hepatology. 1991;14:259A (abstr.).

24. Matoba N, Une M, Hoshita T. Identification of unconjugated bile acids in human bile. J Lipid Res. 1986;27:1154–62.

25. Cowen AE, Korman MG, Hofmann AF, Cass OW. Metabolism of lithocholate in healthy man. I. Biotransformation and biliary excretion of intravenously administered lithocholate, lithocholylglycine, and their sulfates. Gastroenterology. 1975;69:59–66.

26. Hepner GW, Hofmann AF, Thomas PJ. Metabolism of steroid and amino acid moieties of conjugated bile acids in man. II. Glycine-conjugated dihydroxy bile acids. J Clin Invest. 1972;51:1898–1905.

27. Hofmann NE, Hofmann AF. Metabolism of steroid and amino acid moieties of conjugated bile acids in man. IV. Description and validation of a multicompartmental model. Gastroenterology. 1974;67:887–97.

28. Stiehl A. Disturbances of bile acid metabolism in cholestasis. Clin Gastroenterol. 1977;6: 45–67.

29. van Berge Henegouwen GP, Brandt K-H, Eyssen H, Parmentier G. Sulfated and unsulfated bile acids in serum bile and urine of patients with cholestasis. Gut. 1976;17:861–9.

30. Back P. Urinary bile acids. In: Setchell KDR, Kritchevsky D, Nair PP, editors. The bile acids: chemistry, physiology, and metabolism, Vol. 4: Methods and applications. New York: Plenum, 1988:405–40.

31. Takikawa H, Beppu T, Seyama Y. Urinary concentrations of bile acid glucuronides and sulfates in hepatobiliary diseases. Gastroenterol Jpn. 1984;19:104–9.

32. Wietholz H, Marschall HU, Reuschenbach R, Matern H, Matern S. Urinary excretion of bile acid glucosides and glucuronides in extrahepatic cholestasis. Hepatology. 1991;13: 656–62.

33. Hofmann NE, Hofmann AF. Metabolism of steroid and amino acid moieties of conjugated bile acids in man. V. Equations for the perturbed enterohepatic circulation and their applications. Gastroenterology. 1977;72:141–8.

34. Schersten T. Bile acid conjugation. In: Fishman WH, ed. Metabolic conjugation and metabolic hydrolysis, Vol. 2. New York: Academic Press; 1971:75–121.

35. Hardison WGM. Hepatic taurine concentration and dietary taurine as regulators of bile acid conjugation with taurine. Gastroenterology. 1978;75:71–5.

36. Roda E, Mazzella G, Bazzoli F, Villanova N, Minutello A, Simoni P, Ronchi M, Poggi C, Festi D, Aldini R. et al. Effect of ursodeoxycholic acid administration on biliary lipid secretion in primary biliary cirrhosis. Dig Dis Sci. 1989;34:52–58S.

37. LaRusso NF, Hoffman NE, Korman MG, Hofmann AF, Cowen AE. Determinants of fasting and postprandial serum bile acid levels in healthy man. Am J Dig Dis. 1978;23:385–91.
38. Fricker G, Landmann L, Meier PJ. Extrahepatic obstructive cholestasis reverses the bile salt secretory polarity of rat hepatocytes. J Clin Invest. 1989;84:876–85.
39. Yoon YB, Hagey LR, Hofmann AF, Gurantz D, Michelotti EL, Steinbach JH. Effect of side-chain shortening on the physiological properties of bile acids: hepatic transport and effect on biliary secretion of 23-nor-ursodeoxycholate in rodents. Gastroenterology. 1986;90:837–52.
40. Baumgartner U, Feuerstein E, Sellinger H, Gerok W, Farthmann EH, Schölmerich J. Rapid regurgitation of bile acids during short-term cholestasis. J Hepatol. 1991;13:s8 (abstr.).
41. Pertsemlidis D, Kirchman EH, Ahrens EH, Jr. Regulation of cholesterol metabolism in the dog. I. Effects of complete bile diversion and of cholesterol feeding on absorption, synthesis, accumulation and excretion rates measured during life. J Clin Invest. 1973;52:2353–67.
42. Kuipers F, Havinga R, Bosschieter H, Toorop GP, Hindriks FR, Vonk RJ. Enterohepatic circulation in the rat. Gastroenterology. 1985;88:403–11.
43. Harkins RW, Hagerman LM, Sarett HP. Absorption of dietary fats by the rat in cholestyramine-induced steatorrhea. J Nutr. 1965;87:85–92.
44. Moore EW, Celic L, Ostrow JD. Interactions between ionized calcium and sodium taurocholate: bile salts are important buffers for prevention of calcium-containing gallstones. Gastroenterology. 1982;83:1079–89.
45. Sanyal AJ, Shiffman ML, Hirsch JI, Moore EW. Premicellar taurocholate enhances ferrous iron uptake from all regions of rat small intestine. Gastroenterology. 1991;101:382–9.
46. Danzinger RG, Hofmann AF, Thistle JL, Schoenfield LJ. Effect of oral chenodeoxycholic acid on bile acid kinetics and biliary lipid composition in women with cholelithiasis. J Clin Invest. 1973;52:2809–21.
47. Schölmerich J, Becher H-S, Schmidt K, Schubert R, Kremer B, Feldhaus S, Gerok W. Influence of hydroxylation and conjugation of bile salts on their membrane-damaging properties – studies on isolated hepatocytes and lipid membrane vesicles. Hepatology. 1984;4:661–6.
48. Miyazaki K, Nakayama F, Koga A. Effect of chenodeoxycholic and ursodeoxycholic acids on isolated adult human hepatocytes. Dig Dis Sci. 1984;29:1123–30.
49. Quist RG, Ton-Nu H-T, Lillienau J, Hofmann AF, Barrett KE. Activation of mast cells by bile acids. Gastroenterology. 1991;101:446–56.
50. Chadwick VS, Gaginella TS, Carlson GL, Debongnie JC, Phillips SF, Hofmann AF. Effect of molecular structure on bile acid-induced alterations in absorptive function, permeability and morphology in the perfused rabbit colon. J Lab Clin Med. 1979;94:661–74.
51. Miyai K, Price VM, Fisher MM. Bile acid metabolism in mammals. Ultrastructural studies on the intrahepatic cholestasis induced by lithocholic and chenodeoxycholic acids in the rat. Lab Invest. 1971;24:292–02.
52. Palmer KR, Gurantz D, Hofmann AF, Clayton LM, Hagey LR, Cecchetti S. Hypercholeresis induced by norchenodeoxycholate in the biliary fistula rodent. Am J Physiol. 1987;252:G219–28.
53. Heuman DM, Mills AS, McCall J, Hylemon PB, Pandak WM, Vlahcevic ZR. Conjugates of ursodeoxycholate protect against cholestasis and hepatocellular necrosis caused by more hydrophobic bile salts. Gastroenterology. 1991;100:203–11.
54. Galle PR, Theilmann L, Raedsch R, Otto G, Stiehl D. Ursodeoxycholate reduces hepatotoxicity of bile salts in primary human hepatocytes. Hepatology. 1991;12:486–91.
55. Eusafzai S, Ericcson S, Cederlund T, Einarsson K, Angelin B. Effect of ursodeoxycholic acid on ileal absorption of bile acids in man as determined by the SeHCAT test. Gut. 1991;32:1044–8.
56. Stiehl A, Raedsch R, Rudolph G. Acute effects of ursodeoxycholic and chenodeoxycholic acid on the small intestinal absorption of bile acids. Gastroenterology. 1990;98:424–8.
57. Stiehl A, Becker M, Czygan P, Frohling W, Kommerell B, Rotthauwe HW, Senn M. Bile acids and their sulphated and glucuronidated derivatives in bile, plasma, and urine of children with intrahepatic cholestasis: effects of phenobarbital treatment. Eur J Clin Invest. 1980;10:307–16.
58. Lake M. Non-surgical biliary drainage. Med Clin N Am. 1935;19:677–88.
59. Whitington PF, Whitington GL. Partial external diversion of bile for the treatment of

intractable pruritus associated with intrahepatic cholestasis. Gastroenterology. 1988;95:130–6.
60. Hofmann AF, Schteingart CD, Lillienau J. Biological and medical aspects of active ileal transport of bile acids. Ann Med. 1991;23:169–75.
61. Carey JB Jr, Wilson ID, Zaki FG, Hanson RF. The metabolism of bile acids with special reference to liver injury. Medicine. 1966;45:461–70.
62. Greim H, Trulzsch D, Czygan P, Rudick J, Hutterer F, Schaffner F, Popper H. Mechanism of cholestasis. VI. Bile acids in human livers with or without biliary obstruction. Gastroenterology. 1972;63:846–50.

11
Functional considerations in the assessment of therapy of chronic cholestatic diseases

J. REICHEN, F. J. ROOS and H. ZIMMERMANN

Cholestatic liver diseases are heterogeneous not only with respect to aetiology, but also with respect to their natural history. Thus, cholestasis ranges from biochemical abnormalities without any clinical relevance over annoying but benign manifestations such as pruritus, to diseases which progress inexorably to liver failure and death. Even in a given disease, e.g. primary biliary cirrhosis, the natural history is highly variable[1-3]. This heterogeneity in evolution makes any novel form of therapy difficult to assess. This heterogeneity is even more pronounced in paediatric cholestatic liver disease, and clinical trials are difficult if not impossible to perform due to the rarity of some of these cholestatic syndromes.

Conventional liver tests such as alkaline phosphatase or other enzymes indicating cholestasis bear no relation to prognosis. In contrast, serum bilirubin[4] and serum bile acid levels[5] reflect the functional derangement somewhat better. Their serum concentration depends on production, elimination and the volume of distribution:

$$c = (\text{Production} - \text{elimination})/\text{Volume of distribution}.$$

Thus, extrahepatic factors such as bilirubin production, renal excretion of bile acids in cholestasis or ileal bile acid absorption may affect serum levels even when hepatic function is constant. This may explain their limited usefulness in prognostication of chronic cholestatic liver disease[6].

This failure of the easily measurable conventional liver tests has led to the development of composite prognostic indices such as the Mayo[7] or European[8] score, to refine prognostication in primary biliary cirrhosis. Another approach, namely the use of so-called quantitative or dynamic liver function tests, has not been very popular in cholestatic liver disease because of their perceived lack of sensitivity[9,10].

To further investigate whether dynamic liver function tests are affected in

Table 1 Aetiology of cholestasis in 45 consecutive patients presenting with a predominantly cholestatic biochemical profile characterized by dynamic liver function testing

	Extrahepatic		Intrahepatic	
Diagnosis	*Cirrhotic*	*Non-cirrhotic*	*Cirrhotic*	*Non-cirrhotic*
Cholelithiasis	2	3		
Echinococcus	1	5		
Sclerosing cholangitis		3		
Tumours	1			
α_1-Antitrypsin deficiency			1	
Cholestatic hepatitis				9
Cystic fibrosis			8	1
Drug-induced cholestasis				3
Primary biliary cirrhosis			6	2
Total	4	11	15	15

patients with cholestasis we investigated 45 consecutive patients referred for work-up of cholestatic liver disease. All patients had elevated cholestatic enzymes (alkaline phosphatase, γ-glutamyl-transpeptidase and 5′-nucleotidase). Based on the results of appropriate imaging procedures (ultrasound in all patients, followed by nuclear scintigraphy or endoscopic retrograde cholangiography) and liver biopsy, patients were classified as intrahepatic or extrahepatic cholestasis, and as cirrhotic or non-cirrhotic; the diagnoses of these patients are listed in Table 1. Galactose elimination capacity, aminopyrine breath test and sulphobromophthalein retention were determined as previously described[11,12]. The results of these tests are shown in Fig. 1; both the galactose elimination capacity and the aminopyrine breath test showed wide variation and did not discern between cirrhotic and non-cirrhotic disease as assessed by analysis of variance (Fig. 1). Only sulphobromophthalein retention was consistently abnormal in cholestatic patients; this is not surprising since the clearance of this compound depends on hepatic uptake and excretion. However, sulphobromophthalein retention was not able to discriminate between cirrhotic and non-cirrhotic liver disease either (Fig. 1).

The question then arises whether testing of dynamic liver function is of any use in cholestatic liver disease. In Chapter 6 of this volume, V. Desmet makes a clear-cut case that the pathology of cholestasis has to be considered as a highly dynamic process; it stands to reason that the functional sequelae of this dynamic evolution will be reflected in the results of dynamic tests of hepatic function. Indeed, we have shown previously that chronic cholestatic diseases in experimental animals are characterized by a steady decline in cytosolic and microsomal function, and that this decline permits prognostication with appreciable accuracy[13]. The evolution of two aspects of hepatic function, namely microsomal function assessed by the aminopyrine breath test and of cytosolic function assessed by the galactose breath test, in rats with secondary biliary cirrhosis induced by bile duct ligation, is shown in Fig. 2. From a given moment in the evolution of the disease there is a monotonous decline of function.

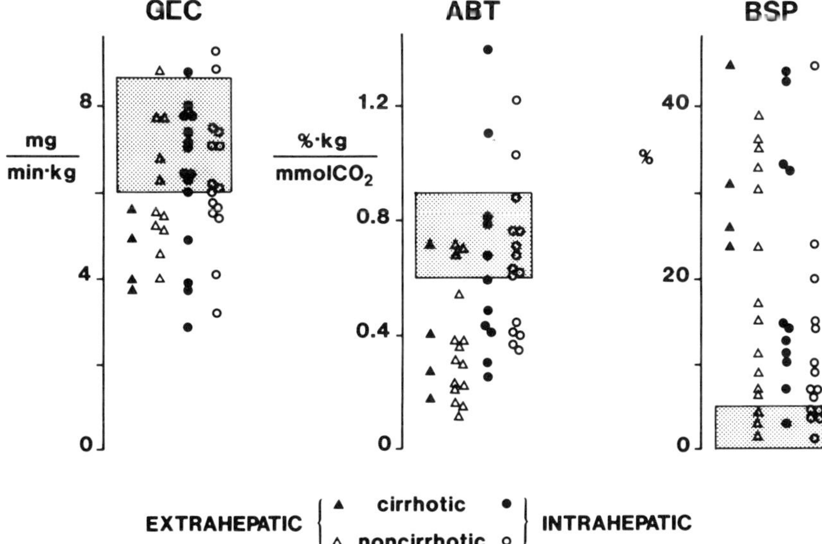

Fig. 1 Results of dynamic liver function testing in 45 patients with extra- or intrahepatic cirrhotic or non-cirrhotic cholestatic liver disease. The diagnoses of the patients are given in Table 1. Galactose elimination capacity (GEC), aminopyrine breath test (ABT) or 45-min retention of sulphobromophthalein (BSP) were determined as a measure of cytosolic, microsomal and excretory hepatic function, respectively. While both ABT and BSP were abnormal in cholestatic liver disease, neither discerned between cirrhotic and non-cirrhotic or intra- and extrahepatic disease

More recently, we have extended this observation to a chronic cholestatic liver disease in humans, namely to patients with primary biliary cirrhosis[3]. Therefore we submit that serial testing of quantitative liver function may permit better prognostication and early appreciation of the value of therapeutic interventions[3,14]. This concept requires a patient to be tested serially with dynamic liver function tests to characterize his or her own natural evolution. A successful therapeutic intervention should then result in an alteration in the slope of the decrease in function or even in recovery of function.

The impact of cholestasis on hepatic function is still controversial (reviewed in ref. 14). However, the use of experimental animal models of chronic cholestatic liver disease, such as secondary biliary cirrhosis induced by bile duct ligation in the rat[13,15], has permitted the generation of testable hypotheses about the impact of chronic cholestasis on hepatic function. A theoretical scenario of how cholestasis could impact on liver function is depicted in Fig. 3. In this scenario cholestasis – the failure to excrete bile or components thereof – leads to retention of different compounds with biological activity; this can induce cell necrosis as exemplified by cholate stasis and feathery degeneration[16]; necrosis in turn leads to fibrosis and regeneration, the two processes if unchecked eventually resulting in cirrhosis. Cirrhosis is obviously a main cause of portal hypertension. The scheme in

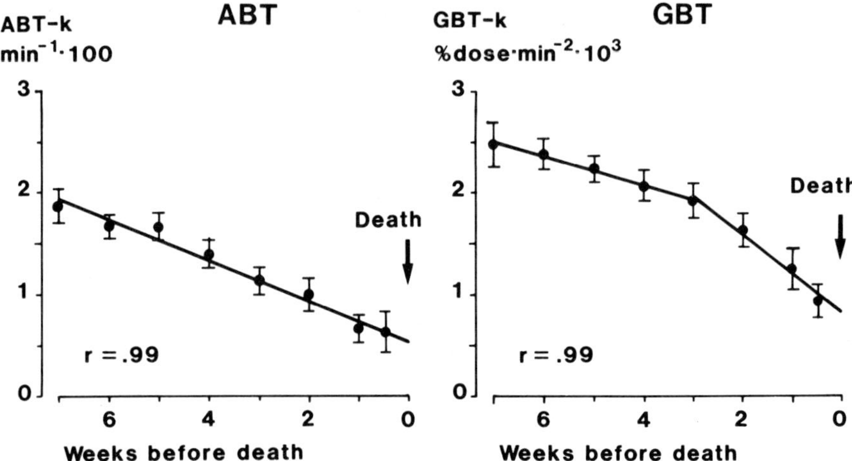

Fig. 2 Evolution of galactose elimination capacity and aminopyrine N-demethylation in rats with secondary biliary cirrhosis as a measure of cytosolic (non-membrane-bound) and microsomal (membrane-bound) liver function ($\bar{x} \pm$ SEM, $n = 8$). There is a monotonous decline in microsomal function suggesting alteration of biomembranes. The biphasic decline in galactose elimination capacity could reflect loss of hepatocellular mass at the break; before the break the decline is due to age-related changes since this is also seen in control animals. Reproduced with permission from the publisher from *Hepatology* 1987;7:457–63

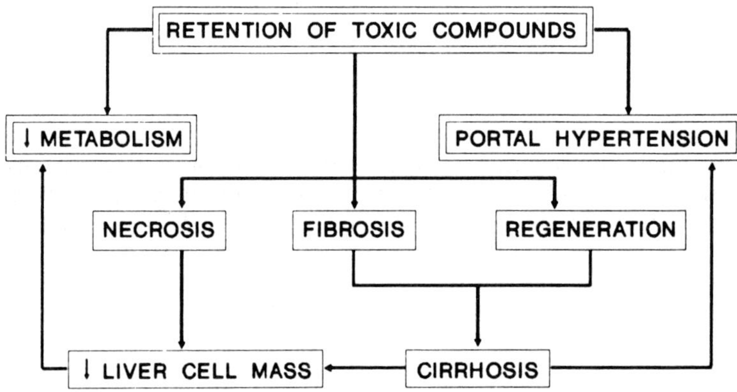

Fig. 3 Hypothetical scenario whereby cholestasis could lead to functional impairment. Cholestasis ('the failure to form bile') leads to retention of compounds which are normally excreted into bile. These set into movement a cascade of events finally leading to biliary cirrhosis. Cirrhosis and decreased metabolism can be ascribed, at least in part, to retention of bile acids, bilirubin, and/or cholesterol, and do not necessitate postulating development of cirrhosis. For further details, see text

Fig. 3 also allows for a direct portal hypertensive effect of biliary toxins. Cell loss can occur either directly as a consequence of necrosis or indirectly in the later stages of cirrhogenesis when the regenerative potential of the liver is exhausted.

Is there evidence for the speculative scenario outlined in Fig. 3? Different compounds normally excreted into bile adversely affect liver function. Thus, bilirubin is an uncoupler of mitochondrial oxidative phosphorylation *in vitro*[17]. Bile acids have many toxic effects on different hepatic and extrahepatic cells (reviewed by the contribution of J. Schölmerich and R. Straub in Chapter 9 of this volume). Bile is the main excretory pathway of leukotrienes, important mediators of inflammation[18]. This list is far from complete, and much work is needed to fill in the gaps outlined in Fig. 3.

We have recently generated some direct proof for the adverse effects of retention of compounds normally excreted into bile[19]. Thus, in rats with a chronic choledochocaval fistula inducing retention of bile in the absence of cholestasis, we observed portal hypertension in the absence of fibrosis, suggesting that some compound(s) normally excreted into bile has vasoactive properties. Good candidates for such an agent are, again, bile acids. Although one investigation cleared bile acids from being involved in the hyperdynamic circulation of cirrhosis of other than biliary origin[20], a more recent study by Bomzon *et al.* demonstrated direct vasoactive actions of bile acids[21].

Another compound involved in the functional alterations in cholestasis could be cholesterol. Cholesterol accumulates in biomembranes in chronic obstruction in experimental animals[22] and in humans[23]. The evolution of liver function in biliary obstructed rats in Fig. 2 demonstrates that the decline is monophasic for a membrane-related function such as the aminopyrine breath test, but biphasic for the cytosolic function of galactokinase measured by the galactose elimination capacity; the first phase of the decline of galactose elimination is an age-related phenomenon, since this decline was also observed in the sham-operated controls[13]. This suggested to us that perhaps the incorporation of cholesterol into biomembranes could be involved in the functional deterioration of cholestasis. Indeed we were able to demonstrate a close correlation between membrane rigidity – owing predominantly to increased cholesterol incorporation but also contributed to by alterations in phospholipid composition – and microsomal membrane function *in vivo* and *in vitro*[24]. An as yet unexplained paradoxical increase in cholesterol and bile acid synthesis leads to aggravation of this phenomenon in biliary cirrhotic rats[25]; whether a similar dysregulation occurs in humans remains to be demonstrated.

We have been interested for some time in the structure–function relationship of the cirrhotic liver. The ideal tool to investigate this is stereological analysis of liver composition. Earlier investigations demonstrated that hepatocyte mass was long maintained in the face of established cirrhosis[13]. This maintenance of hepatocellular mass is demonstrated in Fig. 4: animals with established biliary cirrhosis after bile duct ligation and dissection had decreased volume fraction of hepatocytes as determined stereologically. Hepatocytes were essentially replaced by ductular proliferates and connective tissue. However, due to a marked increase in liver weight absolute hepatocyte volume (volume fraction × liver volume) was maintained. It should also be noted that in these animals microsomal function, as assessed by the aminopyrine breath test *in vivo*, was markedly reduced. This provides further evidence that retention of compounds normally excreted into bile can adversely affect liver function as postulated in Fig. 3. Indeed,

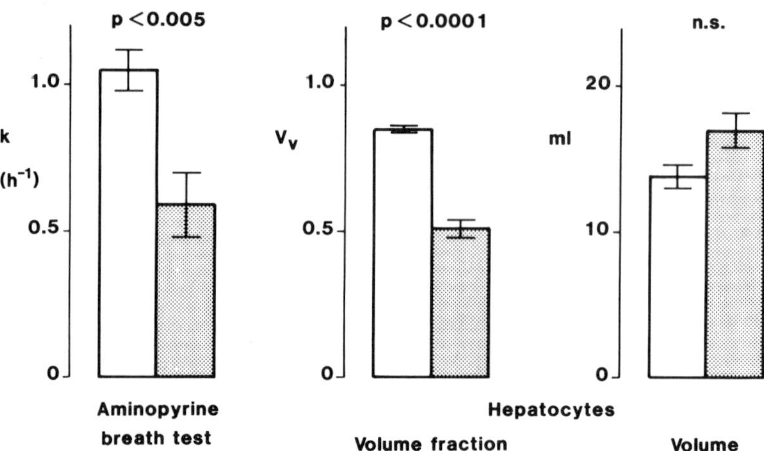

Fig. 4 Maintenance of hepatocellular mass in secondary biliary cirrhosis (hatched panels) in the rat. Microsomal function, measured by the aminopyrine breath test, is markedly reduced. Stereologically determined volume fraction of hepatocytes is reduced owing to replacement of hepatocytes by ductular proliferates and accumulation of connective tissue; however, liver cell volume (volume fraction × liver volume) is maintained. These findings suggest that chronic cholestasis induces a 'sick cell' model of liver disease but can maintain liver cell volume, perhaps due to activation of regenerative stimuli such as epidermal growth factor. For further details see text

such an inhibitory effect has previously been demonstrated for bile acids[26].

In contrast to biliary cirrhosis, hepatocyte mass is reduced in another model of cirrhosis when the disease is further progressed[27]. This observation suggests that at some point in cirrhogenesis the proverbial regenerative potential of the liver could be exhausted. Biliary cirrhosis but not micronodular cirrhosis was characterized by increased nuclear localization of epidermal growth factor (EGF[28,29]), one of the earliest signals for initiation of liver regeneration[30]. This could point to another, this time beneficial, effect of cholestasis. Indeed, EGF is normally excreted into bile[31]. Failure of this excretory pathway could be involved in the maintenance of hepatocellular mass in biliary cirrhosis[13,29].

Are there any practical applications of these concepts besides prognostication? We submit that serial determination of quantitative liver function tests could (a) define patients with a progressive course and (b) once such a decline in function has been defined in an individual patient, to assess the value of therapeutic interventions. This hinges on the premise that (a) a decline in function does occur and that (b) such a decline has elements of reversibility.

The first point has clearly been proven in animal models and patients, as discussed above[3,13]. Recovery of function has been demonstrated after relief of biliary obstruction in paedients[32,33]. We have recently demonstrated that even cirrhosis and portal hypertension are reversible in biliary cirrhotic rat when adequate drainage has been achieved by a choledochojejunal Roux-en-Y anastomosis[34]. This concept could also be applicable to pharmacological interventions as evidenced by the recovery of excretory[35,36] and microsomal[35] function in patients with cholestasis associated with cystic fibrosis and with primary biliary cirrhosis treated with ursodeoxycholate (see also Chapters 34 and 37 in this volume).

The concept of serial testing of dynamic liver function could be particularly useful in children with rare cholestatic diseases, where sufficient patients for formal clinical trials are difficult or impossible to recruit. Tests particularly suited for this purpose are the aminopyrine breath test using stable isotopes[37], and perhaps the lidocaine clearance advocated by M. Burdelski[38]; see also Chapter 22 in this volume. Such an approach could facilitate the assessment of novel therapeutic interventions in small patient groups, and therefore be particularly suitable for paediatric cholestatic disorders.

Acknowledgements

This work was supported by a grant from the Swiss National Foundation for Scientific Research to J.R. (32.30168.90) and H.Z. (32.29977.90). The artwork by Ms M. Kappeler is gratefully acknowledged.

References

1. Sherlock S, Scheuer PJ. The presentation and diagnosis of 100 patients with primary biliary cirrhosis. N Engl J Med. 1973;289:674–8.
2. James O, Macklon AF, Watson AJ. Primary biliary cirrhosis: a revised clinical spectrum. Lancet. 1981;1:1278–81.
3. Reichen J, Widmer T, Cotting J. Accurate prediction of death by serial determination of the galactose elimination capacity in primary biliary cirrhosis: a comparison with the Mayo model. Hepatology 1991;14:504–10.
4. Shapiro JM, Smith H, Schaffner F. Serum bilirubin: a prognostic factor in primary biliary cirrhosis. Gut. 1979;20:137–40.
5. Berry W, Reichen J. Bile acid metabolism: its relation to clinical disease. Sem Liver Dis. 1983;3:330–40.
6. Bremmelgaard A, Alme B. Analysis of plasma bile acid profiles in patients with liver disease associated with cholestasis. Scand J Gastroenterol. 1980;15:593–600.
7. Dickson ER, Grambsch PM, Fleming TR, Fisher LD, Langworthy A. Prognosis in primary biliary cirrhosis: model for decision making. Hepatology. 1989;10:1–7.
8. Christensen E, Neuberger J, Crowe J, Altman DG, Popper H, Portman B, Doniach D, Ranek L, Tiegstrup N, Williams R. Beneficial effect of azathioprine and prediction of prognosis in primary biliary cirrhosis. Gastroenterology. 1985;89:1084–91.
9. Baker AL, Krager PS, Kotake AN, Schoeller DA. The aminopyrine breath test does not correlate with histologic disease severity in patients with cholestasis. Hepatology. 1987;7:464–7.
10. Miguet JP, Vuitton D, Deschamps JP, Allemand H, Joanne C, Bechtel P, Car P. Cholestasis and hepatic drug metabolism. Comparison of metabolic clearance rate of antipyrine in patients with intrahepatic or extrahepatic cholestasis. Dig Dis Sci. 1981;26:718–22.
11. Heri M, Bircher J. Die Galaktose-eliminationskapazitaet, ein zuverlaessiger Test zur quantitativen Erfassung der Leberfunktion. Schweiz Med Wochenschr. 1971;101:735–6.
12. Haecki W, Bircher J, Preisig R. A new look at the plasma disappearance of sulfobromophthalein (BSP): correlation with the BSP transport maximum and the hepatic plasma flow in man. J Lab Clin Med. 1976;88:1019–31.
13. Gross JB, Reichen J, Zeltner T, Zimmermann A. The evolution of changes in quantitative liver function tests in a rat model of cirrhosis. Hepatology. 1987;7:457–63.

14. Reichen J. Liver function in cholestatic liver disease: implications for treatment. Hepatology Rapid Lit Rev. 1991;21:7–14.
15. Kontouras J, Billing BH, Scheuer PJ. Prolonged bile duct obstruction: a new experimental model for cirrhosis in the rat. Br J Exp Pathol. 1984;65:305–11.
16. Desmet VJ. Cholestasis, extrahepatic obstruction and secondary biliary cirrhosis. In: MacSween RNM, Anthony PP, Scheuer PJ, editors. Pathology of the liver. Edinburgh, London and New York: Churchill Livingstone; 1979:272–305.
17. Zettterstrom R, Ernster L. Bilirubin, an uncoupler of oxidative phosphorylation in isolated mitochondria. Nature. 1956;178:1335–7.
18. Wettstein M, Gerok W, Haeussinger D. Characteristics of sinusoidal uptake and biliary excretion of cysteinyl leukotrienes in perfused rat liver. Eur J Biochem. 1990;191:251–5.
19. Zimmermann H, Saegesser H, Tenisch B, Reichen J. Retention of bile induces portal hypertension but not biliary cirrhosis in the rat. Hepatology. 1990;12:854.
20. Genecin P, Polio J, Colombato LA, Ferraioli G, Reuben A, Groszmann RJ. Bile acids do not mediate the hyperdynamic circulation in portal hypertensive rats. Am J Physiol. 1990;259:G21–5.
21. Said O, Shaffer E, Bomzon A. Bile acids and the cardiovascular complications of liver disease. J Hepatol. 1991;13,suppl.2:S67.
22. Kawata S, Chitranukroh A, Owen JS, McIntyre N. Membrane lipid changes in erythrocytes, liver and kidney in acute and chronic experimental liver disease in rats. Biochim Biophys Acta. 1987;896:26–34.
23. Owen JS, McIntyre N. Erythrocyte lipid composition and sodium transport in human liver disease. Biochim Biophys Acta. 1978;510:168–76.
24. Reichen J, Buters JTM, Sojic Z, Roos FJ. Abnormal lipid composition of microsomes from cirrhotic rat liver – does it contribute to decreased microsomal function? Experientia. 1992; (in press).
25. Dueland S, Reichen J, Everson GT, Davis RA. Regulation of cholesterol and bile acid homeostasis in bile obstructed rats. Biochem J. 1992;280:373–7.
26. Hutterer F, Denk H, Bacchin PG, Schenkman JB, Schaffner F, Popper H. Mechanism of cholestasis. 1. Effect of bile acids on microsomal cytochrome P-450 dependent biotransformation systems *in vitro*. Life Sci. 1970;9:977–87.
27. Reichen J, Arts B, Schafroth U, Zimmermann A, Zeltner TB, Zysset T. Aminopyrine N-methylation by rats with liver cirrhosis: evidence for the intact cell hypothesis. A morphometric–functional study. Gastroenterology. 1987;93:719–26.
28. Oguey D, Marti U, Saegesser H, Reichen J. Differential effect of micronodular and biliary cirrhosis on epidermal growth factor receptor binding and expression in the rat. J Hepatol. 1991;13(Suppl.2):S57.
29. Oguey D, Marti U, Reichen J. Epidermal growth factor receptor: Its possible implication in the maintenance of hepatocellular mass in biliary cirrhosis in the rat. (Submitted).
30. Marti U, Burwen SJ, Wells A, Barker ME, Huling S, Feren AM, Jones AL. Localization of epidermal growth factor receptor in hepatocyte nuclei. Hepatology. 1991;13:15–20.
31. Marti U, Burwen SJ, Jones AL. Biological effects of epidermal growth factor with emphasis on the gastrointestinal tract and liver: an update. Hepatology. 1989;9:126–38.
32. Hepner GW, Vessell ES. Assessment of aminopyrine metabolism in man after oral administration of 14C-aminopyrine. Effects of phenobarbital, disulfiram and portal cirrhosis. N Engl J Med. 1974;291:1384–88.
33. Reichen J. Pathophysiology of cholestasis. In: Paumgartner G, Stiehl A, Barbara L, Roda E, editors. Strategies for the treatment of hepatobiliary diseases. Dordrecht: Kluwer, 1990:3–12.
34. Zimmermann H, Reichen J., Zimmermann A, Saegesser H, Thenisch B, Hflin F. Reversibility of the functional and structural sequelae of secondary biliary cirrhosis in the rat by biliodigestive anastomosis. Gastroenterology (Submitted).
35. Cotting J, Lentze MJ, Reichen J. Effects of ursodeoxycholic acid therapy on nutrition and liver function in patients with cystic fibrosis and long-standing cholestasis. Gut. 1990;31:918–21.
36. Poupon R, Chretien Y, Poupon RE, Ballet F, Calmus Y, Darnis F. Is ursodeoxycholic acid an effective treatment for primary biliary cirrhosis? Lancet. 1987;1:834–6.
37. Irving CS, Schoeller DA, Nakamura KI, Baker AL, Klein PD. The aminopyrine breath test as a measure of liver function. A quantitative description of its metabolic basis in normal subjects. J Lab Clin Med. 1982;100:356–73.
38. Oellerich M, Ringe B, Gubernatis G, Pichlmayr R, Burdelski M, Lamesch P, Bunzendahl H, Herrmann H. Lignocaine metabolite formation as a measure of pre-transplant liver function. Lancet. 1989;1:640–2.

Section 3
Clinical Aspects of Paediatric Cholestasis

12
Cholestasis in infancy and childhood: an overview

P. TRIVEDI, G. MIELI-VERGANI and A. P. MOWAT

THE CLINICAL IMPORTANCE OF CHOLESTATIC DISORDERS

Cholestatic disorders recognized in infancy because of jaundice with a conjugated hyperbilirubinaemia account for more than 50% of the work load in tertiary referral centres for paediatric hepatology[1,2]. Many of the infants go on to develop chronic liver disease; they constitute the majority of children requiring liver transplantation[2-6]. Although chronic liver disease presenting as cholestasis in childhood appears to be less common than that following cholestasis in infancy (Table 1), when it does occur treatment is relatively ineffective and cirrhosis and its sequelae are frequent. It is very appropriate that this symposium be devoted to considering in detail the

Table 1 Inpatients, Paediatric Liver Service, King's College Hospital, 1 April 1991–31 July 1991: mode of presentation

Cholestasis in infancy		111
Biliary atresia		60
Portoenterostomy	9	
Transplant-related	12	
2 transplanted		
Complications or colchicine trial	39	
Other surgical disorders		4
α_1-Antitrypsin deficiency		15
Alagille's syndrome		11
Other cholestasis in infancy		21
'Cholestasis' in childhood		11
Autoimmune primary sclerosing cholangitis	6	
Cystic fibrosis	5	
Other liver disorders		75
Total		197

structure and function of the biliary system in health and disease, and reviewing specific cholestatic disorders. In this overview of cholestasis in infancy and childhood three aspects of the problem are highlighted as requiring action to improve the outcome for at least some of our patients.

Area of opportunity: 1

Failure by the primary physician to recognize the true nature of the problem.

In infancy

In infants presenting with a cholestatic syndrome in Britain treatment is often delayed because of failure by the primary health care team to recognize or appreciate the significance of conjugated hyperbilirubinaemia[7,8]. It should be unthinkable to look after an ill, jaundiced infant without measuring the direct or conjugated bilirubin. Nevertheless this is a frequent occurrence. We must teach that in the cholestatic infant with a normal fluid intake the urine is not dark but pale yellow. Our colleagues in neonatology and paediatrics must learn to look at the urine colour. If it is not colourless they must test the urine for bilirubin and measure the direct or conjugated serum bilirubin. Only if this is done will they appreciate that hepatobiliary disease is present and initiate appropriate investigations.

If the infant with jaundice is otherwise well, as are most infants with biliary atresia in the first 4–8 weeks of life, the risk of inappropriate management is perhaps greater. The parents are often advised authoritatively that the jaundice is physiological because it started in the first few days of life. Thus reassured, the inexperienced parent will consider there can be no cause for concern when the jaundice persists beyond 14 days of age. We see infants with biliary atresia whose jaundice has been attributed to breast feeding (a cause of unconjugated hyperbilirubinaemia!). Management may be improved by posters emphasizing the importance of prolonged jaundice, yellow urine and the stool colour as early signs of treatable hepatobiliary disease in antenatal, postnatal and welfare baby clinics, or family practitioner centres in which mothers and babies are seen. A more effective alternative may be systematic screening for hepatobiliary disorders as is done for other relatively rare conditions such as hyperphenylalanaemia or congenital hypothyroidism which have an incidence of approximately 1:4000 live births[9,10]. The estimated incidence of biliary atresia ranges from 1:14000 to 1:21000 live births[11]. The incidence of hepatobiliary disease in early infancy requiring equally early recognition for optimum treatment of infective, metabolic or endocrine causes is at least 5 times higher[12]. If screening (urinalysis for bilirubin and measuring the direct or conjugated serum bilirubin) were limited to infants who remain jaundiced after 14 days of age the number of negative tests would be relatively smaller. Physiological jaundice almost invariably clears by 14 days of age except in a small proportion of breast-fed infants[13]. The cost benefits would be considerable.

If bile is present in the urine, or the conjugated bilirubin is raised, the infant should receive vitamin K and be referred immediately to a paediatric

Table 2 Diagnosis in infants with cholestasis in Paediatric Liver Service, King's College Hospital, 1970–90

Biliary atresia	337
Cryptogenic hepatitis	331
α_1-Antitrypsin deficiency (PIZZ)	189
Other identified associated disorder	94
Alagille's syndrome	61
Choledochal cyst	34
Total	1046

centre for urgent investigation. If the stools do not contain green or yellow pigment over the course of 2–3 days the patient should be referred to a specialist liver centre able to perform portoenterostomy.

In childhood

In childhood the hazard for the child is not a failure to recognize the presence of cholestasis and significant liver disease, but that the primary physician accepts a diagnosis of acute viral hepatitis without serological confirmation. Even worse is the label of non-A–non-B hepatitis. For such children it is mandatory to exclude chronic treatable conditions such as choledochal cyst, Wilson's disease and autoimmune disorders, however mild the illness appears to be or how brief its duration[14]. Continuing education of our colleagues and pressure from parent groups may improve this problem.

Area of opportunity: 2

Diagnostic difficulties within specialist referral units.

In infancy

In referral centres the essentials of management are:

1. Accurate diagnosis including identification of any associated disorder and accurate characterization of the pathological process.
2. Appropriate management of these, including consideration for liver transplantation.
3. Prevention of the complications of cholestasis.

The problem and challenge we face is to develop and maintain the skills and resources to make an accurate diagnosis. We are faced with an ever-growing list of well-defined disorders associated with this syndrome. Identification of any of these is essential and urgent if there is effective treatment. We still have a large proportion with cryptogenic disease (Table 2). Fortunately the majority have self-limiting disease. As discussed below, we can identify some who will have chronic disease. A particularly difficult subgroup are those with fulminant liver failure who in the past may have been allowed to die but are now referred for consideration for transplantation. The increasing availability and acceptance of liver transplantation for fulminant liver failure will bring us more referrals in this category.

Table 3

Abnormal physical signs	Disorders
Skin lesions, purpura, choroidoretinitis, myocarditis etc.	Generalized viral infections
Cataracts	Galactosaemia, hypoparathyroidism
Multiple congenital anomalies	Trisomy 21, 18 or 13
Cystic mass below the liver	Choledochal cyst
Bile-stained herniae	Spontaneous perforation of the bile ducts
Systolic murmur, abnormal facies, embryotoxon	Biliary hypoplasia
Cutaneous haemangiomata	Hepatic or biliary haemangioma
Situs inversus	Extrahepatic biliary atresia
Optic nerve hypoplasia or micro-penis	Septo-optic dysplasia

Table 4 Inherited disorders associated with hepatitis syndrome in infancy

(a)	(b)
Galactosaemia	α_1-Antitrypsin deficiency
Fructosaemia	Cystic fibrosis
Tyrosinaemia	Niemann-Pick disease type 2 (or C)
Defects in synthesis of primary bile acids	Gaucher's disease
Defects in fat oxidation	Wolman's disease
Familial erythrophagocytic reticulosis	Neonatal haemochromatosis
	Zellweger's syndrome
	Infantile polycystic disease

Diagnostic scheme. The clinical history and examination are helpful in the minority. Consanguinity or liver disease in siblings suggests the possibility of familial, genetic, metabolic or haemolytic disease. Review of the perinatal case record and past medical history may reveal features suggesting intrauterine infection, exposure to toxins and drugs or intravenous nutrition. Careful physical examination may reveal features of disorders listed in Table 3. Specimens of all stools passed are saved and looked at for yellow or green pigment: if absent biliary atresia is likely. Changes in standard biochemical tests for liver function are rarely helpful in differential diagnosis. A systematically pursued series of investigations is required[14,15]. In all cases hypoprothrombinaenia due to vitamin K malabsorption must be prevented or treated.

It is important to consider and exclude immediately septicaemia, urinary tract infection, malaria, syphilis, herpes simplex infections, listeriosis, and toxoplasmosis since effective treatment for these is available. Galactosaemia (galactose-1-phosphate uridyl transferase deficiency), fructosaemia (history of dietary exposure and subsequent demonstration of aldolase deficiency in liver biopsy) and tyrosinaemia (increased urinary succinylacetone or δ-aminolaevulinic acid excretion) should be excluded immediately, since dietary measures are required urgently, in the first two particularly. Other treatable genetic or familial disorders are listed in Table 4a. In the past 2 years we have seen three infants with dicarboxylic aciduria (demonstrated by mass spectroscopy) who showed a satisfactory response to a low-fat diet as well

Table 5 Infections associated with conjugated hyperbilirubinaemia in early pregnancy

Septicaemia	Herpes simplex I, II and IV
Urinary tract infection	Cytomegalovirus
Syphilis	Rubella
Listeriosis	Echo virus 9, 11, 14, 19
Tuberculosis	Adenovirus
Toxoplasmosis	Epstein–Barr virus
Malaria	Coxsackie A9, B
	REO virus III
	Hepatitis viruses
	Human immunodeficiency virus (HIV)

as three with primary defects in bile acid metabolism responding in a most encouraging way to administration of cholic and/or chenodeoxycholic acid. Consideration must then be given to excluding common genetic disorders associated with this syndrome (Table 4b). In the United Kingdom, α_1-antitrypsin deficiency, cystic fibrosis and Niemann-Pick type C (also termed type 2) need to be excluded in all instances[16].

An ultrasound examination is performed to identify dilatation of the biliary tree indicating a choledochal cyst. A particular difficulty in some cases is the exclusion of endocrine disorders usually occurring as part of septo-optic dysplasia. The syndrome is frequently incomplete. Both the hepatobiliary picture and the extent of the endocrinopathy are very variable. If there is consanguinity or a positive family history of cholestatic disorders in childhood, or suspicion of undiagnosed metabolic disease, a fibroblast culture should be established for subsequent analysis. This is particularly important in fulminant or fatal cases. Rubella, cytomegalovirus and hepatitis B and other associated infections (Table 5) should be excluded, since the presence of these are important in the future management of the child and its family. The investigations for these infections should not be allowed to delay consideration of genetic or endocrine disorders, biliary atresia or other surgically correctable disorders.

Percutaneous liver biopsy. Accurate characterization of the pathological process is required for both management and prognosis. For this a percutaneous liver biopsy skilfully interpreted by a histopathologist working closely with the clinicians is essential. It is imperative that some of the material obtained is frozen at $-70°C$ for subsequent biochemical analysis for inherited disorders if indicated by the liver histology or other investigations.

The site of the most prominent pathological change has a profound effect on prognosis. It may be on one of four sites:

1. Hepatic parenchyma.
2. Portal tracts.
3. Intrahepatic bile ducts.
4. Extrahepatic bile ducts.

The prognosis in category 1 is dependent on that of any associated disorder and the severity of liver damage. Broad fibrous tracts connecting portal tracts and central veins or cirrhosis leads to chronic liver disease. This occurs rarely in association with infection or where disease remains cryptogenic after full investigation, and there is no positive family history or consanguinity. Categories 2 and 3 are frequently associated with chronic liver disease and may be followed by progressive intrahepatic cholestasis with cirrhosis. Two particular groups with a poor prognosis are those with a normal serum γ-glutamyl transpeptidase activity in the presence of jaundice and abnormal biochemical tests of liver function and those who develop a sclerosing cholangitis[17,18]. Chronic liver disease is inevitable in category 4 if surgical correction is not possible. Radiopharmaceutical tests[19] and cholangiography have a place in selected cases[20].

In childhood

In the older child with a cholestatic disorder as evidenced by jaundice the particular diagnostic difficulty we have highlighted in recent years[21,22] is the marked similarity in childhood between autoimmune active hepatitis and primary sclerosing cholangitis. The clinical, biochemical, liver biopsy appearance and immunological feature may be indistinguishable; so much so that it is now our policy to perform endoscopic cholangiography in all cases. A major problem is identifying progressive biliary pathology in cystic fibrosis before irreversible liver damage has occurred.

Area of opportunity: 3

The prevention of, or control of, progressive hepatic fibrosis and the development of cirrhosis.

As highlighted in the introduction, a large proportion of infants and children with cholestatic disorders develop chronic liver disease with cirrhosis. We need a clearer understanding of factors controlling bile acid metabolism and transport, bile secretion and bile flow. Is (are) there waiting to be identified product(s), e.g. a leukotriene, which is (are) retained because of cholestasis, thereby causing increased connective tissue deposition or decreased connective tissue clearance?

Macromolecules of the extracellular matrix (ECM) and hepatic fibrosis. In recent years there have been exciting developments in our knowledge of the biochemistry, physiology and pathobiological importance of the major macromolecules of the extracellular matrix (ECM), which accumulate in the liver in progressive fibrosis[23-26]. This is a dynamic process, the outcome being dictated by the relative rates of synthesis and degradation.

In the healthy liver the liver cells are supported in single or (under the age of 6 years) double cell plates by a very delicate fine scaffolding of ECM components such as collagens, laminin, undulin and hyaluronic acid. Collagen types I and III are present in healthy liver in a fine fibrillar pattern in the stroma of the portal tracts and around blood vessels. In cirrhotic liver they accumulate in portal tracts, and are found in fibrous bands and around sinusoids. The ratio of type I to III increases. These collagens are synthesized within cells as large precursor procollagen molecules containing additional C and NH propepides; once procollagen leaves the cell, the C propeptide (but not necessarily the NH propeptide) is cleaved, allowing further extracellular processing of collagen. Some aminopropeptide of type III procollagen (PIIINP) remains attached to type III collagen molecules extracellularly, often coating thicker fibres. Thus PIIINP in serum is derived from the breakdown of mature collagen as well as from newly synthesized procollagen. Collagen type IV is a major component of basement membranes, and as such is found in the normal liver in the basement membrane of blood vessels and bile ducts. In cirrhosis it is present in the perisinusoidal region where basement membrane has formed during fibrogenesis. Laminin, a large multifunctional glycoprotein, which is a major component of all basement membranes, anchoring cells to the membrane, is also prominent in perisinusoidal areas only in cirrhosis. Undulin, another large glycoprotein, is located around and between thick collagen type I fibres having a major role in the supramolecular organization of collagen fibrils. In cirrhotic liver undulin is found in fibrous tracts, vessel walls and with a patchy distribution around sinusoids. Hyaluronic acid is a large glycosaminoglycan, essential for the spatial arrangement of the ECM. It is formed by mesenchymal cells, degraded by a specific hydrolase and is of particular interest to hepatologists, since it is cleared from the circulation by a unique receptor on hepatic sinusoidal endothelial cells.

Other actions of macromolecules of the extracellular matrix. Components of the ECM are of biological interest for other reasons[25,27]. They are not inert structures. They control cell movement, adherence and phenotypic expression. They act as major determinants of gene expression and cell differentiation. Their biological effects on cells are mediated via specific receptors which span the cell membrane, thus linking the ECM to cytoskeletal elements within the cell. These actions influence the function of lymphocytes and macrophages as well as hepatic parenchymal cells[28]. The function of these receptors may be affected by other ECM components such as hyaluronic acid. During liver injury, changes in ECM may occur directly as a result of cell damage; in addition, migratory inflammatory cells attracted to the site of injury release cytokines which stimulate local production and degradation of ECM components.

Non-invasive assessment of hepatic fibrosis. To provide an objective, serial non-invasive measure of the progression of hepatic fibrosis and a means of monitoring antifibrotic measures techniques have been developed for measuring metabolites of ECM components in serum[29,30]. We have participated in the development and validation of radioimmunoassays for the aminopropeptide of type III procollagen (PIIINP), the carboxyterminal propeptide of type I procollagen (PICP), the P1 fragment of laminin and hyaluronic acid, and have established normal ranges in healthy infants and children.

We have shown that serial measurement of serum PIIINP is of value in monitoring hepatobiliary disorders in children, such as extrahepatic biliary atresia[31], Indian childhood cirrhosis[32] or veno-occlusive disease[33], conditions in which hepatic fibrogenesis is very rapid with marked accumulation of type III collagen. It does reflect hepatocellular necrosis and inflammatory cell infiltrate as well as hepatic fibrosis[34]. Serum PIIINP is of limited value in assessing other less rapidly progressive liver disorders because any increases in PIIINP released from the liver during hepatic fibrogenesis are masked by the relatively high serum concentrations of PIIINP normally found in growing children[35,36]. Our recent studies suggest that serum concentrations of PICP show a similar pattern of change with growth and with severe liver disease. Since an increased ratio of type I:III collagen in the liver is a feature of cirrhosis, the serum ratio of PICP:PIIINP may be indicative of progressive cirrhosis.

Increases in serum concentrations of hyaluronic acid and laminin have been found in infants and children with progressive liver diseases in which there is on-going fibrogenesis, leading to cirrhosis with normal levels in stable disease[37]. While these results suggest that measurement of serum laminin and hyaluronic acid may provide new information about the fibrogenic process, raised HA and laminin also may reflect sinusoidal endothelial cell insufficiency, since these cells specifically clear these molecules from the circulation. Their serum concentrations may thus serve as a novel means of evaluating and monitoring changes in the sinusoids and the progression of chronic liver disease.

Anti-fibrotic therapy. While we await the identification of a product which will inhibit specifically hepatic fibrosis we are evaluating an old remedy: colchicine; it suppresses collagen biosynthesis directly by inhibiting polymerization of microtubules and blocking transcellular movement of procollagen. Colchicine also has a range of inhibitory effects on inflammatory cells, which reduce their ability to stimulate production of ECM components. In addition, colchicine also accelerates breakdown of collagen by stimulating collagenase activity[38]. We have shown that colchicine inhibits the formation of hepatic collagen and the development of cirrhosis in an experimental model in the rat[39]. In clinical trials in alcoholic cirrhosis and primary biliary cirrhosis, treatment with colchicine resulted in an improvement in biochemical tests of liver function, survival and liver histology[37]. In these trials changes in specific ECM components were not studied.

Since 1985 we have recruited infants with two paediatric liver disorders of different pathogenesis and varying propensity to cirrhosis into a double-blind, randomized clinical trial of colchicine: 85 with extrahepatic biliary atresia (EHBA) and 30 with severe liver disease in infancy in association with genetic deficiency of α_1-antitrypsin (α1ATD; PI ZZ) have completed at least 1 year in the study. Preliminary analysis encourages us to complete the study.

FUTURE RESEARCH

At present, despite exciting advances in understanding of factors controlling the interaction between the specialized liver cells, cells of the reticuloendothelial system, extracellular matrix components (EMC) and cytokines, we are still some way from being able to identify at a cellular or molecular level the pathobiological events leading to abnormal accumulation of ECM and disturbed hepatocyte growth. Given resources further studies are feasible – of factors regulating the expression of cell receptors, of the importance of these in controlling intracellular metabolism and of factors controlling cell regeneration, differentiation and repair particularly in the portal tracts and main intrahepatic and extrahepatic bile ducts. The identification of a liver-specific antifibrotic agent may be a realistic goal[40]. In the meantime as clinicians we must collaborate with basic scientists to exploit the distinct clinical syndromes we encounter, in order to increase our knowledge of factors contributing to intrahepatic fibrosis. The hepatopathy associated with the septo-optic dysplasia syndrome, or an animal model mimicking it, perhaps contrasted with biliary atresia or liver disease associated with parenteral nutrition, may be fruitful fields for study.

References

1. Lloyd-Still JD. Mortality from liver disease in children. Am J Dis Child. 1985;139:381–4.
2. Lloyd-Still JD. Impact of orthotopic liver transplantation on mortality from pediatric liver disease. J Pediatr Gastroenterol Nutr. 1991;12:305–9.
3. Sokal EM, Veyckemans F, de Ville de Goyet J *et al.* Liver transplantation in children less than 1 year of age. J Pediatr. 1990;117:205–10.
4. Starzl TE, Demetris AJ, Van Thiel D. Liver transplantation. N Engl J Med. 1989;321:1014–22.
5. Starzl TE, Demetris AJ, Van Thiel D. Liver transplantation. N Engl J Med. 1989;321:1092–9.
6. Salt A, Barnes ND, Mowat AP, Williams R, Calne RY. Five years experience of liver transplantation in children. Transplant Proc. 1990;22:1514–16.
7. Mieli-Vergani G, Howard ER, Portmann B, Mowat AP. Late referral for biliary atresia – missed opportunities for effective surgery. Lancet. 1989;1:421–3.
8. Hussein M, Howard ER, Mieli-Vergani G, Mowat AP. Jaundice at 14 days of age: exclude biliary atresia. Arch Dis Child. 1991 (in press).
9. Scriver C, Kaufmann S, Woo SLC. The hyperphenylalaninemias. In: Scriver CR, Beaudet AL, Sly WS, Valle D, editors. The metabolic basis of inherited disorders, 6th edn. New York: McGraw-Hill; 1989:495–546.
10. Dumont JE, Vassart G, Refetoff S. Thyroid disorders. In: Scriver CR, Beaudet AL, Sly WS, Valle D, editors. The metabolic basis of inherited disorders, 6th edn. New York: McGraw-Hill; 1989:531, 1872.
11. McClement J, Howard ER, Mowat AP. Results of surgical treatment for extrahepatic biliary atresia in United Kingdom 1980–82. Br Med J. 1985;290:345–7.
12. Dick MC, Mowat AP. Hepatitis syndrome in infancy – an epidemiological study with 10 year follow up. Arch Dis Child. 1985;60:512–16.
13. Maisels MJ, Gifford K. Normal serum bilirubin levels in the newborn and the effect of breast-feeding. Pediatrics 1986;78:837–43.
14. Mowat AP. Liver disorders in childhood, 2nd edn. London: Butterworths; 1987.
15. Fitzgerald JF. Cholestatic disorders in infancy. Ped Clin N Am. 1988;35:357–73.
16. Maconochie IK, Chong S, Mieli-Vergani G, Lake BD, Mowat AP. Fetal ascites: an unusual presentation of Niemann-Pick disease type C. Arch Dis Child. 1989;10:1391–3.
17. Amedee-Manesme O, Bernard O, Brunelle F *et al.* Sclerosing cholangitis with neonatal onset. J Pediatr. 1987;111:225–9.
18. Chobert MN, Bernard O, Bulle F, Lemonnier A, Guellaen G, Alagille D. High hepatic γ-glutamyltransferase activity with normal serum γ glutamyltransferase in children with

progressive idiopathic cholestasis. J Hepatol. 1989;8:22–5.
19. El Tumi MA, Clarke MB, Barrett JJ, Mowat AP. Ten minute radiopharmaceutical test in biliary atresia. Arch Dis Child. 1987;62:180–1.
20. Wilkinson ML, Mieli-Vergani G, Ball C, Portmann B, Mowat AP. Endoscopic retrograde cholangiopancreatography (ERCP) in infantile cholestasis. Arch Dis Child. 1991;66:121–3.
21. El Shabrawi M, Wilkinson M, Portmann B, Mieli-Vergani G, Chong SKF, Williams R, Mowat AP. Primary sclerosing cholangitis in childhood. Gastroenterology. 1987;92: 1226–35.
22. Mieli-Vergani G, Lobo-Yeo A, McFarlane BM, McFarlane IG, Mowat AP, Vergani D. Different immune mechanisms leading to autoimmunity in primary sclerosing cholangitis and autoimmune chronic active hepatitis of childhood. Hepatology. 1989;9:198–203.
23. Bissell DM. Connective tissue metabolism and hepatic fibrosis – an overview. Sem. Liver Dis. 1990;10:iii–iv.
24. Brenner DA, Alcorn JA. Therapy for hepatic fibrosis. Sem Liver Dis. 1990;10:75–83.
25. Schuppan D, Hahn EG. Components of the extracellular matrix. In: Wolff JR, editor. Mesenchymal–epithelial interactions in neural development. Berlin: Springer Verlag; 1987: 3–29. NATO ASI Series.
26. Biagini G, Ballardini G. Liver fibrosis and extracellular matrix. J Hepatol. 1989;8:15–24.
27. Rouslahti E, Pierschbacher MD. Molecular basis of cell–extracellular matrix interactions. In: Arias IM, Jakoby WB, Popper H, Schachter D, Shafritz DA, editors. The liver: biology and pathobiology, 2nd edn. New York: Raven Press; 1987:739–47.
28. Shimizu Y, Shaw S. Lymphocyte interactions with extracellular matrix. FASEB J. 1991;5:2292–9.
29. Risteli J, Risteli L. Non-invasive methods for the detection of organ fibrosis. In: Rojkind M, editor. Focus on connective tissue research in health and disease. Boca Raton, FL: CRC Press; 1990:61–98.
30. Plebani M, Burlina A. Biochemical markers of hepatic fibrosis. Clin Biochem. 1991;24: 219–39.
31. Trivedi P, Cheeseman P, Portmann B, Mowat AP. Serum type III procollagen peptide as a non-invasive marker of liver damage during infancy and childhood. Clin Chim Acta. 1986;161:137–46.
32. Trivedi P, Risteli J, Risteli L, Tanner MS, Bhave S, Pandit A, Mowat AP. Serum type III procollagen peptide and basement membrane proteins as markers of hepatic pathology in Indian Childhood Cirrhosis. Hepatology. 1987;7:1249–53.
33. El-Tumi M, Trivedi P, Cheeseman P et al. Serum type III procollagen peptide predicts and monitors veno-occlusive disease following bone marrow transplantation (Submitted).
34. Trivedi P, Cheeseman P, Portmann B, Hegarty J, Mowat AP. Variation in serum type III procollagen peptide with age and its comparative value in the assessment of disease in children and adults with chronic active hepatitis. Eur J Clin Invest. 1985;15:69–74.
35. Calcado A, Trivedi P, Portman B, Mowat AP. Serum concentrations of ECM components: novel markers of metabolic control and hepatic pathology in glycogen storage disease? J Ped Gastroenterol Nutr. 1991;13:1–9.
36. Trivedi P, Risteli J, Risteli L, Hindmarsh P, Brook CGD, Mowat AP. Serum concentrations of the type I and III procollagen peptides as biochemical markers of growth velocity in healthy children and children with growth disorders. Ped Res. 1991;30:276–80.
37. Trivedi P, Portmann B, Mowat AP. Serum hyaluronic acid as a marker of progressive liver damage in extrahepatic biliary atresia. J Hepatol. 1988(Suppl. 1 to Vol 1):s82.
38. Warnes TW. Colchicine in primary biliary cirrhosis. Aliment Pharmacol Ther. 1991;5:321–9.
39. Tanner MS, Jackson D, Mowat AP. Hepatic collagen synthesis and its modification by colchicine in a rat model of cirrhosis of the liver. J Pathol. 1981;135:179–87.
40. Lie TS, Lacina T. Prevention of cirrhosis by anti-fibrotic liver factor from perfused liver. J Hepatol. 1991;13:S2:s43.

13
Congenital ductopenia

M. ODIÈVRE

A paucity of interlobular bile ducts has been described in association with an inborn error of metabolism such as α_1-antitrypsin deficiency[1], a congenital infection (rubella, cytomegalovirus)[2,3] or a chromosomal abnormality[4]; it frequently appears after birth so that its congenital nature is not proven.

In this paper, description of congenital ductopenia will be restricted to the paucity of interlobular bile ducts associated with multiple congenital abnormalities, a condition described under various names (syndromic paucity of interlobular bile ducts, arteriohepatic dysplasia, Alagille syndrome, etc.).

Many cases have been reported in children and adults since the first description of this syndrome in 1975[5]. The largest series was reviewed in 1987 by Alagille et al.[6], enabling them to distinguish five major features among many abnormalities in 80 patients.

MAJOR FEATURES (Table 1)

Chronic cholestasis

This was observed in 73 patients. Jaundice developed within the first 3 months of life in 32 and before the third year of life in the others; it was associated with pale or acholic stools and dark urine. Pruritus, present in the majority of patients, was never seen before the age of 4–6 months of life. The liver was enlarged in all cases. Xanthomas were seen in the 22 patients

Table 1 Frequency of the five main abnormalities

	No. of patients examined	No. present	Percentage
Cholestasis	80	73	91
Characteristic facies	80	76	95
Cardiac murmur	80	68	85
Vertebral abnormalities	80	70	87
Posterior embryotoxon	62	55	88

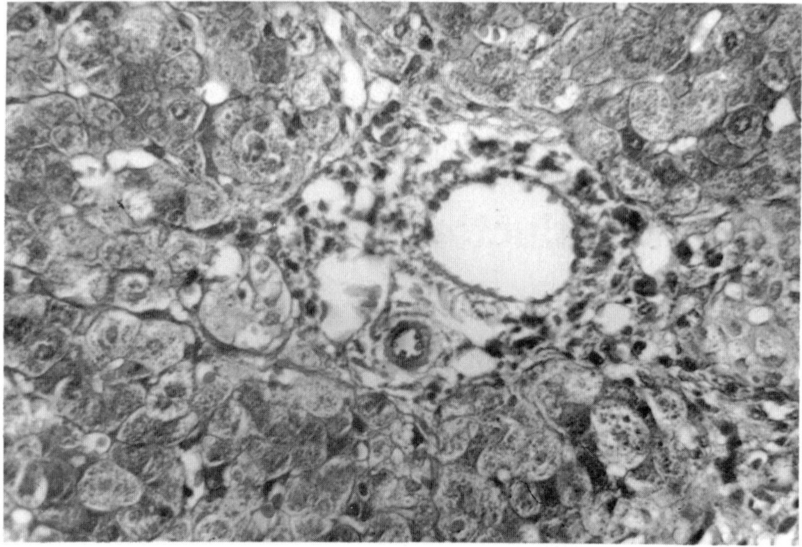

Fig. 1 Liver biopsy from a 6-month-old infant showing a large portal area without an interlobular bile duct (Trichome Masson × 160)

with a prolonged and severe cholestasis, more often after the age of 4 years.

All the constituents of bile showed an increased level in serum: conjugated bilirubin, bile acids and cholesterol; these two last constituents were often markedly elevated.

Liver biopsy in the first months of life usually showed intrahepatic cholestasis and sometimes some giant cell transformation and portal inflammation; but the most prominent finding was the absence or paucity of interlobular bile ducts in the portal areas which themselves seemed reduced in number (Fig. 1)[7].

Facies appearance

This was characteristic (Fig. 2). The forehead is prominent, the eyes are deeply set and somewhat widely separated, the nose is straight, the chin is small and pointed. These features were present in 76 of the 80 patients but were not always evident during the early infancy.

Cardiovascular abnormalities

These were seen in 68 of the 80 patients. In 56 patients, there was a moderate degree of hypoplasia and stenosis of the peripheral pulmonary arteries with a harsh systolic murmur, heard in the third intercostal space at the left sternal border, sometimes audible posteriorly. This vascular abnormality

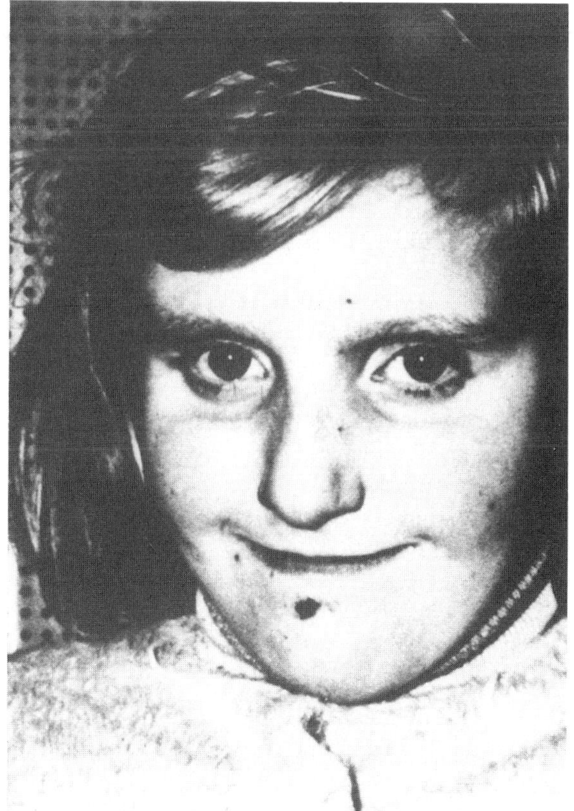

Fig. 2 Congenital ductopenia. Characteristic facies at 12 years

may be documented by angiography. In the other patients, the pulmonary stenosis was a part of an extremely severe form of tetralogy of Fallot with cyanosis.

Vertebral arch defects

These were seen in 70 of the 80 patients. They consisted of an absence of fusion of the anterior arch of one or several dorsal vertebrae, resulting in a 'butterfly-like' appearance (Fig. 3). These abnormalities were more easily recognized after a few months of life.

Embryotoxon

A posterior embryotoxon was present in 55 of the 62 examined patients; this abnormality, which represents one of the anterior chamber cleavage syndromes, is found in only about 10% of the normal subjects[8].

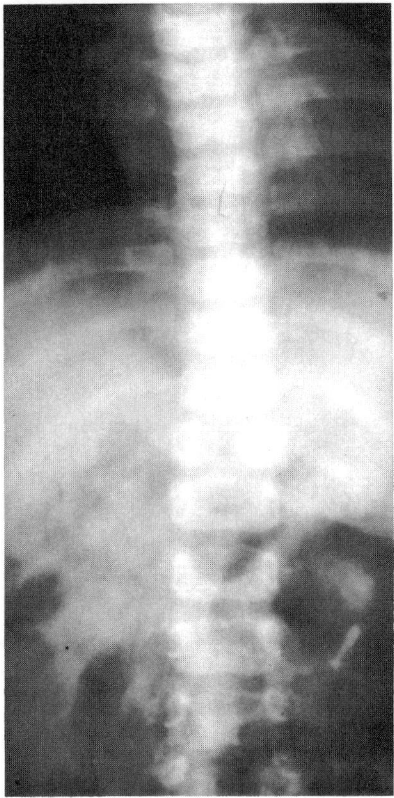

Fig. 3 Congenital ductopenia. Vertebral arch defects: absence of fusion of the anterior arch of D_{12}

LESS FREQUENT ABNORMALITIES

Renal involvement

Cholestyramine is often badly tolerated by these patients; it is responsible for the development of renal acidosis with hyperchloraemia which requires adjunction of sodium bicarbonate. Since 1960, pathological examinations of the kidneys have been performed in 26 of the 80 patients[9]. Although only one of those had clinically severe renal symptoms, it was possible to demonstrate characteristic glomerular changes in 18. At light microscopy there was a fibrillar appearance of the mesangium, and electron microscopy showed lipid vacuoles widely distributed in the mesangial matrix and sometimes presence of mesangial foam cells. These lesions of mesangio-lipidosis were not clearly related to the age of patients, the most severely affected of them being between 3 months and 2 years of age. The lesions, similar to those seen in familial lecithine–cholesterol acyltransferase deficiency, were positively correlated with the degree of cholestasis and the abnormalities of lipid metabolism.

Mental retardation

An IQ less than 80 was observed in 16% of the patients.

Skeletal abnormalities[8]

An abnormally narrow interpedicular distance in the lumbar spine was seen in 23 of the 43 patients examined. Short distal phalanges and short ulnae have been occasionally seen, possibly developing with increasing age.

Voice

In many patients, the voice is high-pitched without laryngeal abnormality at laryngoscopy.

CLINICAL DIAGNOSIS

Clinical diagnosis of Alagille syndrome may be missed, especially in infancy when the facies and vertebral arch defects are not yet characteristic, or when the syndrome is incomplete. We consider the diagnosis if at least three of the five main features are present, or if only two are present but associated with familial evidence of the disease. This point is important, since in early infancy the relative frequency of cholestasis can indicate extrahepatic biliary atresia[10], a condition that must be operated on before the age of 2 months.

COURSE

The clinical course is usually characterized by recurrent episodes of cholestasis often associated with common respiratory tract infection. The cholestasis gradually subsides within a few years and the prognosis for prolonged survival is good. Several adults with normal serum bilirubin and bile acid concentrations are now reported[11].

However, cholestasis can remain severe and permanent for many years; this was the case in 28 of our patients. Malnutrition was an important risk. Portal fibrosis progressively developed in 11 of the patients and cirrhosis was the cause of death in four of them before the age of 10 years.

Seven patients died at a mean age of 9 months from infection, a complication which was essentially seen in the 1970s.

Six other patients died at a mean age of 6 months from severe cardiac or vascular abnormality similar to tetralogy of Fallot. The peripheral pulmonary lesion seen in the other patients was well tolerated and did not progress.

Another cause of death, still insufficiently documented, was represented by systemic arterial complications; one of our patients recently died after cerebral haemorrhage a few days after liver transplantation.

Finally, the overall prognosis is perhaps not so good as initially reported, since 21 patients died in our series of 80.

TREATMENT

The cholestatic patients are given low-fat diets with medium-chain triglyceride supplementation. Additional calories must be given to malnourished children. Intramuscular injections of fat-soluble vitamins are necessary during the cholestatic period, including vitamin A, E, D_3 and K_1. After clinical disappearance of cholestasis, blood vitamin levels (E, D) and prothrombin time should be carefully monitored. The first cases of Alagille syndrome developed a disabling neuromuscular degeneration due to prolonged vitamin E deficiency; this syndrome, initially considered as a part of the abnormalities associated with congenital ductopenia, can be prevented by vitamin E administration.

Patients with pruritus and hypercholesterolaemia are given cholestyramine. More recently, ursodeoxycholic acid has been given in patients who did not respond to cholestyramine[12]. In our short experience, such a drug is effective only in patients with incomplete cholestasis.

INHERITANCE PATTERN

An autosomal dominant transmission with reduced penetrance and variable expressivity has been suggested from familial pedigrees. This pattern was well illustrated by Labrecque *et al.*[13], who documented the presence of the syndrome in four successive generations of a single kindred. A partial deletion of the short arm of chromosome 20 has been reported in about 10 patients in the literature. Only one patient among 30 in our series has this deletion (M. Hadchouel, personal communication).

References

1. Hadchouel M, Gautier M. Histopathologic study of the liver in the early cholestatic phase of alpha-1-antitrypsin deficiency. J Pediatr. 1976;89:211–15.
2. Heathcote J, Deodhar KP, Scheuer PJ, Sherlock S. Intrahepatic cholestasis in childhood. N Engl J Med. 1976;295:801–5.
3. Finegold MJ, Carpenter RJ. Obliterative cholangitis due to cytomegalovirus: a possible precursor of paucity of intrahepatic bile ducts. Hum Pathol. 1982;13:662–5.
4. Alpert LI, Strauss L, Hirschhorn K. Neonatal hepatitis and biliary atresia associated with trisomy 17-18 syndrome. N Engl J Med. 1969;280:16–20.
5. Alagille D, Odièvre M, Gautier M, Dommergues JP. Hepatic ductular hypoplasia associated with characteristic facies, vertebral malformations, retarded physical, mental and sexual development and cardiac murmur. J Pediatr. 1975;86:63–71.
6. Alagille D, Estrada A. Hadchouel M, Gautier M, Odièvre M, Dommergues JP. Syndromic paucity of interlobular bile ducts (Alagille syndrome of arteriohepatic dysplasia): review of 80 cases. J Pediatr. 1987;110:195–200.
7. Hadchouel M, Hugon RN, Gautier M. Reduced ratio of portal tracts to paucity of intrahepatic bile ducts. Arch Pathol Lab Med. 1978;102:402.
8. Riely CA, Cotlier E, Jensen PS, Klatskin G. Arteriohepatic dysplasia: a benign syndrome of intrahepatic cholestasis with multiple organ involvement. Ann Intern Med. 1979;91: 520–7.
9. Habib R, Dommergues JP, Gubler MC, Hadchouel M, Gautier M, Odièvre M, Alagille D. Glomerular mesangiolipidosis in Alagille syndrome (arteriohepatic dysplasia). Pediatr Nephrol. 1987;1:455–64.

10. Markowitz J, Daum F, Kahn EI, Scheider KM, So HB, Altman RP, Aiges HW, Alperstein G, Silverberg M. Arteriohepatic dysplasia. 1. Pitfalls in diagnosis and management. Hepatology. 1983;3:74–6.
11. Riely CA, Labrecque DR, Ghent C, Horwich A, Klatskin G. A father and son with cholestasis and peripheral pulmonic stenosis. A distinct form of intrahepatic cholestasis. J Pediatr. 1978;92:406–11.
12. Balistreri WF, A-Kader HH, Heubi JE, Setchell KDR. Effect of ursodeoxycholic acid on pruritus and serum cholesterol levels in patients with cholestasis associated with syndromic paucity of intrahepatic bile ducts (Alagille syndrome). Hepatology. 1990;12:994 (abstr.).
13. Labrecque DR, Mitros FA, Nathan RJ, Romanchuk KG, Judisch GF, El-Khoury GH Four generations of arteriohepatic dysplasia. Hepatology. 1982;2:467–74.

14
α_1-Antitrypsin deficiency

B. STRANDVIK and A. NEMETH

DEFINITIONS AND INCIDENCE

Homozygous PiZ α_1-antitrypsin deficiency (ATD) is the most common metabolic disease associated with neonatal cholestasis and general liver disease in Caucasian children, and the most common metabolic cause for liver transplantation in childhood[1]. It is an autosomal inherited disorder with the gene localized on chromosome 14[2]. α_1-Antitrypsin (AT) expression is controlled by more than 30 codominant alleles, the most common being designated PiM, and the deficiency alleles PiZ and PiS[3]. The Z-mutation involves a substitution of glutamine for lysine in 342 position[4]. The deficiency genotypes are associated with reduced serum concentrations of AT to 10–15% of the normal. The incidence and prevalence of the deficiency depend on the population studied. It seems to be more common in northern Europe, with an incidence in Sweden of about 1 in 1600 live births[5].

EXPRESSION AND FUNCTION

The AT gene encodes for a single-chain glycoprotein. The molecular structure and functional characteristics are similar to a group of other glycoproteins, the serpins, exemplified by antithrombin III, ovalbumin, angiotensinogen and corticosteroid binding globulin, with which genes the AT gene has at least 25–40% structural homology[6]. The gene is expressed in macrophages, intestinal cells and hepatocytes, the major synthesis considered to occur in the liver. In transgenic mice the human AT gene is shown to be expressed in liver, kidney, stomach, proximal and distal intestine, pancreas and adrenal glands. Hybridization was further present in total RNA in brain, lung, female reproductive system, testes, spleen, thymus and colon[7]. It is not known how and why the defective gene product accumulates in the endoplasmic reticulum and does not reach the Golgi[8]. It has been suggested that the PiZ substitution results in an abnormal folding, giving an abnormal tertiary structure of the protein thereby affecting its secretion. Some recent observations suggest that misfolded proteins are selectively retained within the endoplasmic reticulum by interaction with members of the heat-shock/stress protein family. Such a hypothesis is supported by the fact that shock/stress protein synthesis is markedly increased in monocytes from PiZZ individuals with liver disease but not in PiZZ individuals without evidence of tissue damage[9].

AT is an inhibitor of serine proteases in general, but the most important target is neutrophil elastase to which AT binds directly[10]. The plasma concentration of AT increase 3–4-fold during inflammation/tissue injury[11]. Bacterial lipopolysaccharide mediates a 5–10-fold increase in synthesis, not only by stimulating macrophage synthesis but more heavily by stimulation of liver synthesis mediated by interferon-2/interleukin-6 from the macrophages[12]. The half-life of AT in plasma is about 5 days and the daily production rate is 34 mg per kg body weight, with 33% of the intravascular pool being degraded daily. There is a slight increase in the rate of clearance of radiolabelled PiZZ AT compared with PiMM AT[13].

CLINICAL DISEASE

ATD was first described about 30 years ago related to early pulmonary emphysema[14], later to liver disease[15] and membranoproliferative mesangionephritis[16]. Pancreatitis[17] and panniculitis[18] have also been described.

The close association between liver disease and ATD was first described by Sharp et al. in 1969[15]. Liver disease usually starts as neonatal hepatitis or smouldering fibrosis–cirrhosis, which sometimes does not give symptoms until in adult life[19], sometimes remains benign but sometimes proceeds to fulminant liver disease as early as the first months of life[20]. Extrahepatic biliary atresia has in some cases been reported to be associated with ATD[21]. In adults there is an increased risk of hepatocarcinoma in those with abnormal liver, and heterozygotes have been reported to run an increased risk of liver malignancy[22,23]. Also, in infants with neonatal cholestasis of unknown aetiology, there is an increased frequency of heterozygoty for the PiZ allele (Strandvik, unpublished observation).

Sveger in Sweden prospectively screened 200 000 newborns and found 127 PiZZ infants, who have now been followed for more than 12 years[5]. Fourteen of the 127 infants developed neonatal cholestasis and about 50% had pathological serum concentrations of transaminases. In his prospective study death due to liver failure was found only in the group with neonatal cholestasis. During a 25-year period we have followed 50 infants and children, 28 of whom presented with neonatal cholestasis, and all but six of the others were identified due to abnormal liver function tests or hepatomegaly. In this selected group of referred patients seven died of liver failure; five of these had had neonatal cholestasis (Fig. 1). Two have undergone successful liver transplantation. In our series we found the typical male predominance[5] but no influence on birth weight or HLA status[24] or the presence or absence of perinatal virus infection. Two patients have had pancreatitis and one has chronic arthritis.

The characteristic – although not pathognomonic – histological features of PiZ homozygous ATD are periodic-Schiff-positive, diastase-resistant

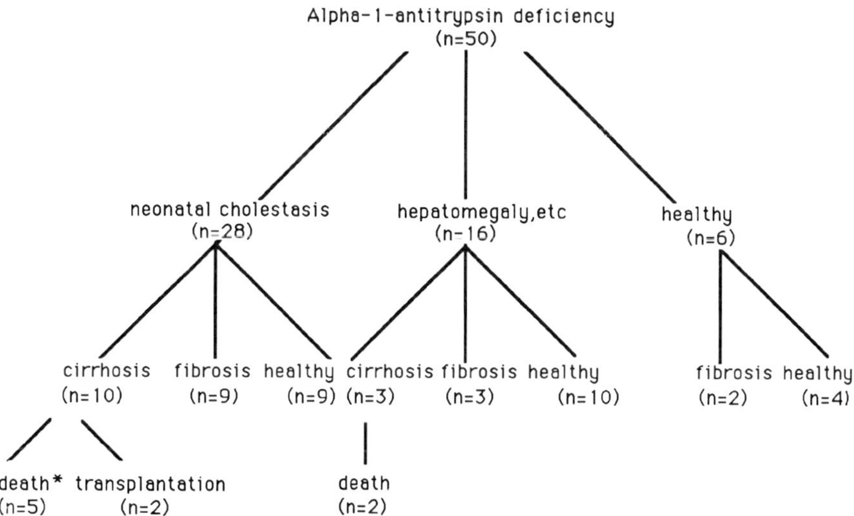

Fig. 1 Natural history of infants with α_1-antitrypsin deficiency, followed by the authors, and presenting with neonatal cholestasis (28 cases) or with increased serum concentrations of transaminases or hepatomegaly (16 cases) or found as healthy siblings to the patients presenting with symptoms of liver disease (six cases). *Out of the five deceased patients in the group of neonatal cholestasis, three died in infancy. The liver-transplanted patients are alive and well

globules in the endoplasmic reticulum of, preferentially, the periportal hepatocytes[25,26]. They have also been described in liver biopsies from heterozygous patients[27]. The globules are eosinophilic, round to oval and $1-40\,\mu m$ in diameter. They may be seen in Kupffer cells, and cells that have the appearance of bile duct epithelial origin. There is usually a varying degree of inflammatory cells, hepatocellular necrosis, periportal fibrosis and/or cirrhosis. There is no clear explanation why some patients develop a severe liver disease early in life and some will continue to have normal livers into adulthood. That the low level of AT itself should give liver damage is unlikely, since patients with Pi null, i.e. without serum levels of AT, do not develop liver disease[28]. Further evidence that it is the accumulation of defective AT in the liver cells which causes liver damage comes from the experiments in transgenic mice performed by Joyce Carlsson and co-workers[29]. In this animal model the mutant human protein was abundantly synthesized in the livers of the transgenic animals and accumulated within the rough endoplasmic reticulum of the hepatocytes. There was significantly more inflammation and liver cell necrosis in PiZ mice than in PiM transgenic mice or control litter mates. Although only slight fibrosis was seen, and no development to cirrhosis noticed during 20 months follow up, the degree of liver damage was correlated to the amount of PiZ AT retained in the liver. They also found that the degree of liver damage was not influenced by positive serology to mouse hepatitis virus, an observation in accordance with our clinical material[30].

NATURAL HISTORY

Since the progression of liver disease is so unpredictable[31,32], also in those infants presenting with neonatal cholestasis or abnormal serum transaminases, we have searched for tests which could be of prognostic value. We prospectively followed our patients with standard liver function tests, serum and urinary bile acids and liver biopsy. The results of liver function tests did not differ from those of infants with other chronic liver disease and were not prognostic until late stage of liver damage[33]. Standard serum bile acids were also similarly insensitive[34]. In the acute phase the primary urinary bile acid concentrations, including ratios between cholic and chenodeoxy-cholic acids and elimination of radiolabelled bile acids, did not differ from patients with cholestasis of other known or unknown causes[30,35]. Unusual bile acids gave some more information. The persistence of bile alcohols after the neonatal period indicated a severe liver disease with cirrhosis[36]. The major bile alcohol, 27-nor-5β-cholestan-3,7,12,24,25-pentol was a good marker of bad prognosis, more sensitive than the occurrence of toxic monohydroxy bile acids. A favourable sign was the finding of large amounts of tetrahydroxylated bile acids in urine[37]. This could be interpreted as meaning that those patients who managed to polyhydroxylate their bile acids could increase the urinary excretion of bile acids. All these patients recovered, but those with a low percentage of tetrahydroxylated bile acids in the acute phase all died or developed cirrhosis early. Thus, more unusual bile acids may be used as prognostic markers in this disease.

TREATMENT

Due to the fact that hepatic accumulation of abnormal AT could damage the liver, there is at present no indication to supply infants with ATD with AT as has been suggested for the treatment of the pulmonary symptoms[38]. The disease can be treated with transplantation of a normal liver which, performed at end-stage liver disease, has given a 15-year survival in some cases[39]. Since a family with one infant with liver disease seems to have an increased risk of having more affected siblings, prenatal diagnosis should be offered to parents with an affected child[40].

CONCLUSION

ATD is one of the most common causes of liver disease in infancy, especially related to the neonatal cholestasis syndrome. The explanation why some of these infants develop cirrhosis during infancy, like some of those without neonatal cholestasis, remains obscure, and association with a viral infection seems not to be crucial. No therapy is at present available, but liver transplantation at end-stage liver disease will substitute the deficiency and give possibilities of long-term survival of high quality.

Acknowledgement

This work was supported by grants from the Swedish Medical Research Council (44995).

References

1. Starzl TE. Surgery for metabolic liver disease. In: McDermott WV Jr, editor. Surgery of the liver. Oxford: Blackwell Scientific Publications; 1989:127–36.
2. Lai EC, Kao F-T, Law ML, Woo SLC. Assignment of the α_1-antitrypsin gene and sequence-regulated gene to human chromosome 14 by molecular hybridization. Am J Hum Genet. 1983;35:385–92.
3. Fagerhol MK. The genetics of alpha-1-antitrypsin and its implications. Postgrad Med J. 1976(Suppl.2):72–83.
4. Jeppsson JO. Amino acid substitution Gln-Lys in alpha-1-antitrypsin PiZ. FEBS Lett. 1976;65:195–6.
5. Sveger T. Liver disease in α-1-antitrypsin deficiency detected by screening of 200 000 infants. N Engl J Med. 1976;294:1316–21.
6. Carrell RW. α-1-antitrypsin: molecular pathology, leukocytes and tissue damage. J Clin Invest. 1986;78:1427–31.
7. Carlson JA, Rogers BB, Sifers RN, Hawkins HK, Finegold MJ, Woo SLC. Multiple tissues express alpha-1-antitrypsin in trangenic mice and man. J Clin Invest. 1988;82:26–36.
8. Feldmann G, Bignon J, Chahinian R, Degott C, Benhamou J-P. Hepatocyte ultrastructural changes in α_1-antitrypsin deficiency. Gastroenterology. 1974;67:1214–24.
9. Perlmutter DH, Schlesinger M, Pierce JA, Punsal PI, Schwartz AL. Synthesis of stress proteins is increased in individuals with homozygous PiZZ α_1-antitrypsin deficiency and liver disease. J Clin Invest. 1989;84:1555–61.
10. Gadek JE, Fells GA, Zimmerman RL, Rennard SI, Crystal RG. Antielastase of the human alveolar structures. Implications for the protease-antiprotease theory of emphysema. J Clin Invest. 1981;68:889–98.
11. Dickson I, Alper CA. Changes in serum proteinase inhibitor levels following bone surgery. Clin Chem Acta. 1974;54:381 5.
12. Barbey-Morel C, Pierce JA, Campbell EJ, Perlmutter DH. Lipopolysaccharide modulates the expression of α_1-proteinase inhibitor and other serine proteinase inhibitors in human monocytes and macrophages. J Exp Med. 1987;166:1041–54.
13. Glaser CB, Karic L, Fallat RJ, Stockert R. Plasma survival studies in rat of the normal and homozygote deficient forms of α_1-antitrypsin. Biochim Biophys Acta. 1977;495:87–95.
14. Eriksson S. Pulmonary emphysema and alpha-1-antitrypsin deficiency. Acta Med Scand. 1964;175:197–201.
15. Sharp HL, Bridges RA, Krivit W, Freier EF. Cirrhosis associated with alpha-1-antitrypsin deficiency: a previously unrecognized inherited disorder. J Lab Clin Med. 1969;73:934–9.
16. Moroz SP, Cutz E, Balfe JW, Sass-Kortsak A. Membranoproliferative glomerulonephritis in childhood cirrhosis associated with alpha-1-antitrypsin deficiency. Pediatrics. 1976;57:232–8.
17. Freeman HJ, Weinstein WM, Shnitka TK, Crockford PM, Herbert FA. Alpha-1-antitrypsin deficiency and pancreatic fibrosis. Ann Intern Med. 1976;85:73–6.
18. Hendrick SJ, Silverman AK, Solomon AR, Headington JT. α-1-Antitrypsin deficiency associated with panniculitis. J Am Acad Dermatol. 1988;18:684–92.
19. Schwarzenberg SJ, Sharp HL. Pathogenesis of α-1-antitrypsin deficiency-associated liver disease, 1990. J Pediatr Gastroenterol Nutr. 1990;10:5–12.
20. Gishan FK, Gray GF, Greene HL. α-1-Antitrypsin deficiency presenting with ascites and cirrhosis in the neonatal period. Gastroenterology. 1983;85:435–8.
21. Crest L, Chapuis Collier C, Arnaud P, Berger C, Creyss R. Atresie des voies biliares extrahepatiques associée a un deficit en alpha-1- antitrypsine. Coll Inst Natl RS Med INSERM. 1975;40:121–30.
22. Carlson J, Eriksson S. Chronic 'cryptogenic' liver disease and malignant hepatoma in intermediate alpha$_1$-antitrypsin deficiency identified by a PiZ-specific monoclonal antibody.

Scand J Gastroenterol. 1985;20:835–42.
23. Eriksson S, Carlsson J, Velez R. Risk of cirrhosis and primary liver cancer in alpha-1-antitrypsin deficiency. N Engl J Med. 1986;314:736–9.
24. Nemeth A, Möller E. HLA in juvenile liver disease with alpha-one-antitrypsin deficiency. Acta Paediatr Scand. 1987;76:603–7.
25. Palmer PE, Delellis RA, Wolfe HJ. Immunohistochemistry of liver in alpha-1-antitrypsin deficiency. Am J Clin Pathol. 1974;62:350–4.
26. Nemeth A, Glaumann H, Strandvik B. Alpha-1-antitrypsin deficiency and juvenile liver disease. Virchows Arch (Cell Pathol). 1983;44:15–33.
27. Hultcrantz R, Jelf E, Nilsson LH. Minimal liver disease in young persons with homozygous and heterozygous alpha-1-antitrypsin deficiency. Scand J Gastroenterol. 1984;19:389–93.
28. Courtney M, Crystal RG. α-1-antitrypsin null$_{\text{Granite Falls}}$, a non-expressing α-1-antitrypsin gene associated with a frameshift to stop mutation in a coding exon. J Biol Chem. 1987;262:1999–2004.
29. Carlson JA, Rogers BB, Sifers RN, Finegold MJ, Clift SM, DeMayo FJ, Bullock DW, Woo SLC. Accumulation of PiZ α_1-antitrypsin causes liver damage in transgenic mice. J Clin Invest. 1989;83:1183–90.
30. Strandvik B. Natural history of cholestatic liver disease in Sweden. In: Javitt NB, editor. Neonatal hepatitis and biliary atresia. Bethesda: US DHEW Publ (NIH) 79-1296;1979: 151–62.
31. Nemeth A, Strandvik B. Natural history of children with alpha-1-antitrypsin deficiency and neonatal cholestasis. Acta Paediatr Scand. 1982;71:993–9.
32. Nemeth A, Strandvik B. Liver disease in children with alpha-1-antitrypsin deficiency without neonatal cholestasis. Acta Paediatr Scand. 1982;71:1001–5.
33. Nemeth A. Alpha-1-antitrypsin deficiency in juvenile liver disease. A clinical and histological study on pathogenesis and clinical course with special reference to bile acid metabolism (dissertation). Stockholm: Karolinska Institutet; 1982.
34. Nemeth A, Samuelson K, Strandvik B. Serum bile acids as markers of juvenile liver disease in alpha-1-antitrypsin deficiency. J Pediatr Gastroenterol Nutr. 1982;1:479–83.
35. Norman A, Strandvik B. Excretion of bile acids in extrahepatic biliary atresia and intrahepatic cholestasis of infancy. Acta Paediatr Scand. 1973;62:253–63.
36. Karlaganis G, Nemeth A, Hammarskjöld B, Strandvik B, Sjövall J. Urinary excretion of bile alcohols in normal children and patients with alpha-1-antitrypsin deficiency during development of liver disease. Eur J Clin Invest. 1982;12:399–405.
37. Nemeth A, Strandvik B. Excretion of tetrahydroxylated bile acids in children with alpha-1-antitrypsin deficiency and neonatal cholestasis. Scand J Clin Lab Invest. 1984;44:387–92.
38. Wewers MD, Casolaro A, Sellers SE, Swayze SC, McPhaul KM, Wittes JJ, Crystal RG. Replacement therapy for alpha-1-antitrypsin deficiency associated with emphysema. N Engl J Med. 1987;316:1055–62.
39. Starzl TE, Demetris AJ, van Thiel D. Liver transplantation (first of two parts). N Engl J Med. 1989;321:1014–22.
40. Cox DW, Mansfield T. Prenatal diagnosis of α-1-antitrypsin deficiency and estimates of fetal risk for disease. J Med Genet. 1987;24:52–9.

15
Inborn errors of bile acid metabolism

K. D. R. SETCHELL, D. PICCOLI, J. HEUBI and W. F. BALISTRERI

INTRODUCTION

Cholestasis in the newborn has a multitude of origins[1]. Some of these are clearly definable, such as known infections, anatomical variants and well-delineated metabolic errors. Other causes are less well defined and may represent inherited or acquired defects in hepatobiliary structure and function. Although the list of disorders associated with cholestasis is long, most of the conditions are rare[1]. The most frequently occurring are the entities classified as idiopathic neonatal hepatitis, which often demonstrate a pattern of intrafamilial recurrence suggesting an underlying genetic basis and generally have a poor prognosis. This has consequently led to the suggestion that some of the patients within this category may have an inborn error in bile acid synthesis which would lead to an under-production of primary bile acids that are essential for the promotion and secretion of bile and to a concomitant over-production and accumulation of atypical bile acids which may have the potential for causing cholestasis and liver injury.

DEFECTS IN BILE ACID BIOSYNTHESIS

The classical pathway for bile acid synthesis from cholesterol involves at least nine steps catalysed by 15 different enzymes that are located within various subcellular fractions of the hepatocyte[2,3]. There are now *four* recognized disorders affecting this biosynthetic pathway[3,4]. The first to be identified, the rare lipid storage disease of cerebrotendinous xanthomatosis and the peroxisomal disorder of Zellweger, involve defects in the latter steps in the pathway, i.e. side-chain oxidation. More recently two new defects have been characterized involving the enzymes responsible for catalysing the initial reactions in the metabolism of cholesterol. These two defects (Fig. 1), the 3β-hydroxy-C_{27}-steroid dehydrogenase/isomerase deficiency[5,6] and the Δ^4-3-oxosteroid 5β-reductase deficiency[7] are clinically manifest by progressive

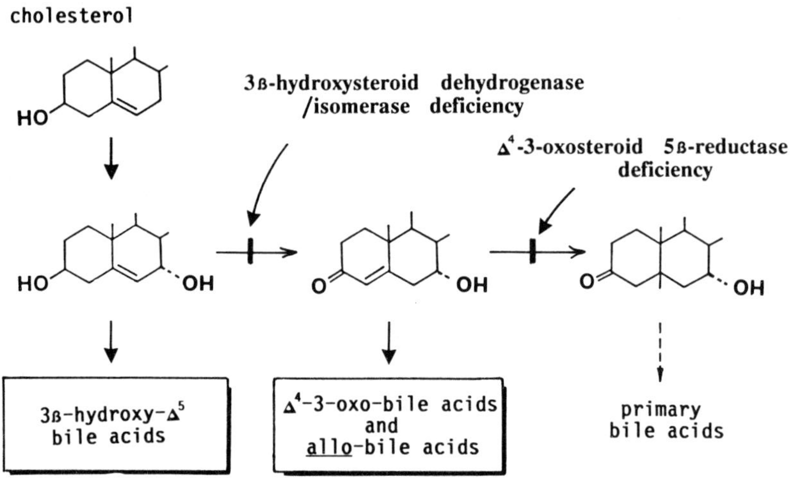

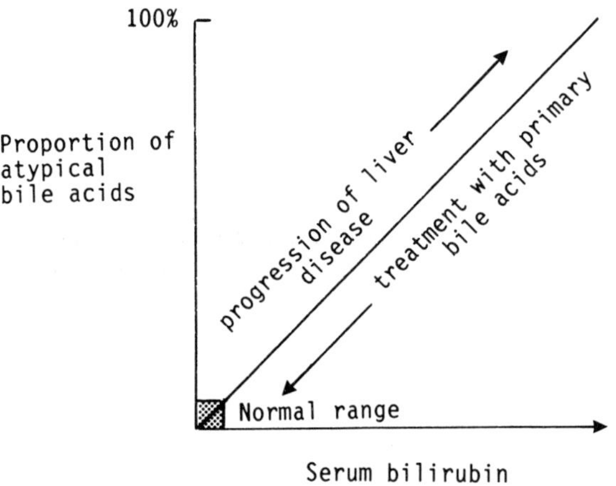

Fig. 1 Metabolic defects in bile acid synthesis affecting early steps in the conversion of cholesterol to the primary bile acids, cholic and chenodeoxycholic acids. For simplicity only the AB-ring structures of the steroid nucleus is indicated, and the boxes highlight the atypical bile acids that result from each specific enzyme deficiency

Fig. 2 Clinical manifestation of inborn errors in bile acid synthesis and effect of primary bile acid therapy

neonatal hepatitis, although in a number of patients diagnosis was not made until infancy and in one patient as old as 10 years of age[5], suggesting late-onset chronic cholestasis may be explained by these inborn errors. At the time of diagnosis all cases had evidence of hepatic disease with jaundice and a moderate conjugated hyperbilirubinaemia and elevated transaminases.

Confirmation of the biochemical defect was established from urinary bile acid analysis using the technique of fast atom bombardment ionization mass spectrometry (FAB-MS)[3,4], which provides a definitive screening procedure

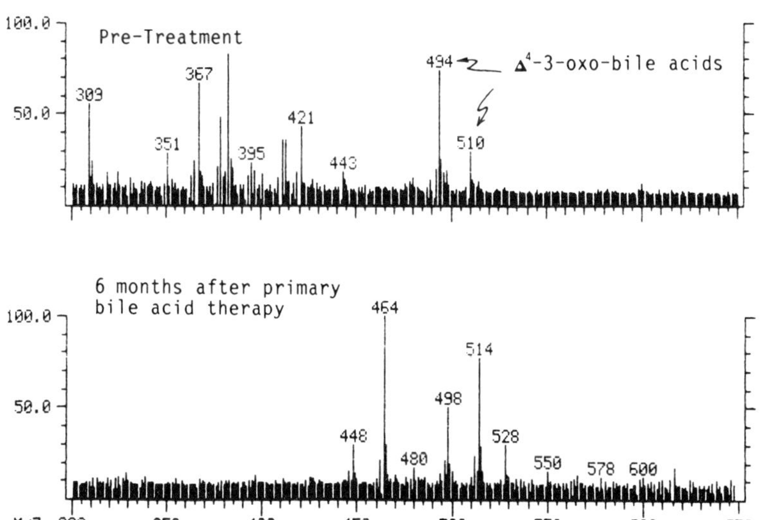

Fig. 3 FAB-MS analysis of the urine of a patient (SG) diagnosed with a Δ^4-3-oxosteroid 5β-reductase deficiency treated with bile acids

for the presence of elevated levels of the atypical bile acids that are synthesized and accumulate in response to the enzyme deficiency. In all cases primary bile acid synthesis was absent or markedly diminished.

The 3β-hydroxy-C_{27}-steroid dehydrogenase/isomerase deficiency is characterized by the production of large amounts of C_{24} bile acids retaining the 3β-hydroxy-5-ene structure characteristic of 7α-hydroxycholesterol, the precursor for the enzyme. The lack of expression of the enzyme in cultured human fibroblasts from one of the patients provided evidence for a primary enzyme defect[8].

The Δ^4-3-oxosteroid 5β-reductase deficiency was recognized by the presence of C_{24}-bile acids having a Δ^4-3-oxo structure characteristic of the sterol intermediates 7α-hydroxy- and 7α,12α-dihydroxy-4-cholesten-3-one. This defect has now been recognized in 11 infants, seven of whom died before diagnosis was established. Following our description of this inborn error[7] it was reported that many patients with cholestatic liver disease excrete Δ^4-3-oxo bile acids[9], and that this might suggest the defect could be acquired rather than being a primary enzyme defect. While oxo-bile acids are found in the urine of many patients with cholestatic liver disease, the striking feature of the patients with a Δ^4-3-oxosteroid 5β-reductase deficiency is the presence almost exclusively of the unsaturated oxo-bile acids, the frequent occurrence of *allo*-(5α-H) bile acids and the virtual absence of primary bile acids. The formation of *allo*-bile acids, which are usually considered to occur mainly in the gastrointestinal tract as a result of bacterial action[2], takes place in the hepatocyte and presumably because the sterol intermediates accumulate in sufficient concentrations to exceed the K_m for the enzyme reaction. Although the Δ^4-3-oxosteroid 5β-reductase enzyme is not expressed

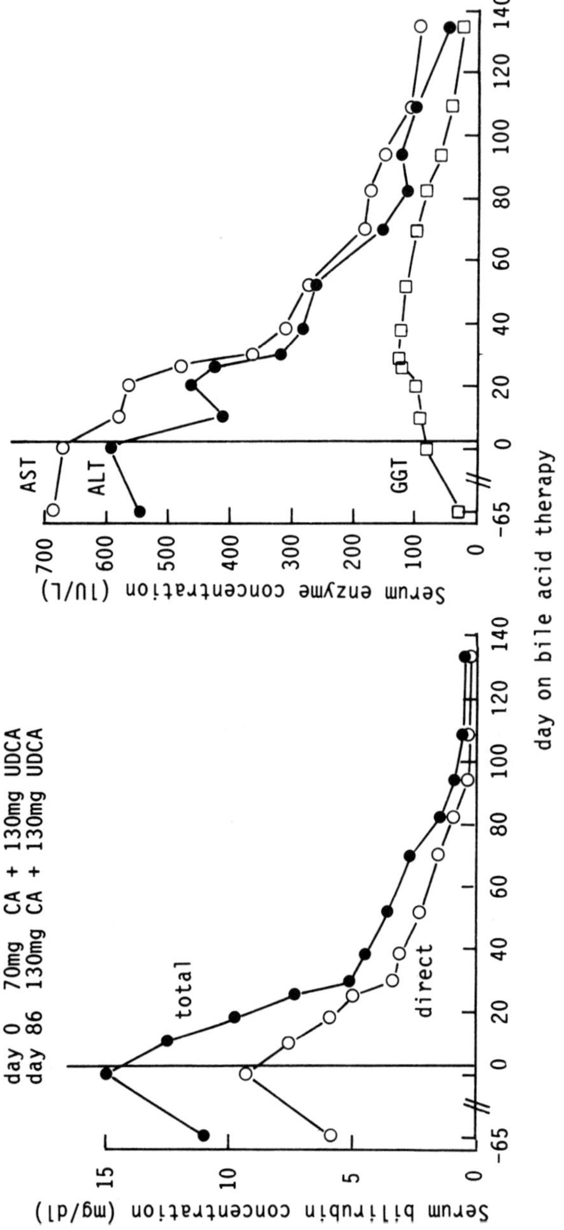

Fig. 4   Patient DM. Δ^4-3-oxosteroid 5β-reductase deficiency – oral bile acid therapy started at age 1 year

in fibroblasts, a primary enzyme defect was recently confirmed from the failure to detect the 38 kD protein in the liver tissue from one of the patients using monoclonal antibodies to the Δ^4-3-oxosteroid 5β-reductase enzyme and immunoblot analysis.

MECHANISM OF CHOLESTASIS AND LIVER INJURY AND TREATMENT

The cholestasis and liver injury in these patients is considered to occur either because of the lack of primary bile acids that are essential to facilitate bile-flow and/or the accumulation of atypical bile acids that are potentially hepatotoxic.

The increasing accumulation of atypical bile acids which appear to be poorly transported at the canalicular level into bile probably leads to cholestasis and liver injury. As the proportions of these bile acids increase, particularly in the absence of the normal primary bile acids that might otherwise provide a compensatory choleresis, progression of liver injury occurs (Fig. 2).

For these reasons we have used primary bile acids to treat these conditions[10] in the expectation that this would facilitate bile flow and down-regulate endogenous synthesis of the atypical bile acids, thereby leading to improved liver function in what appear to be otherwise fatal conditions.

FAB-MS analysis of the urine has been used to monitor the disappearance of the atypical bile acid metabolites (Fig. 3), and although complete suppression in synthesis is difficult to achieve, there occurs a significant reduction in its absolute levels and proportions of these metabolites after primary bile acid therapy. This appears to be accompanied by a normalization in liver function tests (Fig. 4) and an improvement in liver histology. The clinical improvement in these patients was striking, and indicates the importance of early diagnosis of this new category of metabolic liver diseases.

References

1. Balistreri WF. Neonatal cholestasis: lessons from the past, issues for the future. Sem Liver Dis. 1987;7(2) (Foreword).
2. Björkhem I. Mechanism of bile acid biosynthesis in mammalian liver. In: Dannielson H, Sjövall J, editors. Sterols and bile acids. Amsterdam: Elsevier; 1985:231–78.
3. Setchell KDR. Disorders of bile acid synthesis. In: Walker WA, Durie PR, Hamilton JR, Walker-Smith JA, Watkins JA, editors. Pediatric gastrointestinal disease, pathophysiology, diagnosis, management. Toronto and Philadelphia: BC Decker, vol. 2; 1990:992–1013.
4. Setchell KDR, Street JM. Inborn errors of bile acid synthesis. Sem Liver Dis. 1987;7: 85–99.
5. Clayton PT, Leonard JV, Lawson AM, Setchell KDR, Andersson S, Egestad B, Sjövall J. Familial giant cell hepatitis associated with synthesis of $3\beta,7\alpha$-dihydroxy- and $3\beta,7\alpha,12\alpha$-trihydroxy-5-cholenoic acid. J Clin Invest. 1987;79:1031–8.
6. Setchell KDR, Flick R, Watkins JB, Piccoli D. Chronic hepatitis in a 10-year-old due to an inborn error in bile acid synthesis – diagnosis and treatment with oral bile acid. Gastroenterology. 1990;98(5):A631 (abstr.).
7. Setchell KDR, Suchy FJ, Welsh MB, Zimmer-Nechemias L, Heubi J, Balistreri WF. Δ^4-3-

Oxosteroid 5β-reductase deficiency described in identical twins with neonatal hepatitis – a new inborn error in bile acid synthesis. J Clin Invest. 1988;82:2148–57.
8. Buchmann MS, Kvittingen EA, Nazer H, Gunasekaran T, Clayton PT, Sjövall J. Lack of 3β-hydroxy-Δ^5-C$_{27}$-steroid dehydrogenase/isomerase in fibroblasts from a child with urinary excretion of 3β-hydroxy-Δ^5-bile acids – a new inborn error of metabolism. J Clin Invest. 1990;86:2034–7.
9. Clayton PT, Patel E, Lawson AM, Carruthers RA, Tanner MS, Strandvik B, Egestad B, Sjövall J. 3-Oxo-Δ^4-bile acids in liver disease. Lancet. 1988;1:1283–4 (Letter).
10. Setchell KDR, Balistreri WF, Piccoli DA, Clerici C. Oral bile acid therapy in the treatment of inborn errors in bile acid synthesis associated with liver disease. In: Paumgartner G, Stiehl A, Gerok W, editors. Bile acids as therapeutic agents. Dordrecht/Boston/London: Kluwer; 1990:367–73.

16
Cholestasis in cystic fibrosis

M. J. LENTZE

INTRODUCTION

Cholestatic liver disease is a common manifestation of cystic fibrosis in adolescence and adulthood. As the percentage of patients with cystic fibrosis (CF) surviving childhood becomes larger and reaches about 66%[1], the involvement of the hepatobiliary tract in these patients with CF has become a predominant clinical problem[2]. Twenty-five per cent of patients with CF are developing progressive biliary cirrhosis in adulthood[3], in 18% we find a microgallbladder, 7% suffer from biliary colics and cholecystitis and 12% present with cholesterol gallstones. The first description of liver disease in cystic fibrosis by Andersen in 1978 (cited in ref. 3) was followed by a number of confirming reports of clinical liver disease in this condition[4–9]. Pathological findings of liver disease in CF are reported up to 50%[8]. Cholestasis is present in end-stage liver disease in these patients, but may be present earlier before biliary cirrhosis develops. In neonates and young infants cholestasis has been described associated with excessive biliary mucous and mild periportal changes[7,10–15].

DEVELOPMENT AND INCIDENCE OF HEPATOBILIARY DISEASE IN CYSTIC FIBROSIS

Early involvement of the liver in cystic fibrosis was described as focal biliary cirrhosis by Bodian in 1952[4]. The changes are characterized by inspissated granular eosinophilic material in portal ducts associated with proliferations of bile ducts and fibrosis. The mucus accumulation in the intra- and extrahepatic ducts was found to be the cause of obstructive lesions as well as transient jaundice in these patients[12]. If focal obstruction persists, focal biliary cirrhosis follows and may progress into multilobular cirrhosis which then presents with clinical signs of cholestasis. Although cholestatic changes are visible within the regions of focal biliary cirrhosis the overall bile secretion might be sufficient to avoid clinical signs of cholestasis in the patient. The aetiology of cholestasis and jaundice in CF, however, is variable. It is associated with meconium ileus[10,14] or with intestinal atresia[7], as well as with volvulus[17]. Congenital cytomegalovirus infection was found in two patients with CF and neonatal jaundice[17]. The pathogenesis of cholestasis in cystic fibrosis is a matter of dispute. As most authors agree upon the focal biliary cirrhosis as the first developmental step towards liver disease in CF, the transition into multilobular cirrhosis in these patients remains controversial. Mucous plugging occurs in young infants with CF leading to 10.8% of focal biliary cirrhosis in infants below 3 months to 15% in infants from 3 to 12 months and to 26.8% in children over 1 year of age[12]. From this study it was suggested that cholestatic liver disease was dependent upon age of the patient. Which of the pathogenetic factors were involved from focal into multilobular cirrhosis remained unclear. Gaskin *et al.*[18] found, in their series of 92 patients with CF, evidence of biliary obstruction in 96%, and speculated whether this condition could be a pathogenetic factor in the development of liver disease in CF. However, this finding was not confirmed by others. In contrast, in a small study of five children with CF and mild or absent clinical liver disease investigated by percutaneous liver biopsy, light microscopy showed changes in the livers with slight fibrosis or focal cirrhosis but no signs of cholestasis within the hepatocytes[16]. Hultcrantz *et al.* speculate that the ultrastructural findings cannot explain the basis for liver cell damage, and moreover that cholestasis does not seem to be a presumable aetiological factor for the changes in the liver of CF patients[16]. As liver needle biopsies were the only source for the assessment of liver pathology in this study, the conclusions drawn by the findings may be limited by the fact that sampling errors occur in 66% of needle biopsies in determining the presence of liver cirrhosis[19]. In some cases other factors have been implicated in the occurrence of cholestasis in CF. Neonatal hepatitis syndrome as a cause for cholestasis in a newborn infant with CF has been described[20] with the typical clinical and pathological picture of paucity of interlobular bile ducts associated with conjugated hyperbilirubinaemia. Similar changes have been described previously in CF patients[5,13]. Inspissated bile within extrahepatic biliary tissue was also found as a manifestation of cholestasis in cystic fibrosis. In a 3.5-month-old infant with CF associated with meconium ileus, peritonitis and jejunal atresia, extrahepatic biliary obstruction was found during surgery due to inspissated bile, which was relieved by hydrostatic infusion of 2% *N*-acetylcysteine into the biliary tree over a 6-day period[21].

Gallstones composed of cholesterol are a well-known complication of CF[22–26]. The routine ultrasonographic investigation demonstrates that the incidence of gallstones in CF patients is higher than initially thought. Exocrine pancreatic insufficiency in CF is associated with large losses of faecal bile salts[27], which leads to a decreased bile salt pool size[28], low duodenal bile salt concentration[29] and lithogenic bile[24]. The supersaturation of bile with cholesterol was suggested to be coupled with an interruption of the enterohepatic circulation of bile salts[2].

TREATMENT OF HEPATOBILIARY DISEASE IN CYSTIC FIBROSIS

Cholestatic liver disease due to multilobular cirrhosis in cystic fibrosis caused by the accumulation of inspissated bile in the interhepatic ducts has recently

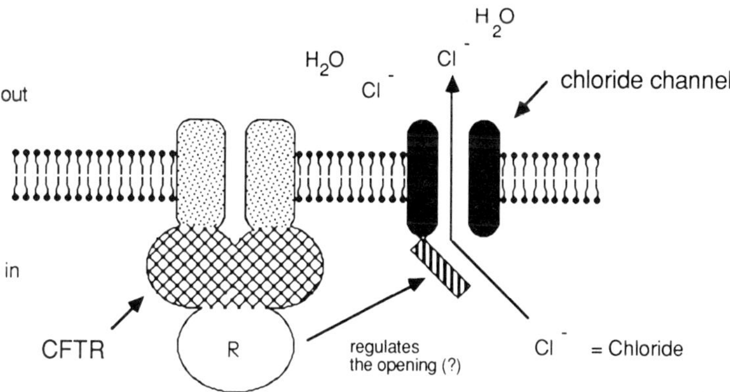

Fig. 1   Regulation of the chloride channel. It remains controversial whether CFTR regulates the chloride channel or serves as chloride channel itself

been treated by ursodeoxycholic acid. In open trials patients with liver disease and CF have been shown to improve under treatment with the tertiary choleretic bile acid ursodeoxycholic acid by better liver functions such as biochemical parameters, as well as quantitative liver function tests[30,31]. In addition the patients gained weight and showed an increased body mass index. The rationale for such a treatment derived from studies in patients with primary biliary cirrhosis[32] where a beneficial effect upon cholestasis was found, and from patients with extrahepatic biliary atresia which demonstrated an improvement of their nutritional status[33]. However, it remains to be established whether a long-term treatment with ursodeoxycholic acid can improve cholestatic liver disease in these patients or whether an early start with this tertiary bile acid can even prevent cholestasis.

THERAPEUTIC IMPLICATIONS OF THE DETECTION OF THE GENE DEFECT IN CYSTIC FIBROSIS WITH CHOLESTATIC LIVER DISEASE

With detection of the cystic fibrosis transmembrane conductance regulator (CFTR) as the gene product being defective in cystic fibrosis with the locus upon chromosome 7[34-36], the understanding of the disease has reached a stage whereby for the first time a potential curing therapy is in sight, namely gene therapy. Whether CFTR is controlling the chloride channel or whether it serves as the channel itself has not been clarified completely, and remains controversial (Fig. 1). CFTR has been shown to be located in the human pancreas[35] and in a variety of tissues in the rat, i.e. intestinal mucosa, testis, lung and uterus[37]. The hepatobiliary tree has not been investigated in human tissue for the presence of CFTR. It is suggested that CFTR is located with the bile canaliculi regulating chloride transport. In cystic fibrosis a defect within the CFTR could lead to a defect in chloride transport leading to a more viscous bile which finally is followed by bile plugs, bile retention and bile obstruction (Fig. 2). Any restoration of chloride movements within the

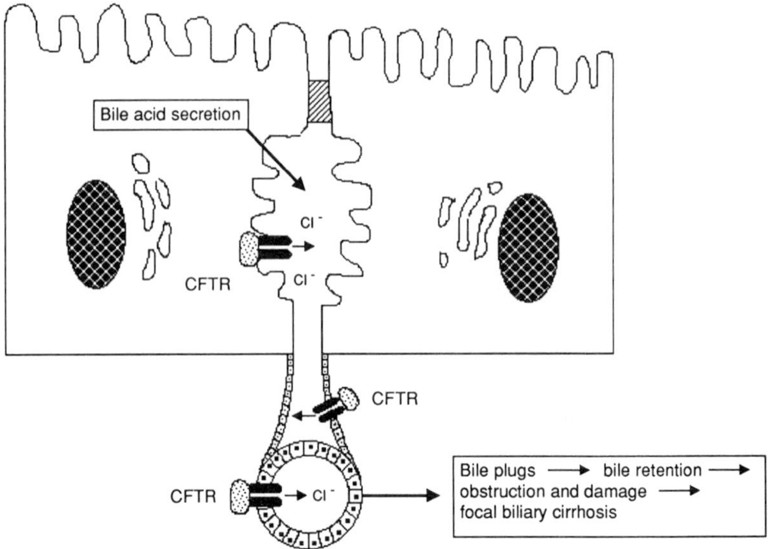

Fig. 2 Disregulation of chloride into the canaliculi and/or in the bile ductules by a defective CFTR could lead to increased viscosity of bile followed by bile plugs, bile retention and consecutive obstruction and damage

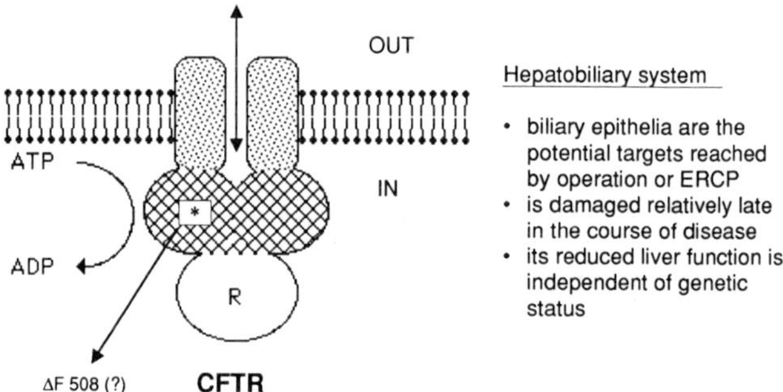

Fig. 3 Potential of CFTR restoration in the hepatobiliary tract by gene therapy

bile canaliculi would reverse the viscosity and prevent cirrhosis. For this goal biliary epithelial cells would need to be transduced by exposure to retroviral vectors bearing the correct CFTR gene during instillation of the biliary tree, for example by ERCP. However, at the present time no *in vitro* and *in vivo* data are available which demonstrate that this target can be reached. Preliminary data suggest that the crypt cells of the intestine can be reached and transduced by this route of instillation[38]. Difficult to understand is the fact that within the context of potential gene therapy the incidence of liver disease in adolescents and adults with cystic fibrosis is not correlated with the classical ΔF 508 defect. Factors other than the genetic defect in cystic fibrosis obviously contribute to the viscous bile and consecutive liver damage. In this perspective it will be difficult to determine the right time at which patients should undergo such a therapeutic approach. Until this potential cure can be applied broad evaluation of ursodeoxycholic acid therapy has to be studied in long-term multicentre prospective studies.

References

1. Corey ML. Longitudinal studies in cystic fibrosis. In: Sturgess JM, editor. Perspectives in cystic fibrosis: proceedings of the 8th international cystic fibrosis congress held in Toronto, Canada, 26–30 May 1980. Missisauga, Ont: Imperial Press; 1980:246–55.
2. Roy CC, Weber AM, Morin CL, Lepage G, Brisson G, Yousef I, Lasalle R. Hepatobiliary disease in cystic fibrosis: a survey of current issues and concepts. J Pediat Gastroenterol Nutr. 1982;1:469–78.
3. Park RW, Grand RJ. Gastrointestinal manifestations of cystic fibrosis: a review. Gastroenterology. 1981;81:1143–61.
4. Bodian M. Fibrocystic disease of the pancreas. A congenital disorder of mucus production – mucosis. London: William Heinemann Medical Books; 1952.
5. Di Sant'Agnese PA, Blanc WA. A distinct type of biliary cirrhosis of the liver in cystic associated with cystic fibrosis of the pancreas. Pediatrics. 1957;18:387–409.
6. Feigelson J, Pecau Y, Sauvegrain J. Liver function studies and biliary tract investigations in mucoviscidosis. Acta Paediatr Scand. 1970;59:539–44.
7. Gatzimos C, Jowitt R. Jaundice in mucoviscidosis (fibrocystic disease of pancreas). Am J Dis Child. 1955;89:182–6.
8. Stern RC, Stevens DP, Boat TF, Doershuk CF, Izant RJ, Matthews LW. Symptomatic hepatic disease in cystic fibrosis: incidence, course, and outcome of portal systemic shunting. Gastroenterology. 1976;70:645–9.
9. Wilroy RS, Crawford SE, Johnson WW. Cystic fibrosis with extensive fatty replacement of the liver. J Pediatr. 1966;68:67–73.
10. Bernstein J, Vawter G, Harris G, Young V, Hillman LS. The occurrence of intestinal atresia in newborn with meconium ileus. Am J Dis Child. 1960;99:804–18.
11. Craig M, Haddad H, Schwachman H. The pathological changes in the liver in cystic fibrosis of the pancreas. Am J Dis Child. 1957;93:357–69.
12. Oppenheimer E, Esterly J. Hepatic changes in young infants with cystic fibrosis: possible relation to focal biliary cirrhosis. J Pediatr. 1975;86:683–9.
13. Shier K, Horn R. The pathology of liver cirrhosis in patients with cystic fibrosis of the pancreas. Can Med Assoc J. 1963;89:645–51.
14. Talamo R, Hendren WH. Prolonged obstructive jaundice, report of a case in a neonate with meconium ileus and jejunal atresia. Am J Dis Child. 1968;115:74–79.
15. Taylor W, Qaqundah B. Neonatal jaundice associated with cystic fibrosis. Am J Dis Child. 1972;123:161–2.
16. Hultcrantz R, Mengarelli S, Strandvik B. Morphological findings in the liver of children with cystic fibrosis: a light and electron microscopic study. Hepatology. 1986;6:881–9.
17. Valman HB, France, Wallis PG. Prolonged neonatal jaundice in cystic fibrosis. Arch Dis Child. 1972;46:805–9.
18. Gaskin KJ, Waters DLM, Howman-Giles R, de Silva M, Earl JW, Martin HCO, Kan AE, Brown JM, Dorney SFA. Liver disease and common-bile-duct stenosis in cystic fibrosis. N Engl J Med. 1988;318:340–6.
19. Soloway RD, Baggenstoss AH, Schoenfield LJ, Summerskill WHJ. Observer error and sampling variability tested in evaluation of hepatitis and cirrhosis by liver biopsy. Am J Dig Dis. 1971;16:1082–6.
20. Furuya KN, Roberts EA, Canny GJ, Philips MJ. Neonatal hepatitis syndrome with paucity of interlobular bile ducts in cystic fibrosis. J Pediat Gastroenterol Nutr 1991;12:127–30.
21. Evans JS, George DE, Mollit D. Biliary infusion therapy in inspissated bile syndrome of cystic fibrosis. J Pediat Gastroenterol Nutr. 1991;12:131–5.
22. Feigelson J, Mareschal JL, Sauvegrain J. Anomalies of the gallbladder in mucoviscidosis: à propos of 57 cases. Med Chir Dig. 1975;4:121–4.

23. Isenberg J, L'Heureux P, Warwick W, Sharp H. Clinical observations on the biliary system in cystic fibrosis. Am J Gastroenterol. 1976;65:134–41.
24. Roy CC, Weber AM, Morin CL, Combes JC, Nüsslé D, Megevand A, Lasalle R. Abnormal biliary lipid composition in cystic fibrosis. Effect of pancreatic enzymes. N Engl J Med. 1977;297:1301–5.
25. Hubbard VS, Head GL, Shawker TH, Di Sant'Agnese PA. Radiological and ultrasound evaluation of the gallbladder in patients with cystic fibrosis. Pediatr Res. 1978;12:437 (abstr.).
26. Goriup W, Rickham PP, Deyhle P, Shmerling DH. Cholelithiasis als Erstmanifestation der zystischen Pankreafibrose. Helv Paediatr Acta. 1980;35:177–84.
27. Weber AM, Roy CC, Chartrand L, Lepage G, Dufour OL, Morin CL, Lasalle R. Relationship between bile acid malabsorption and pancreatic insufficiency in cystic fibrosis. Gut. 1976;17:295–9.
28. Watkins JB, Tercyak AM, Szczepanik P, Klein PD. Bile salt kinetics in cystic fibrosis: influence of pancreatic enzyme replacement. Gastroenterology. 1977;73:1023–8.
29. Harries JT, Muller DPR, McCollum JPK, Lipson A, Roma E, Norman AP. Intestinal bile salts in cystic fibrosis. Arch Dis Child. 1979;54:19–24.
30. Cotting J, Lentze MJ, Reichen J. Effects of ursodeoxycholic acid treatment on nutrition and liver function in patients with cystic fibrosis and longstanding cholestasis. Gut. 1990;31:918–21.
31. Colombo C, Setchell KDR, Podda M et al. Effects of ursodeoxycholic acid therapy for liver disease associated with cystic fibrosis. J Pediatr. 1990;117:482–9.
32. Poupon R, Chretien Y, Poupon RE, Ballet F, Calmus Y, Darnis F. Is ursodeoxycholic acid an effective treatment for primary biliary cirrhosis? Lancet. 1987;1:834–6.
33. Ullrich D, Rating D, Schroeter W, Hanefeld F, Bircher J. Treatment with ursodeoxycholic acid renders children with biliary atresia suitable for liver transplantation. Lancet. 1987;2:1324.
34. Rommens JM, Iannuzzi MC, Kerem B, Drumm ML, Melmer G, Dean M, Rozmahel R, Cole JL, Kennedy D, Hidaka N, Zsiga M, Buchwald M, Rioradan JR, Tsui LC, Collins FS. Identification of the cystic fibrosis gene: chromosome walking and jumping. Science. 1989;245:1059–65.
35. Riordan JR, Rommens JM, Kerem B, Alon N, Rozmahel R, Grzelczak Z, Zielinski J, Lok S, Plavsic N, Chou J, Drumm ML, Iannuzzi MC, Collins FS, Tsui LC. Identification of the cystic fibrosis gene: cloning and characterization of complementary DNA. Science. 1989;245:1066–72.
36. Kerem B, Rommens JM, Buchanan JA, Markiewicz D, Cox D, Cox TK, Chakravarti A, Buchwald M, Tsui LC. Identification of the cystic fibrosis gene: genetic analysis. Science. 1989;245:1073–80.
37. Trezise AEO, Buchwald M. *In vivo* cell-specific expression of the cystic fibrosis transmembrane conductance regulator. Nature. 1991;353:434–7.
38. Soriano-Brucher H, Lau C, Hourigan T, Finegold M, Ledley FD, Henning SJ. Gene transfer in to the intestinal epithelium. Gastroenterology. 1991;100:A252.

17
Progressive familial intrahepatic cholestasis (Byler's disease)

P. F. WHITINGTON, D. K. FREESE, E. M. ALONSO, M. H. FISHBEIN and J. C. EMOND

INTRODUCTION

The first detailed description of hereditary hepatocellular cholestasis was provided by Clayton *et al.* in 1965 and involved the members of an Amish kindred, the members of which were descended from Jacob Byler[1]. Affected individuals of the Byler kindred had severe intrahepatic cholestasis, usually beginning in the first months of life. The disease progressed to cirrhosis almost always before the end of the second decade. The pattern of appearance within the kindred was consistent with autosomal recessive inheritance. The name 'Byler's disease' has been used subsequently to describe this condition.

We prefer the descriptive term 'progressive familial intrahepatic cholestasis' (PFIC), which we define by the following criteria: chronic unremitting cholestasis, a thorough examination that excludes any known metabolic or anatomical aetiology, and a combination of clinical and biochemical characteristics that we have found distinguishes PFIC from other chronic cholestatic conditions. It is clear that not all hereditary hepatocellular cholestasis fits into the mould of PFIC, as we will describe. Two reports involving native Arctic Indians, one by Weber *et al.*[2] and one by Ornvold *et al.*[3], present distinct groups with progressive childhood cholestasis that differs significantly from PFIC. Byler's disease deserves to be looked at more critically to determine how it fits into the definition of PFIC, but at this time the term should be restricted to the Amish kindred in which it was described.

Overall, somewhat fewer than 100 cases meeting the general description of PFIC have been reported[4-17]. Our experience, which involves 33 well-studied patients[18], suggests that PFIC may be a relatively common cause for chronic intrahepatic cholestasis in children. In this report we will detail the clinical and histological characteristics of PFIC. Further, we will present an approach to surgical management of these patients, which can interrupt the cycle of disease. Finally, we present results of investigation into the cellular mechanism of disease.

CLINICAL FINDINGS AND COMPLICATIONS

We have studied 33 patients with PFIC. Thirty of the patients were examined by the authors at one of three medical centres (University of Chicago Wyler Children's Hospital, $n = 17$; University of Minnesota Medical Center, $n = 7$; and University of Tennessee LeBonheur Children's Medical Center, $n = 6$) when they presented for evaluation of cholestasis or for management of advanced liver disease. Siblings of children evaluated at our centres were included when we had clinical and histological data documenting progressive cholestasis ($n = 3$). In addition, two siblings of one patient died in Bolivia and two first cousins of another died in Iran, but were not included because no records were available.

Age of onset

All patients with one exception presented at less than 12 months of age, with an average of 3 months. The exceptional patient presented at 17 years of age when he developed unremitting progressive cholestasis. He had undergone cholecystectomy for idiopathic cholecystolithiasis at 2 years of age, but had no clinical cholestasis in the intervening 15 years. He would not have been included in the series except that his female sibling presented with cholestasis at 5 months of age and had developed cirrhosis by 2 years of age.

Age at death or liver transplantation

Six patients have died at an average age of 3 years. Two died in liver failure, two died with hepatocellular carcinoma, and two died from complications of orthotopic liver transplantation. Ten patients have had successful liver transplants at an average age of 4 years.

Presenting symptoms

The predominant presenting symptom in PFIC is pruritus, which is often very severe and out of proportion to the level of jaundice. Seven patients presented with cutaneous mutilation (4+ pruritus) and another 19 had persistent itching with significant excoriations (3+ pruritus). All patients had jaundice, varying from mild to severe. Thirty-two had significant hepatomegaly, while splenomegaly occurred only in patients with advanced fibrosis or cirrhosis.

Growth failure, defined as height less than the fifth percentile for age, was observed in 31 patients. The weight is relatively preserved, until the onset of cirrhosis-related cachexia producing a 'short and stocky' appearance. Intellectual development has been normal in all patients except one, who had mild mental retardation dating from birth.

Symptoms referable to the airway have been prominent. Ten patients experienced asthma-like disease, perennial wheezing and cough most prominent at night and in the early morning. These symptoms resolved in nine of nine patients receiving effective therapy. Seventeen patients had recurrent epistaxis in the absence of coagulopathy or thrombocytopenia. Again, these symptoms resolved in all patients receiving effective therapy.

Most adolescent patients had disturbed development of secondary sexual characteristics. Three of three adolescent females had amenorrhoea, and two of three had delayed sexual development prior to therapy. Three of four adolescent males experienced delayed development of secondary sexual characteristics. The one male with late onset of disease experienced secondary impotence.

Familial pattern

The pattern of occurrence definitely suggests autosomal recessive inheritance. In our series there were 35 affected individuals among 67 children at risk in 26 families. Nineteen cases came from families in which there was repeated incidence in the sibships, but no consanguinity among the parents. Two additional cases presented in families with no other affected siblings, but with consanguineous parents. Fourteen cases were sporadic, presenting in families with no other affected siblings and with no consanguinity among parents. There was no other clinical liver disease in any family, except two. In one family the parents of the proband were first cousins, who themselves had two first cousins who died of progressive cholestatic liver disease in Iran. In the other, the mother and the maternal grandmother had both experienced cholestasis of pregnancy. Unaffected siblings and parents in 11 families were screened for subclinical cholestasis by measuring total fasting serum bile salt concentration, all of which proved normal.

Complications

Fat-soluble vitamin deficiency states were observed in most patients. Twenty-eight patients had vitamin D deficiency with rickets and/or severe osteopenia. Eight patients had vitamin K-sensitive hypoprothrombinaemia. Seventeen patients had biochemical evidence of vitamin E deficiency, and 13 had clinical neuropathy.

Cholelithiasis was identified in nine patients, four by ultrasonography or cholecystography and five during laparotomy.

Serum biochemistries

Patients with PFIC have distinctly different values for γ-glutamyl transpeptidase (GGTP) and serum cholesterol, as compared to most if not all other chronic cholestatic conditions (Table 1). Values for alkaline phosphatase, aminotransferases, serum bilirubin, and serum bile salt concentrations are not different from several other childhood cholestatic disorders.

Serum GGTP values are distinctly low in PFIC. In our patients they

Table 1 Clinical biochemistry values in 33 PFIC patients and children with other cholestatic diseases

Patient no.	GGTP[a] (IU/l)	GGTP[b] (IU/l)	SGPT (IU/l)	5'NT (U/l)	Cholesterol (mg/dl)	Bilirubin high[c] (mg/dl)	Bilirubin low[d] (mg/dl)	Alkaline phosphatase (IU/l)	Bile salt (μmol/l)
PFIC	15 ± 12	34 ± 21	241 ± 218	29 ± 13	155 ± 65	13.0 ± 7.9	4.5 ± 4.3	1074 ± 872	226 ± 87
Sclerosing cholangitis[e]		2138 ± 1477	277 ± 163		737 ± 495	8.6 ± 2.7		1418 ± 1056	346 ± 93
Arteriohepatic dysplasia[f]		1893 ± 1534	390 ± 191		773 ± 439	10.7 ± 5.4		1148 ± 466	206 ± 123
Biliary atresia[g]		1135 ± 307	214 ± 41		266 ± 105	12.3 ± 1.6		855 ± 118	117 ± 16

[a]GGTP value before phenobarbital.
[b]Value after phenobarbital.
[c]Lowest bilirubin value recorded.
[d]Highest value recorded.
[e]Patient $n = 10$.
[f]$n = 14$.
[g]$n = 23$.

averaged 14 IU in 14 patients in which they were measured prior to the initiation of phenobarbital therapy. There is approximately a two-fold increase after therapy with phenobarbital; in 30 patients being treated with phenobarbital the average GGTP was 34 IU.

The cholesterol level in PFIC patients is also somewhat lower than in other cholestatic disorders. Thirty-three PFIC patients showed an average cholesterol value of 156 mg/dl.

Bile acid analyses

The qualitative and quantitative patterns of bile acids in urine, serum and bile have been measured in 15 patients by gas chromatography/mass spectroscopy or fast atom bombardment mass spectroscopy. The cholic acid to chenodeoxycholic acid ratio in urine from PFIC patients was elevated, in excess of 3.5:1 in most and as high as 9:1 in one patient. The cholic acid predominance was even more striking in bile, where cholic acid routinely constituted about 90% of the bile acids present. We did not find large quantities of lithocholic acid in urine or bile of patients with PFIC, as has been previously observed in patients with 'Byler's disease'[4], although lithocholic acid and another monohydroxy bile acid, 3β-OH-Δ5-cholenoic acid, were present in concentration of 1–5% of total bile acids in urine. This was not different from that found in patients with other cholestatic diseases. Several unusual bile acids, including hyocholic acid, ursodeoxycolic acid and tetrahydroxylated bile acids, were present in minute quantities in the urine of PFIC patients and in patients with other cholestatic diseases, but no abnormal bile acids indicative of an intrinsic defect in bile acid metabolism were found. Conjugation of bile acids was predominantly with glycine, and the majority of urinary bile acids were present in the monosulphate form.

HISTOLOGICAL PATHOLOGY IN PFIC

Ninety tissue samples from 28 patients were examined in blinded review. Seventeen patients had biopsies during the first year of life. Twenty-six patients had multiple biopsies (range 2–7).

Findings in the lobule

Hepatocyte and canalicular cholestasis was evident in all biopsies from untreated patients. Cholestasis predominantly involved zone 3 hepatocytes, which contained flocculent bile pigment. The hepatocytes in zone 3 often formed pseudoacini, often containing bile plugs (Fig. 1). There was distinct disruption of the liver cell plate arrangement. Zone 3 hepatocytes demonstrated ballooning and feather degeneration in all untreated patients. Giant cell transformation was observed in 56% of initial biopsies, but often persisted in biopsies obtained after 3 years of age (Fig. 2). Mallory hyalin was observed only in advanced cases, being present in eight of the 11 specimens obtained

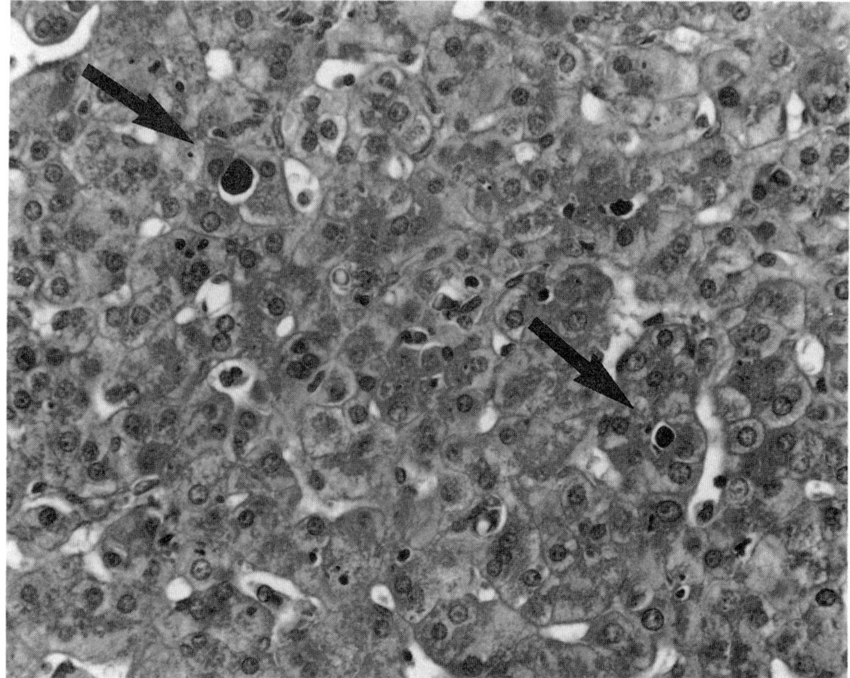

Fig. 1 Hepatocanalicular cholestasis with pseudo-acinus formation. Needle biopsy from a 19-month-old demonstrates generalized cellular cholestasis. Canalicular cholestasis and formation of pseudo-acini are evident throughout the lobule (arrows). (H&E; × 240)

at the time of transplantation (Fig. 3). Figure 4 shows the frequency of hepatocellular histological abnormalities in biopsies with respect to the patients' ages.

Findings in portal spaces

Loss of interlobular bile ducts was prominent; 70% of patients developed paucity of interlobular bile ducts (defined as < 0.6 ducts per portal space) at some time during the course of disease (Fig. 5). Smaller ducts were lost preferentially. In some biopsies with complete absence of small interlobular ducts, ducts remained in portal areas that spanned across the biopsy. Epithelial injury, consisting of attenuated cell cytoplasm, nuclear change (small, hyperchromatic) and loss of lumina, preceded duct loss. No inflammation was associated with the epithelial injury. Proliferating ductules (tubules) were observed at the edges of portal tracks in 21 patients, and were especially prominent in end-stage biopsies (Fig. 6).

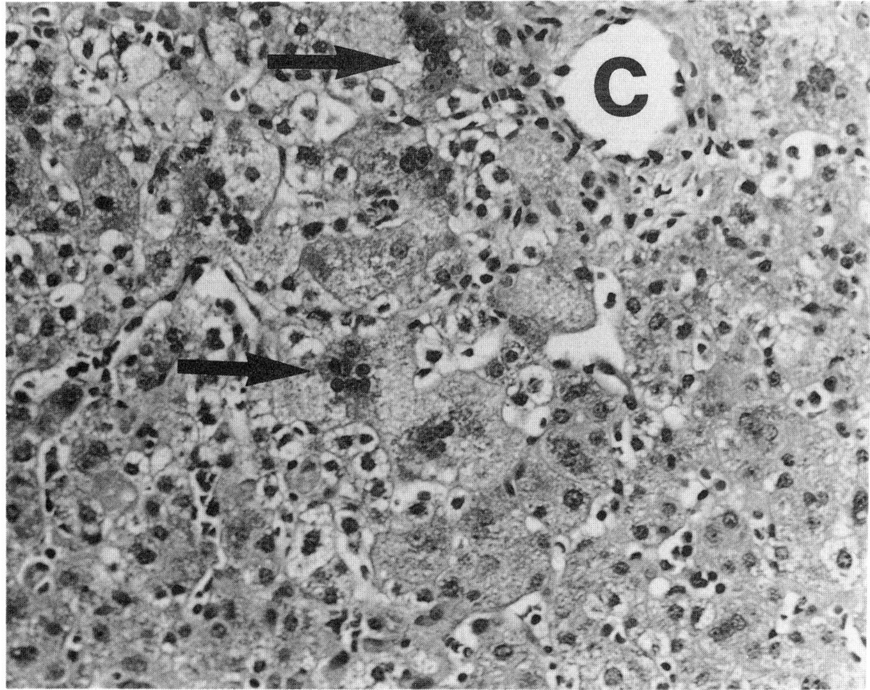

Fig. 2 Hepatocellular cholestasis and giant cell transformation. Needle biopsy from a 6-month-old demonstrates diffuse cellular cholestasis. Multiple giant cells (arrows) surround central vein (C) that shows early pericentral sclerosis. (H&E; × 300)

Fibrosis and cirrhosis

The disease characteristically resulted in fibrosis and cirrhosis if untreated. Fibrosis was an early finding, present in 76% of biopsies obtained before 2 years of age (Fig. 7). The earliest finding in many cases was pericentral sclerosis (Fig. 8), which often extended peripherally, resulting in central to portal bridging. Sixteen of 27 patients with multiple biopsies developed advanced fibrosis with bridging. In six cases this occurred before 2 years of age. Nine of 16 patients developed cirrhosis. The cirrhosis in PFIC is characterized by micronodular biliary cirrhosis with diffuse stellate and lacy fibrosis in the lobule, associated with severe cholestasis and pseudoacinar change (Fig. 9).

Two patients developed well-differentiated hepatocellular carcinoma before 3 years of age.

SURGICAL THERAPY FOR PFIC

Medical therapy, in our experience, has been unsuccessful. Virtually all patients have been administered the combination of phenobarbitol and bile

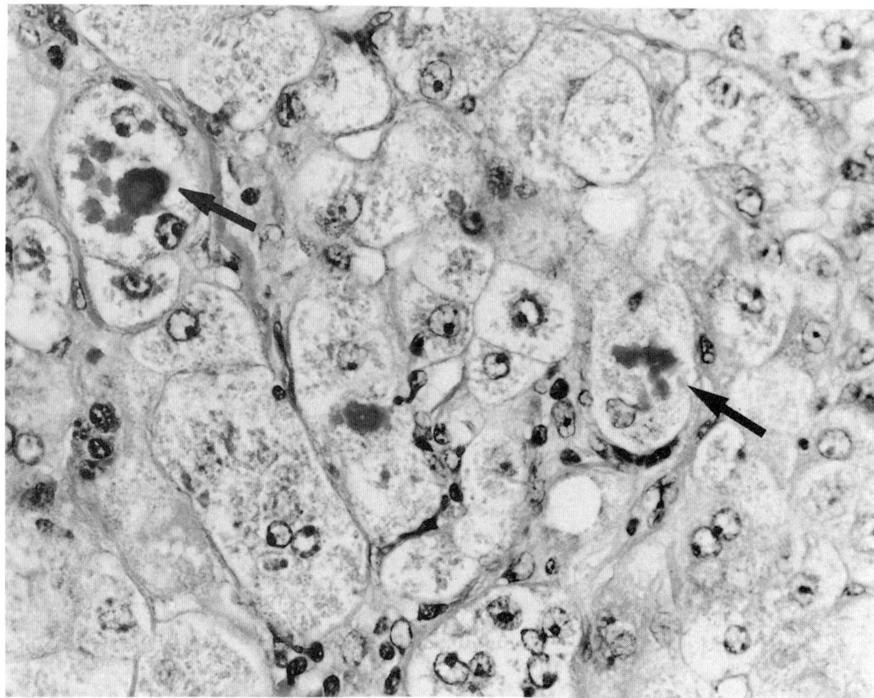

Fig. 3 Mallory's hyalin. This late finding is clearly seen (arrows) in material obtained at the time of liver transplantation of a 5-year-old with cirrhosis. (H&E; × 480)

salt binding resins, with no effect on symptoms or serum biochemistries. Antihistamines have been used for therapy of pruritus with no effect. Nine patients were administered rifampin, two of whom had minimal transient improvement. Six patients were administered ursodeoxycholic acid (10–20 mg/kg per day), one of whom had definite transient improvement. Two patients were administered chenodeoxycholic acid (10 mg/kg per day) with no improvement. Three patients have received UV-B therapy with no improvement and three patients have received courses of plasmapheresis, two of whom experienced transient improvement.

Fourteen patients have received surgical therapy with partial cutaneous biliary diversion. In this procedure a 10–15 cm jejunal conduit is swung up to the right upper quadrant on its vascular pedicle. The distal end is prepared as a cutaneous stoma and the proximal end is closed. The gallbladder is anastomosed to this conduit, side to side. This produces a partial diversion of bile. The flow of bile into the stoma is regulated by the spiral sphincter of the gallbladder and the sphincter of Oddi. Most patients drain 1–4 ounces (28–113 g) of bile per day, which is discarded. Of the 14 patients thus treated, eight achieved complete relief from symptoms. Their serum bilirubin and serum bile salt concentrations are normal, as are their liver enzymes. Two other patients experienced complete relief with the addition of ursodeoxy-

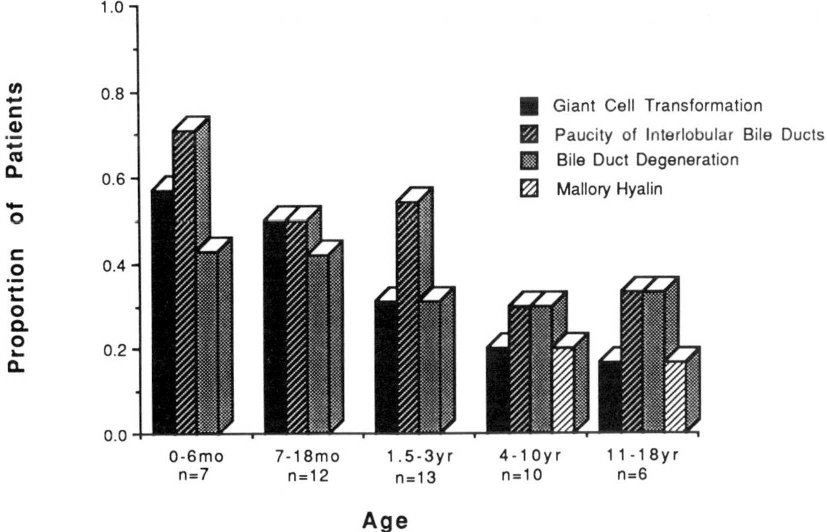

Fig. 4 Frequency histogram of various histological evidence of hepatocyte and ductal injury versus patients' ages at time of biopsy. If any biopsy obtained from a given patient during any age range contained the finding in question, the patient was tallied as having the finding. Biopsies obtained after surgical intervention have been excluded. The frequency of findings (giant cell transformation, ductal paucity, degenerative changes of bile duct epithelium and Mallory's hyalin) are given as a proportion of patients for whom biopsy material was available ('n' at bottom)

cholic acid at a dose of 8–10 mg/kg per day. All patients treated with partial cutaneous biliary diversion have had follow-up histological evaluation. The six patients with no fibrosis at the time of the procedure have had resolution of histological cholestasis and their histology is now normal. Four patients with fibrosis at the time of the procedure have had symptomatic relief. Three have had no resolution of fibrosis, two from bridging fibrosis to nil and one with pericentral sclerosis to nil. One has had worsening of the fibrosis from pericentral and portal fibrosis to bridging. Four patients have had no benefit from partial cutaneous biliary diversion. Three of these had cirrhosis at the time of procedure and one had bridging fibrosis. All of these patients subsequently had liver transplantation.

Patients with PFIC have often presented to us after cholecystectomy because of the frequent incidence of cholelithiasis. Cholecystectomy presents a significant impediment to the comprehensive surgical management of these patients and should be avoided. We have treated two patients with previous cholecystectomy by performing a limited ileal diversion. These patients, both teenagers, had more than 100 cm of distal ileum removed from the intestinal mainstream. The bowel was divided 110–150 cm proximal to the ileal caecal valve, and the distal bowel closed. The proximal bowel was anastomosed end-to-side to the terminal ileum 3–4 cm proximal to the ileocaecal valve, producing a self-emptying ileal blind loop. Both patients have had complete relief from symptoms of PFIC. Both experience modest diarrhoea which was

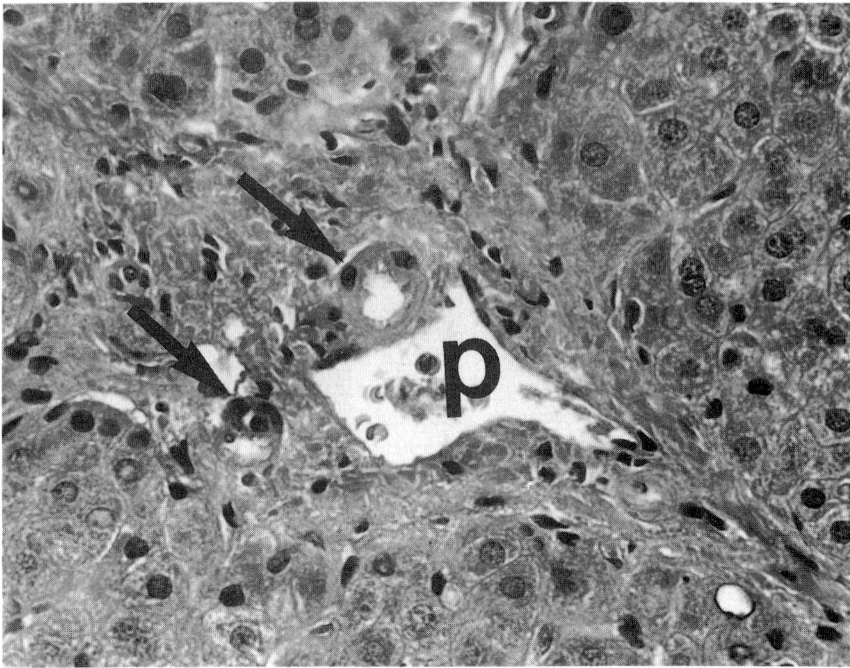

Fig. 5 Paucity of interlobular bile ducts. A needle biopsy specimen from a 4-year-old contains a portal tract with minimal fibrosis, portal vein (P) and two arterioles (arrows), but without a bile duct. Bile ducts were absent in five of the six portal tracts in this biopsy. (H&E; × 370)

controlled with cholestyramine. Both have normal serum bilirubin and serum bile acid concentrations as well as normal liver enzymes. One had no fibrosis at the time of the procedure and one had bridging fibrosis. Both now have normal histology.

STUDIES OF HEPATIC ENZYMOLOGY AND BILE ACID TRANSPORT

Liver tissue obtained at the time of transplantation was used to test two hypotheses regarding the mechanism of disease in PFIC[19]. The first hypothesis is that a synthetic or processing defect of GGTP results in disordered glutathione homeostasis, which in turn is important in the genesis of cholestasis. Low plasma GGT activity is the clue to this possible mechanism of disease. The second hypothesis is that the disease represents a generalized defect in bile acid transport at the canalicular level. It would appear from the response to partial cutaneous biliary diversion that the defect is only partial, and results in accumulation of bile acids when the preload for transport is excessive. The consequence of retained bile acids is a generalized injury to membranes and impairment of other excretory processes.

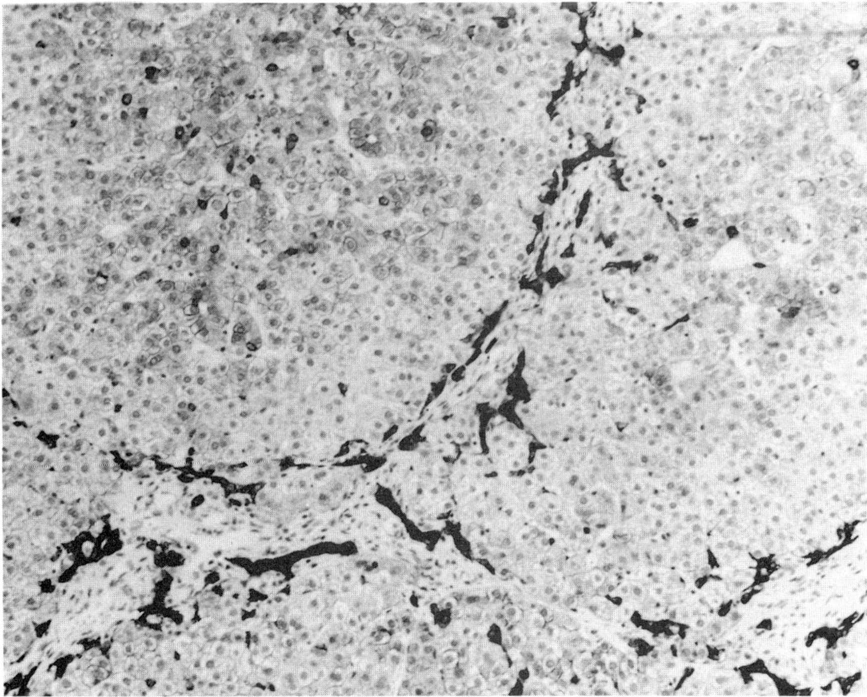

Fig. 6 Proliferation of bile ductules. This is a needle biopsy from 1-year-old, showing portal areas with minimal expansion but portal-to-portal bridging fibrosis. Proliferating ductules are difficult to appreciate along the margins of the portal areas (H&E; × 175)

Five livers from patients with PFIC were compared to 10 normal livers obtained at the time of segmental liver transplantation, five from patients with biliary atresia, and five from α_1-antitrypsin deficiency. Normal and diseased livers were treated in an identical fashion.

Twenty-five per cent homogenates of liver were made in iced buffer (10 mmol/l HEPES-Tris, pH 7.4, 0.25 mol/l sucrose, 0.2 mmol/l $CaCl_2$) in a Sorvall Omnimixer. The homogenate was filtered through cheesecloth and homogenized with a Dounce glass tissue homogenizer with a loose-fitting pestle for 10 strokes. Whole homogenate was retained for enzyme analysis. Canalicular membrane vesicles were prepared by differential centrifugation and calcium precipitation. Both whole homogenate and membrane vesicle preparations were stored frozen at $-80°C$ for up to 30 days before analysis.

The following enzyme activities were measured using kinetic, spectrophotometric methods: NA^+,K^+-ATPase, Mg^+-ATPase, alkaline phosphatase, GGTP, NADH dehydrogenase and succinic dehydrogenase. Protein content was determined and activities were expressed as units of activity per protein content. Bile salt concentrations of liver homogenates were measured using an enzymatic 3α-hydroxysteroid dehydrogenase method.

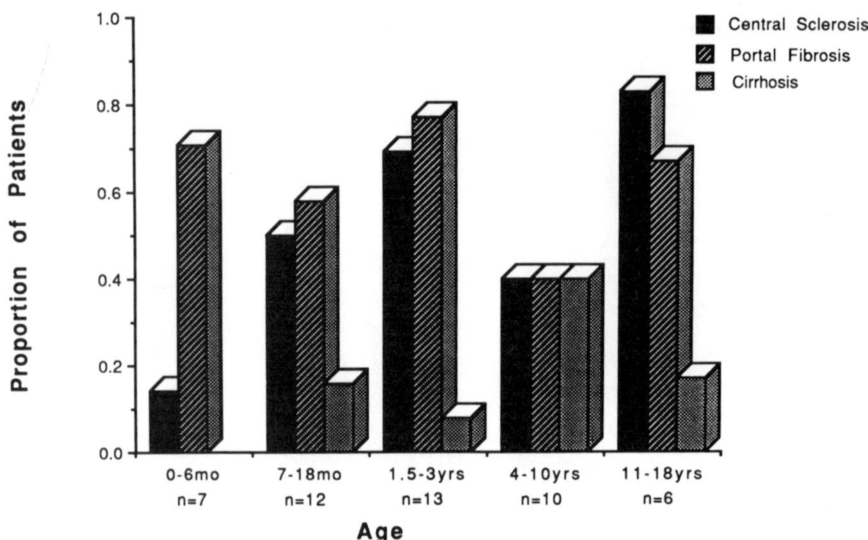

Fig. 7 Frequency histogram of histological findings of fibrosis versus the patients' ages at the time of biopsy. The frequency was tallied as in Fig. 1. The frequency is expressed as the proportion of patients in each age group whose biopsies demonstrated central sclerosis, +1– +3 fibrosis and cirrhosis

RESULTS

Whole liver homogenate bile salt concentrations were increased in patients with PFIC and biliary atresia as compared to normal liver and liver from patients with α_1-antitrypsin deficiency. The increase was by one log order in PFIC and by nearly two log orders in biliary atresia. Whole homogenate alkaline phosphatase activity was significantly increased in livers from patients with biliary atresia as compared to normal liver. Alkaline phosphatase activities in livers from patients with PFIC and α_1-antitrypsin deficiency were higher than normal, though not significantly so. There were no significant differences in homogenate GGTP activity among the groups. The livers from patients with PFIC had the lowest average value for GGTP (13 units/mg protein) as compared to an average of 17 units/mg in normal livers and 20 units/mg in livers from patients with biliary atresia. This is in contrast to the findings from Alagille's group, but the cause for the difference is not clear[20].

We were able to demonstrate adequate purity of canalicular membrane preparations from the livers of PFIC patients. Canalicular membrane alkaline phosphatase activity and GGTP activity were not different in the livers from PFIC patients as compared to normal livers. Alkaline phosphatase activity averaged 40 units/mg in both preparations while GGTP activity averaged 1200 units/mg in normal livers and 800 in patients with PFIC. The step-up enrichment of GGTP activity in canalicular membranes from normal and PFIC livers was identical, and the reduced GGTP activity in the canalicular membranes reflects an overall reduction in the mass of canalicular membrane

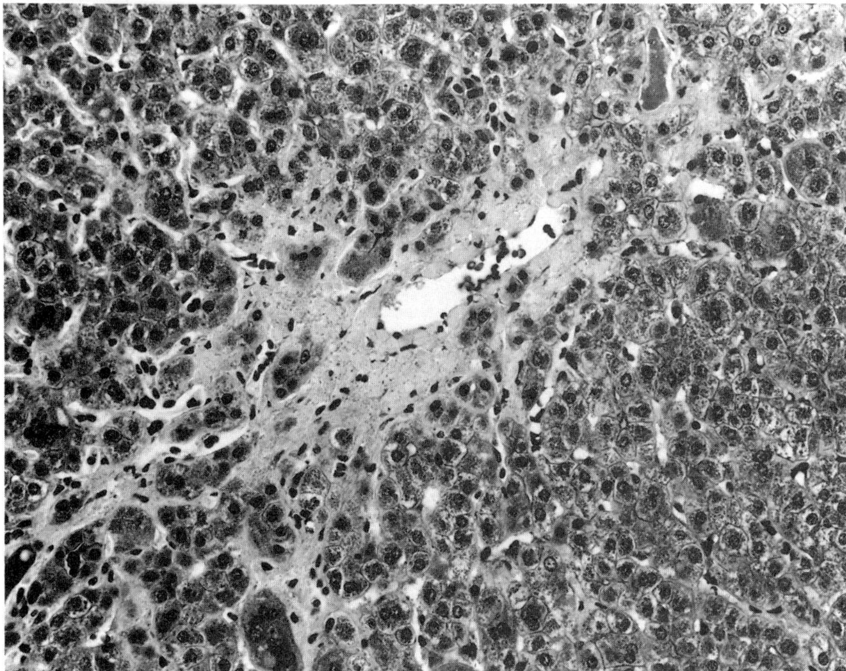

Fig. 8 Pericentral sclerosis. Needle biopsy from a 5-year-old boy demonstrates sclerosis surrounding a central vein. This type of fibrosis was frequently seen in biopsies without significant portal fibrosis and is one of the earliest findings in PFIC. (Masson's trichrome; × 233)

in these livers.

The kinetics of taurocholate uptake were studied in the canalicular membranes from normal and PFIC livers using a rapid filtration technique. Transport kinetics were determined by measuring initial rates of uptake at 25°C using taurocholate concentrations between 1 and 300 μmol/l in the presence of a 100 mmol/l sodium gradient. The initial uptakes of taurocholate in canalicular membrane vesicles were not different between PFIC and normal livers (Fig. 10). The K_m for the transport process was 141 μmol/l in normal livers and 138 in PFIC livers, and V_{max} was 1.46 nmol/mg per minute in the normal livers and 1.41 in the PFIC livers. In summary of the preliminary studies involving PFIC livers, we were unable to prove either hypothesis related to the pathogenesis of this disease.

SUMMARY AND CONCLUSIONS

We conclude from our studies that PFIC is a distinct clinical entity that produces progressive cholestatic liver disease of childhood. The pathogenesis of the disease is unknown, although it appears to be inherited. As with other autosomal recessive diseases, it is reasonable to assume that this disease

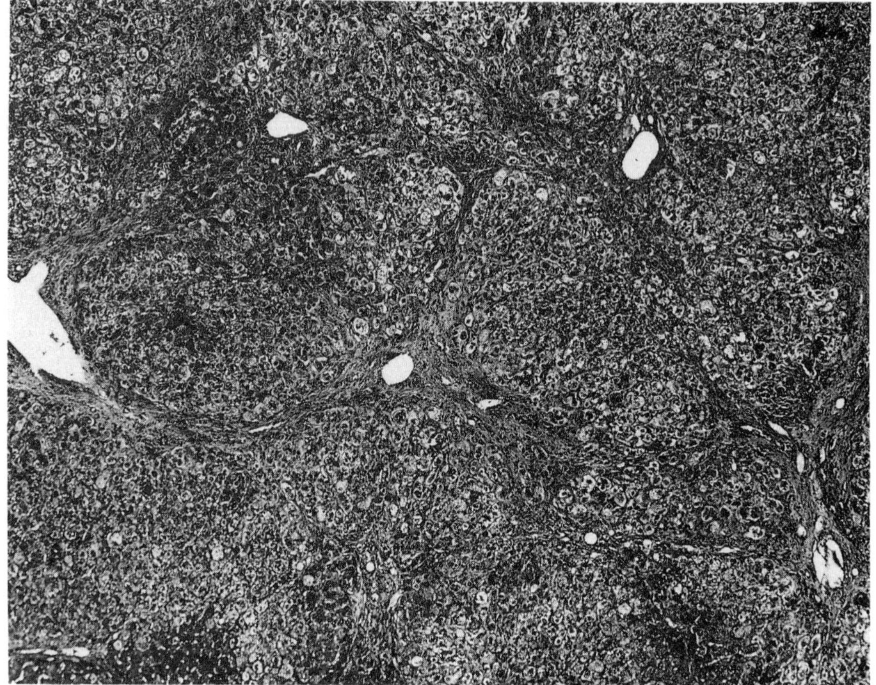

Fig. 9 End-stage liver pathology. Material obtained at the time of liver transplantation in the patient in Fig. 8 at 10 years of age shows the typical end-stage pattern, which consists of a feathery mesh of lobular fibrosis, severe cholestasis, portal-to-portal and portal-to-central bridging fibrosis. Regenerating nodules are evident. (H&E; × 45)

represents the expression of a base deletion or substitution in a gene encoding for a single protein essential for the maintenance of bile flow. Patients suffering from the disease have severely diminished quality of life secondary to their unusually severe pruritus, delayed growth and development, and from complications of progressively worsening liver disease. The diagnosis can be suspected in a cholestatic infant in whom pruritus is prominent and in whom laboratory evaluation reveals relatively low levels of GGTP and cholesterol. Other known disorders resulting in intrahepatic cholestasis should be specifically excluded. At present the only known effective treatments of PFIC are partial bile diversion or orthotopic liver transplant. Although few patients with this disorder have been reported, it is expected that better characterization of this syndrome will result in increased recognition of PFIC by physicians treating children with liver disease, increased understanding of its pathogenesis and development of alternative therapies.

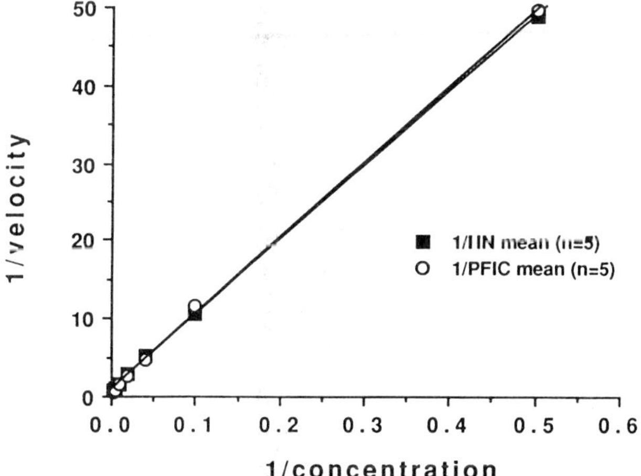

Fig. 10 Lineweaver–Burk transformation of initial uptake of Na$^+$ taurocholate at 25°C performed with canalicular membrane vesicles prepared from five livers from patients with PFIC and five human cadaver liver donors. The points are average values for triplicate uptake studies of all livers. The regression lines are virtually identical. The computed K_m for transport in the PFIC livers was 138 μmol/l as compared to 141 μmol/l for the normal livers. The V_{max} for the PFIC livers was 1.41 nmol/mg per min, and for the normal was 1.46

Acknowledgements

This work was supported in part by the Pediatric Liver Research Fund (University of Chicago), the Johnny Genna Foundation (Chicago), the March of Dimes National Research Foundation and the Center for Study of Advanced Liver Disease P30-DK34931 (University of Minnesota).

References

1. Clayton RJ, Iber FL, Ruebner BH, McKusick VA. Fatal familial intrahepatic cholestasis in an Amish kindred. J Pediatr. 1965;67:1025–8.
2. Weber AM, Tuchweber B, Yousef I, Brochu P, Turgeon C, Gabbiani G, Morin CI, Roy CC. Severe familial cholestasis in North American Indian children: a clinical model of microfilament dysfunction? Gastroenterology. 1981;81:653–62.
3. Ornvold K, Nielson I-M, Poulsen H. Fatal familial cholestatic syndrome in Greenland Eskimo children. Virchows Archiv A Pathol Anat. 1989;415:275–81.
4. Linarelli LG, Williams CN, Phillips MJ. Byler's disease: fatal intrahepatic cholestasis. J Pediatr. 1972;81:484–92.
5. Williams CN, Kaye R, Baker L, Hurwitz R, Senior JR. Progressive familial cholestatic cirrhosis and bile acid metabolism. J Pediatr. 1972;81:493–500.
6. Odievre M, Gautier M, Hadchouel M, Alagille D. Severe familial intrahepatic cholestasis. Arch Dis Child. 1973;48:806–12.
7. Ballow M, Margolis CZ, Schachtel B, Hsia YE. Progressive familial intrahepatic cholestasis. Pediatrics. 1973;51:998–1007.
8. de Vos R, de Wolf-Peters C, Desmet V, Eggermont E, Van Acker K. Progressive intrahepatic cholestasis (Byler's disease): case report. Gut. 1975;16:943–50.

9. Jones EA, Rabin L, Buckley CH, Webster GK, Owens D. Progressive intrahepatic cholestasis of infancy and childhood; clinicopathological study of a patient surviving to the age 18 years. Gastroenterology. 1976;71:675–82.

10. Van Acker KJ, Eggermont E, Deprettere A, Marien P. Fatal familial intrahepatic cholestasis (Byler disease). Acta Paediatr Belg. 1977;30:157–63.

11. Ugarte N, Gonzalez-Crussi F. Hepatoma in siblings with progressive familial cholestatic cirrhosis of childhood. Am J Clin Pathol. 1981;76:172–7.

12. Tazawa Y, Konno T. Familial cholestasis with gallstone, ataxia and visual disturbance. Tohoku J Exp Med. 1982;137:137–44.

13. Nakagawa M, Tazawa Y, Kobayashi Y, Yamada M, Suxuki H, Konno T, Tada K. Familial intrahepatic cholestasis associated with progressive neuromuscular disease and vitamin E deficiency. J Pediatr Gastroenterol Nutr. 1983;3:385–9.

14. Pincon JA, Chatelain P, Mallet-Guy Y, Bouvier R, de Parscau L, Francois R. Maladie de byler etude ultrastructurale; A propos d'une observation chez nourrisson. Pediatrie. 1984;4:279–88.

15. Haratake J, Horie A, Nobuyoshi I, Okuno F. Familial intrahepatic cholestatic cirrhosis in young adults. Gastroenterology. 1985;89:202–9.

16. Riely C. Familial intrahepatic cholestatic syndromes. Sem Liv Dis. 1987;7:119–33.

17. Whitington PF, Whitington GL. Partial external diversion of bile for the treatment of intractable pruritus associated with intrahepatic cholestasis. Gastroenterology. 1988;95:130–6.

18. Whitington PF, Freese DK, Alonso EM, Snover D, Montag A, Sharp HL, Schwarzenberg SJ. Progressive familial intrahepatic cholestasis. Clinical and histologic findings in thirty-three children and young adults. Gastroenterology. 1991 (In review).

19. Fishbein MH, Choe D, Whitington SH, Whitington PF. Progressive familial intrahepatic cholestasis: Serum and hepatic gamma glutamyl transpeptidase (GGTP) and canalicular membrane bile salt transport. Pediatr Res. 1991;29:102A.

20. Chobert MN, Barnard O, Bulle F, Lemonnier A, Guellaen G, Alagille D. High hepatic γ-glutamyltransferase (γ-GT) activity with normal serum γ-GT in children with progressive idiopathic cholestasis. J Hepatol. 1989;8:22–5.

18
Defect of biliary chenodeoxycholate secretion in Byler's disease

E. JACQUEMIN, O. BERNARD, M. DUMONT, S. ERLINGER and
M. HADCHOUEL

INTRODUCTION

Byler's disease, a familial intrahepatic cholestasis of childhood[1], has been attributed to a defect in bile acid metabolism, involving a primary bile acid secretion defect[2]. To pursue this hypothesis we tested the bile acid composition of serum and bile in five patients with Byler's disease.

PATIENTS

Criteria for Byler's disease have been described previously[3] (see also preceding chapter). Three of the five children had a sibling with the same disease. Serum and gallbladder bile samples were obtained at the time of percutaneous cholecystography or operative cholangiography after an overnight fast. Seven children with other types of liver diseases were studied as controls (Alagille syndrome $n = 2$, choledochal cyst $n = 1$, neonatal common bile duct lithiasis $n = 1$, sclerosing cholangitis $n = 1$, idiopathic gallbladder lithiasis $n = 1$, congenital hepatic fibrosis $n = 1$).

METHODS

Total bile acid concentration in bile and serum was measured by an enzymatic technique using 3α-hydroxysteroid dehydrogenase. Bile acid composition of bile and serum was analysed by high-pressure liquid chromatography. Bile acids were identified and quantified as their amidated conjugates.

RESULTS

In serum, total bile acid concentration (normal $< 6\,\mu\text{mol/l}$) was markedly increased in patients with Byler's disease (mean $\pm$ SD: $271 \pm 34\,\mu\text{mol/l}$)

as well as in control patients $(204 \pm 52\,\mu mol/l)$. Cholic acid (CA) and chenodeoxycholic acid (CDC) comprised the major proportion of bile acids (BA) in patients with Byler's disease (CA = 38% of total BA; CDC = 46%) as well as in control patients (CA = 66%; CDC = 23%). Hyocholic acid (HC) was found in all patients with Byler's disease (HC = 16%) and lithocholic acid (LC) was present only in control patients (LC = 16%).

In bile, total bile acid concentration (normal = 20–30 mmol/l) was very low in patients with Byler's disease $(0.8 \pm 1.0\,mmol/l)$ compared to control patients $(67 \pm 60\,mmol/l)$. Cholic acid and CDC were the major BA in control patients (CA = 66%; CDC = 34%), whereas CA and HC comprised the major proportion of BA in patients with Byler's disease (CA = 66%, HC = 30%). Of note, CDC was either absent from bile or detected in very low amount, varying from 0% to 8% of total BA, in patients with Byler's disease.

SUMMARY

In these patients with Byler's disease the bile acid composition of serum and bile was characterized by (1) the presence of a very low total bile acid concentration in bile, and a high total bile acid concentration in serum; (2) the absence, or a very low amount, of chenodeoxycholate in bile, despite its presence in considerable amount in serum; (3) the presence of hyocholate in serum and bile and the absence of lithocholate. Such a bile acid composition was not found in serum and bile of control patients.

CONCLUSION

Taken together these results suggest that: (1) patients with Byler's disease have a defect in biliary bile acid secretion, affecting mainly the biliary secretion of chenodeoxycholate; (2) the formation of hyocholate seems related to this defect and may prevent further hepatic accumulation of chenodeoxycholate.

We hypothesize that these patients with Byler's disease have an inborn error impairing the biliary secretion of chenodeoxycholate. A molecular step involved either in intracellular transport or canalicular secretion of bile salts might be related to this defect[4,5].

Acknowledgements

The authors thank Dr C. Juste for the supply of hyocholate.

References

1. Clayton RJ, Iber FL, Ruebner BH, McKusick VA. Byler disease. Fatal familial intrahepatic cholestasis in an Amish kindred. Am J Dis Child. 1969;117:112–24.

2. Tazawa Y, Yamada M, Nakagawa M, Konno T, Tada K. Bile acid profiles in siblings with progressive intrahepatic cholestasis: absence of biliary chenodeoxycholate. J Pediatr Gastroenterol Nutr. 1985;4:32–7.
3. Maggiore G, Bernard O, Riely CA, Hadchouel M, Lemonnier A, Allagile D. Normal gamma-glutamyl transpeptidase activity identifies groups of infants with idiopathic cholestasis with poor prognosis. J Pediatr. 1987;111:251–2.
4. Lamri Y, Roda A, Dumont M, Feldmann G, Erlinger S. Immunoperoxidase localisation of bile salts in rat liver cells. Evidence for a role of the Golgi apparatus in bile salt transport. J Clin Invest. 1988;82:1173–82.
5. Nishida T, Gaitmaitan Z, Che M, Arias IM. Rat liver canalicular membrane vesicles contain an ATP-dependent bile acid transport system. Proc Natl Acad Sci USA. 1991;88:6590–4.

19
Initial presentation of Byler's disease with profuse watery diarrhoea – involvement of regulatory gut peptides?

B. M. WINKLHOFER-ROOB, D. H. SHMERLING, W. H. HÄCKI and J. BRINER

INTRODUCTION

In 1965 Clayton and co-workers originally described a syndrome of familial intrahepatic cholestasis in an Amish family named Byler, that frequently led to death in early childhood[1,2]. The main clinical and laboratory features are quoted from this first description in Table 1. Since then, further cases have been documented and it became obvious that the clinical expression of the underlying disease, whose pathogenesis is still not fully understood, varies quite substantially. Undoubtedly, it may be a question of definition which cases are to be considered for inclusion in this entity. Conversely, more sophisticated methods will probably differentiate several more distinct entities within this syndrome.

The clinical course of a patient with Byler's disease recently treated in our

Table 1 First description of Byler's disease, by Clayton *et al.*

Clinical features
1   Loose, foul-smelling stools
2   Jaundice
3   Hepatosplenomegaly
4   Failure to thrive
5   Death

Laboratory findings
1   Hyperbilirubinaemia
2   Elevated serum alkaline phosphatase
3   Normal or low serum cholesterol
4   Hypoprothrombinaemia

"

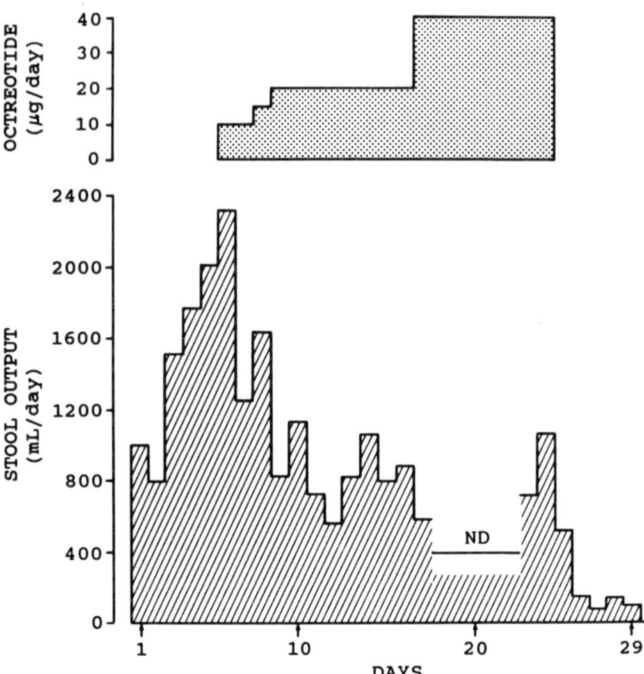

Fig. 1 Stool output (ml/day) during octreotide treatment (10–40 µg/day). ND = Stool output not determined

hospital focused our interest on diarrhoea as a significant presenting feature of the disease. The detailed case report is published elsewhere[3], and we restrict our description here to this particular aspect of the disease.

CASE REPORT

R.P., born 1986 as the second child of healthy unrelated parents, presented at 2 months of age with diarrhoea, elevated bilirubin, aspartate aminotransferase, and alanine aminotransferase. Cow's milk protein intolerance was suggested, but none of several dietary regimes was successful. Recurrent diarrhoeal episodes followed during the further course.

At 13 months of age, severe watery diarrhoea (> 2.5 l/day) ensued, which persisted under total parenteral nutrition and loperamide. Weight and height dropped below the 3rd percentile. Severe metabolic deficiencies were found. Usual causes of chronic infantile diarrhoea were excluded. Finally, treatment with daily 10–40 µg s.c. of a long-acting somatostatin analogue (octreotide, Sandostatin®, Sandoz, Basle, Switzerland) led to a substantial decrease in stool output after 4 days treatment (Fig. 1). In an endeavour to further reduce stool output the octreotide dosage was doubled, yet normalization was achieved only after complete cessation of the treatment. A further episode of watery diarrhoea 2 weeks later responded promptly to octreotide.

Table 2 Regulatory gut peptides (pmol/l) in plasma at three occasions with (*) and without octreotide treatment

Age (months)	VIP	Gastrin	GRP	NT	SMS	PP
14.0*	36	90	30	21	28	12
14.5	58	78	71	22	38	20
15.0	41	55	100	18	42	18
Normal†	< 40	< 25	< 50	< 40	< 50	< 50

†Normal values from our laboratory. Abbreviations: VIP = vasoactive intestinal polypeptide, GRP = gastrin-releasing peptide, NT = neurotensin, SMS = somatostatin, PP = pancreatic polypeptide. Data obtained from ref. 3 with permission

Vasoactive polypeptide (VIP), gastrin-releasing peptide (GRP), and gastrin were elevated in the untreated patient. Under octreotide, VIP and GRP were normal, yet gastrin was elevated on each occasion. Neurotensin (NT) and pancreatic polypeptide (PP) were normal (Table 2). Later on the child did not exhibit any further similar episodes of diarrhoea.

At 1 year 10 months, increasing jaundice with acholic stools and pruritus appeared. γ-Glutamyltransferase remained normal in contrast to other laboratory indices for cholestasis. Mild diarrhoea alternated with acholic fatty stools. Repeated infections occurred throughout the course. At 3 years 6 months the boy died of fulminant purulent meningitis. Liver histology (intra-acinar and intracellular cholestasis, bile duct paucity, bile duct proliferation, slight fibrosis of the portal area) as well as the clinical and laboratory findings are in agreement with the very first description of Byler's disease by Clayton and co-workers[2].

DISCUSSION

The presentation of our patient with severe and persistent diarrhoeal episodes has attracted our attention and prompted a comparison with the clinical course of patients documented in the literature. In four of the seven cases documented by Clayton and co-workers[1,2] 'loose, foul-smelling stools', which are considered as one of the main features of the disease, were followed by diarrhoea. For case 3 'worsening diarrhoea during 6 years' is reported, case 4 'developed severe haemorrhagic gastroenteritis at 31 mo. and died', case 5 showed 'worsening of diarrhoea', and in case 6 'milk allergy was suspected, but frequent formula changes did not influence the character of the stools'. Linarelli and co-workers[4] reported for their patient that 'loose bowel movements became profuse and persistent by 6 weeks of age'. The latter patient presented with bloody diarrhoea besides all the other main features of the disease and 'both diarrhoea and jaundice persisted over 5 months'. Another patient described by Van Acker et al.[5] exhibited an 'abrupt deterioration with rapidly progressive jaundice and abundant watery stools'. Other groups, however, did not describe diarrhoea as a prominent feature in their cases with Byler's disease[6,7]. This possibly could indicate that different entities within this syndrome should be considered.

There is no evidence that severe and persistent diarrhoea is directly linked, as a consequence, to cholestatic liver disease. In this context it is an essential observation that diarrhoea persists even after successful liver transplantation (personal communication, M. Burdelski).

Persisting stool outputs up to 2.5 l/day, even under total parenteral nutrition and loperamide, have been attributed to secretory diarrhoea in our patient. Unfortunately, stool osmolality and stool electrolytes have not been monitored, neither before nor under treatment with octreotide, so that there is no direct proof whether the mechanisms causing diarrhoea did actually involve secretory processes. Yet neurotensin, which is secreted in the distal ileum and stimulated by intraluminal nutrients in malabsorptive states, was not elevated. These normal concentrations, even without somatostatin treatment, are an argument against malabsorption as a cause of the observed diarrhoea. There is also no evidence for an involvement of cholinergic mechanisms, because pancreatic polypeptide concentrations were within the normal range.

As can be seen from Fig. 1, stool output decreased drastically under octreotide, a long-acting octapeptide analogue of somatostatin, which inhibits experimentally induced intestinal secretion. It has been successfully used in the treatment of patients with secretory diarrhoea. Although the mechanism for the inhibitory effect on intestinal secretion is not fully understood, it is suggested to involve an inhibition of the adenyl-cyclic adenosine mono-phosphate system as well as an interference with calcium as an intracellular mediator of enterocyte secretion[8]. The reduction of plasma levels of regulatory peptides may contribute to the efficacy, but therapeutic effects in non-endocrine secretory diarrhoea have also been documented[8]. The effective dose is considered to be 0.7–2.8 µg per kg given twice or three times daily subcutaneously. There was no evidence in our patient that the higher dosage (2.1 µg/kg twice daily) exhibited a further beneficial effect. So far, there is no explanation for the observation that only the cessation of the medication was followed by a normalization of stool output.

Determinations of regulatory gut peptides in the plasma, one during octreotide treatment and two in the untreated patient, yielded elevated concentrations for gastrin on all occasions. GRP was substantially, and VIP slightly elevated without treatment, yet, as expected, was normal under octreotide. GRP has been proposed to play a local role in stimulating the release of antral mucosal gastrin[9]. In addition, there is evidence that somatostatin plays an inhibitory role in the regulation of gastrin release[10]. In our patient, however, gastrin was still elevated under octreotide therapy, and interestingly, in the presence of normal GRP. Obviously, more data are needed to draw any conclusions for pathophysiological considerations.

So far, it is not quite clear whether these findings are indicative of a particular involvement of regulatory gut peptides in Byler's disease, or otherwise represent an unspecific and epiphenomenal finding within a complex syndrome. Further investigations of regulatory gut peptides in patients with Byler's disease exhibiting diarrhoea are warranted to confirm these findings and to elucidate possible implications for pathogenetic mechanisms of the disease.

References

1. Clayton RJ, Iber FL, Ruebner BH, McKusick VA. Byler's disease: Fatal familial intrahepatic cholestasis in an Amish kindred. Am Pediatr Soc. 1965;67:1025–8 (abstr.).
2. Clayton RJ, Iber FL, Ruebner BH, McKusick VA. Byler disease. Fatal familial intrahepatic cholestasis in an Amish kindred. Am J Dis Child. 1969;117:112–24.
3. Winklhofer-Roob BM, Shmerling DH, Solèr R, Briner J. Progressive idiopathic cholestasis presenting with profuse watery diarrhoea and recurrent infections (Byler's disease). Acta Paediatr Scand. 1992 (In press).
4. Linarelli LG, Williams CN, Phillips MJ. Byler's disease: fatal intrahepatic cholestasis. J Pediatr. 1972;81:484–92.
5. Van Acker KJ, Eggermont E, Deprettere A, Marien P. Fatal familial intrahepatic cholestasis (Byler disease). Acta Paediatr Belg. 1977;30:157–63.
6. Williams CN, Kaye R, Baker L, Hurwitz R, Senior JR. Progressive familial cholestatic cirrhosis and bile acid metabolism. J Pediatr. 1972;81:493–500.
7. Razemon-Pinta M, Lecomte-Houcke M, Mary JP, Loreille GA. La maladie de Byler (cholestase familiale fibrogène de l'enfant). A propos de 7 cas. Pédiatrie. 1988;43:361–70.
8. Gaginella TS, O'Dorisio TM, Fassler JE, Mekhjian HS. Treatment of endocrine and nonendocrine secretory diarrheal states with Sandostatin®. Metabolism. 1990;39(Suppl. 2):172–5.
9. McGuigan JE. Hormones of the gastrointestinal tract. In: DeGroot LJ, editor. Endocrinology. Philadelphia: W.B. Saunders; 1989;2741–68.
10. Wolfe MM, Reel GM, McGuigan JE. Inhibition of gastrin release by secretin is mediated by somatostatin in cultured rat antral mucosa. J Clin Invest. 1983;72:1586–93.

20
Total parenteral nutrition-associated cholestasis: factors responsible for the decreasing incidence

W. F. BALISTRERI, J. C. BUCUVALAS, M. K. FARRELL and
K. E. BOVE

INTRODUCTION

When *enteral* alimentation is not possible, sufficient calories and essential
nutrients can be infused intravenously to sustain growth of an infant[1]. The
documented efficacy of this route of nutrient delivery as the only source of
calories allowed total parenteral nutrition (TPN) to gain wide acceptance.
However, the intravenous route of nutrition administration has been associated with a wide spectrum of adverse hepatobiliary consequences including
asymptomatic abnormalities in biochemical indicators of hepatobiliary integrity, biliary sludge, fatty liver, and *cholestasis*, with the potential for
progression to end-stage liver disease[1-8]. TPN-associated cholestasis (TPN-
AC) was most frequently documented in infants, especially those born
prematurely, in whom the exclusive intravenous infusion of nutrients presumably catalysed deleterious intrahepatic reactions[1,2]. In recent years the
incidence of TPN-AC has apparently decreased; however, this enigmatic and
potentially fatal complication remains the limiting factor in the effective *long-
term* use of TPN as a nutritional modality in low birth weight infants,
supplanting sepsis and malnutrition as the leading cause of death in this
population[9]. While the pathogenesis of TPN-AC in infants remains poorly
defined, an analysis of factors associated with the declining incidence has
offered new clues.

HISTORICAL PERSPECTIVE

TPN-associated liver dysfunction was most frequently noted in small,
critically ill neonates whose clinical picture was dominated by hypotension,
hypoxaemia, sepsis and/or failure or dysfunction of multiple organ sys-

tems[1,2,10]. TPN-AC was first described in a premature infant who had received lifelong parenteral nutrition; postmortem findings (71 days) included prominent bile duct proliferation with centrilobular cholestasis and cirrhosis[7]. Subsequent studies documented the *reproducibility* of TPN-AC as a major complication of exclusive long-term TPN without enteral feeding[1,48].

Historically, the incidence of TPN-AC was noted to correlate inversely with gestational age and birth weight[1,2,8,11–16]. Cholestasis occurred in 20–25% of low birth weight infants who received TPN, progressed as long as the infant continued to receive exclusive parenteral nutrition, and persisted for a variable period following discontinuation[11]. The incidence of cholestasis was as high as 50% in infants whose birth weight was less than 1000 g[11]. The incidence of TPN-AC also correlated with the *duration* of administration of the infusate[11,13], becoming more frequent in those infants who received TPN for more than 2 weeks[11,17,18]. In recent years the incidence of TPN-AC has decreased substantially; at present, hepatobiliary injury appears to occur only in infants who require *prolonged* TPN.

The role of other factors in the incidence of TPN-AC, such as the route of administration, comorbidity (pre- or perinatal), and the precise composition and balance of the individual constituents, is less clear[19]. Cholestasis has been noted to be associated with neonatal insults associated with *hypoxia* (respiratory distress or bleeding), *gastrointestinal* conditions requiring surgery, or *sepsis*; these factors may not only contribute to the development of TPN-AC, but also enhance the severity[1,2,19]. The precise contribution of factors such as the concomitant medication administration and delayed enteral feedings are difficult to separate as individual variables, since each is influenced by the indication for the use of TPN and the severity of the illness[1,2].

CLINICAL FEATURES

Although diminishing in frequency, TPN-AC may be noted at some point in the clinical course of infants who are unable to tolerate even small amounts of enteral feedings and cannot ingest sufficient calories to sustain life or promote growth[1,2]. The onset is insidious – during routine serial monitoring the infant most often is noted to have a progressive rise above baseline of biochemical markers of cholestasis, such as serum bilirubin or serum bile acid levels, often without an increase in aminotransferase values[1,2,11–13,20]. We believe that serum bile acid concentrations may be a sensitive indicator of hepatic dysfunction[12,21–23]; an elevated serum bile acid concentration was the initial biochemical abnormality in infants receiving TPN for more than 2 weeks[23,24]. Later in the course of TPN, serum aminotransferase activity may be mildly to moderately elevated. Hepatic synthetic function is normal.

TPN-AC remains a diagnosis of exclusion since specific clinical biochemical or histological criteria are lacking. Consideration of other causes of conjugated hyperbilirubinaemia is the first priority[1,2,24]. Every infant with cholestasis should be evaluated for the possibility of an alternative cause of hepatobiliary dysfunction, otherwise readily reversible disorders may be overlooked or the parenteral nutrition may inappropriately be discontinued. If the clinical and/or biochemical features are not typical, or remain enigmatic, needle biopsy of the liver may help to clarify the nature of the hepatobiliary disorder. In older patients hepatomegaly may occur due to excessive deposition of glycogen and/or fat[25-38]. Hepatomegaly without cholestasis is not associated with progressive liver disease[25,27,28,39].

Despite reports of distinct elevations in aminotransferase and alkaline phosphatase levels in older children or adults receiving long-term TPN, there are few data which correlate these biochemical changes with hepatic histology since biopsies are rarely performed[18,25-35]. The histological changes that have been noted in adults consisted primarily of *steatosis*; true cholestasis, as seen in the newborn patients, is uncommon[1,2,25,29]. In adults the serum bilirubin levels are typically not elevated, further suggesting an alternative genesis and pathophysiology from infantile TPN-AC[34-38].

There are also multiple reports of specific *biliary* complications of intravenous nutrition, namely, the development of cholelithiasis and acalculous cholecystitis[40-45]; however, the relationship to TPN-AC is unclear. Gallstones, composed predominantly of calcium bilirubinate, may develop in up to 40% of children requiring TPN for a minimum of 3 months[44]. Risk factors that predispose to cholelithiasis include ileal disease, lack of an ileocaecal valve, short bowel syndrome, furosemide administration (especially common in the low birth weight infant), an increased number of abdominal operative procedures, and a longer duration of parenteral feeding; there is a higher coincidence of both cholestasis and necrotizing enterocolitis[40-45]. These specific biliary complications might be readily susceptible to treatment with choleretic agents, such as ursodeoxycholic acid.

PATHOLOGY

The histological changes noted in the liver of infants receiving prolonged TPN are non-specific and highly variable[1-3,46-49]. The major component is intralobular cholestasis, alone or in conjunction with an inflammatory portal tract lesion, which may be suggestive of biliary obstruction and may be accompanied by progressive portal fibrosis. Canalicular and cytoplasmic bile stasis are found with a predilection to severe expression in the central lobular region[1,2,47]. Giant cell transformation of hepatocytes is rarely prominent. Fatty change in hepatocytes is an inconstant finding in infants; this feature has been attributed to adults to an unbalanced composition of the infusate[1,50-52]. Kupffer cells and portal macrophages are often hyperplastic, containing abdundant, brown-staining lipofuscin pigment. Persistent sinusoidal erythropoiesis may be prominent; however, stimulation of extramedullary haematopoiesis by underlying conditions cannot be clearly distinguished from a direct effect of the infusate. Portal inflammation (mononuclear cells and neutrophils) is often accompanied by mild to moderate bile duct proliferation with occasional evidence of ductular bile plug formation in those patients with TPN-AC of longer duration[47]. This persistent portal reaction may be followed by creeping portal fibrosis and, in some instances, cirrhosis[27,47,48].

Table 1 Correlation of postmortem hepatic histological features with coexisting morbidity in infants who had received TPN (Children's Hospital Medical Center, Cincinnati, OH, 1971–87)

Liver lesion	No. of patients	Mean age at death (days)	Co-morbidity*
Intralobular cholestasis alone	5	42	0
No chronic lesion	18	57	6
Portal triaditis/variable fibrosis	9	82	8
Cirrhosis	8	225	7
Portal fibrosis (late death)	1	225	1
Central fibrosis	2	30/300	2

*Asphyxia, necrotizing enterocolitis, or other gastrointestinal disease
Modified from ref. 1.

Despite the coexistence of asphyxial episodes in the perinatal period of infants who eventually develop TPN-associated liver injury, hepatic changes typical of poor perfusion are not seen.

CHILDREN'S HOSPITAL MEDICAL CENTER EXPERIENCE

In order to assess the severity of liver injury or exclude an alternative diagnosis, liver biopsies were performed in 20 TPN recipients with prolonged cholestasis over a 15-year period at Children's Hospital Medical Center, Cincinnati, Ohio; this represents a minute subset of the numerous babies who received TPN in our own institution[1,2]. All of these patients were infants who had received TPN for several weeks in the absence of enteral feedings. Intralobular cholestasis and portal triaditis with variable fibrosis was present in virtually all specimens. Subsequent progression of portal fibrosis to cirrhosis was documented in several patients. Proliferative changes in small bile ducts were common, simulating obstruction; however, the presence of ductular bile plugs seemed to have no relationship to progressive liver disease.

During the same period, a group of 43 infants died of their underlying disease, after having received TPN for variable periods (2 weeks to 10 months) (Table 1)[1]. We noted that the severity of liver histological changes was strongly associated with age at death and with antecedent asphyxia and/or neonatal gastrointestinal catastrophes[1]. These findings suggest that the vulnerability of infants to TPN-associated progressive liver disease is not only a function of the time of exposure but may also be a sequel to liver injury due to hypoperfusion, alone or in conjunction with byproducts of intestinal injury or stasis such as bacterial toxins or monohydroxy bile acids. This observation offers insight into the pathophysiology as well as the factors responsible for the recent decline in the incidence of TPN-AC, as discussed below.

Table 2 Multifactorial genesis of TPN-cholestasis

A. Immature hepatic function
  1. Low rates of bile flow
  2. Production of abnormal (? toxic) bile acids
     (a) Intrahepatic (altered biosynthesis)
     (b) Intraintestinal (bacterial biotransformation)

B. Toxicity
  1. Amino acids
     (a) Specific toxic components
     (b) Photo-oxidation products
     (c) Imbalance
  2. Improper caloric (dextrose) and protein loads
  3. Bile acid (monohydroxy)
  4. Lipids
  5. Trace elements
  6. Other constituents (e.g. aluminium)

C. Specific deficiencies (e.g. antioxidants and essential nutrients)
  1. Taurine
  2. Glutathione
  3. Vitamin E/selenium
  4. Trace elements
  5. Essential fatty acids
  6. Carnitine

D. Perinatal insults
  1. 'Enteral starvation' (NPO)
     (a) Output of gastrointestinal hormones decreased
     (b) Decreased vagal stimulation
     (c) Specific trophic effect of intraluminal nutrients absent
  2. Free-radical stress
  3. Hypoxia/hypoperfusion (and reperfusion injury)
  4. Intestinal disease (e.g. necrotizing enterocolitis, bacterial overgrowth, factors enhancing translocation)
  5. Sepsis (endotoxaemia)
  6. Exposure to hepatotrophic virus (especially transfusion-related)
  7. Drugs

Modified from ref. 1.

PATHOPHYSIOLOGY

The pathogenesis of liver injury during TPN in infants is presumably *multifactorial*, as outlined in Table 2[1,2,27,53,54]. The administration of a nutrient solution, which may be directly damaging to hepatocyte structure and function, occurs in a clinical milieu complicated by *confounding* features – the patient is often of low birth weight, is receiving nothing by mouth, may have sepsis, is exposed to multiple medications, may have cardiopulmonary failure, and often has serious gastrointestinal disease. This clinical setting may be compounded by potential toxicities and deficiencies engendered by the infusion. There may also be limited capacity for the infantile liver to resist *oxidant* stress due to a relative antioxidant deficiency[55,56].

Despite the frequency of hepatobiliary dysfunction in low birth weight infants during TPN infusion, there are few prospective or controlled studies addressing the disorder. In part this is due to the fact that confounding

Table 3 'Physiological cholestasis' – experimental evidence indicating a decreased capacity for bile acid transport and metabolism in early life[21,22,56,59]

1. ↑ Serum bile acid concentrations (human neonates and rats)
2. ↓ Uptake of bile acids (isolated rat hepatocytes, basolateral membrane vesicles)
3. Altered intracellular binding or transport
4. ↓ Biotransformation (conjugation and sulphation) and low levels of specific enzyme activity (ligase, N-acyltransferase) in rat hepatocytes
5. Altered bile acid synthesis (quantitative and qualitative)
6. Low bile flow rates
7. Contracted bile acid pool size
8. ↓ Intraluminal bile acid levels
9. ↓ Ileal active bile acid transport

variables are often not readily susceptible to analysis; for example, although the high prevalence of TPN-AC in premature infants would suggest that immaturity of hepatic excretory function is a prime factor in pathogenesis, it is this group of patients who usually require prolonged parenteral nutrition.

The most obvious predisposing factor (Table 2) is *immaturity of hepatic excretory function* (bile formation), a state of 'physiological cholestasis'[1,2,21,22]. The primary motive force in bile formation is the efficient enterohepatic circulation of bile acids; therefore, altered bile acid metabolism and transport by the immature hepatocytes (Table 3) may initiate the cholestatic tendency in a low birth weight infant[1,21,22,57]. Amino acid administration may further imbalance this precarious, vulnerable situation[58]. There is discordance between the ontogeny of bile acid and amino acid transport mechanisms; therefore the elevated plasma amino acid concentrations in early life enhance the inhibitory effects of amino acids on bile acid uptake by the developing liver[59,60]. The net effect may be a diminished bile acid excretion and therefore decreased bile flow[1,60,61].

The immature hepatocyte also produces abnormal, potentially toxic, bile acids, such as monohydroxy bile acids (lithocholate) via fetal bile acid pathways[21,22,59,62,63]. The hepatic histological alterations noted in TPN-AC resemble the changes induced by lithocholate infusion to experimental animals[1,2,62].

The exclusive intravenous infusion of a nutrient solution predicted to meet all requirements might engender specific *deficiencies*[1,2]; for example, hepatic glutathione depletion in the presence of a relative deficiency of antioxidants may render the infantile liver more suceptible to oxidant (free-radical)-induced hepatocellular injury[55,56].

Other perinatal factors (Table 2) may interact to further exacerbate hepatic dysfunction in a sick premature infant who requires TPN[1]. The mandated 'enteral starvation' and deprivation of intraluminal nutrients further decreases the enterohepatic recirculation of bile acids, thereby decreasing bile flow. Enteral starvation blunts the output of gastrointestinal hormones normally released by oral nutrient intake, such as cholecystokinin, secretin, gastrin, neurotensin, and glucagon, which are normal stimulants to bile flow[64-70]. Gut hypomotility, which also attends enteral starvation, may contribute to hepatic injury and elevated bilirubin levels[71]. Alterations in motility are associated with *bacterial overgrowth* of the small intestine; the abundant flora may produce hepatotoxic agents, such as bacterial byproducts, endotoxin and lithocholate. Fasting may also decrease the inactivation of chemically reactive metabolites by glutathione and increase their hepatotoxicity[72].

Sepsis also exacerbates these cholestatic tendencies of the low birth weight infant; in fact, cholestasis has been detected in neonates with bacterial sepsis *not* receiving parenteral alimentation[73]. Intrahepatic cholestasis associated with inspissated bile within dilated and proliferated portal and periportal bile ductules has been attributed to sepsis[73,74]. TPN may contribute by promoting bacterial translocation from the gut via impairment of intestinal defence mechanisms and induction of small bowel bacterial overgrowth[75]. Absorbed bacterial endotoxins, such as those produced by *Escherichia coli*, are capable of inhibiting bile flow[76-78]. In fact the *serum* of a patient who became jaundiced while receiving long-term TPN caused a decrease in bile flow in rats; the suspected toxic circulating factor was neutralized with antiserum to *E. coli* endotoxin[79].

Intestinal bacteria and their byproducts have been associated with extraintestinal inflammation; however, the potential mechanisms, other than molecular mimicry, are not understood[80-85]. Poorly degradable bacterial cell wall polymers derived from the enteric flora may exert potent immunostimulatory and inflammatory effects[80-82]. Lichtman *et al.* have developed an animal model of hepatobiliary injury (portal inflammation and bile duct proliferation) associated with small bowel bacterial overgrowth and defined the mechanism and the site of injury[81-84]. In this model there was no evidence of previously postulated factors such as specific direct hepatic infection, portal vein bacteraemia, or toxic bile acids[81]. The hepatobiliary lesions were *not* prevented by the prior administration of ursodeoxycholic acid, prednisone, cyclosporin or methotrexate[81-84]. The authors concluded that mucosal absorption of bacterial cell wall polymers from intraluminal anaerobic bacteria was responsible for the hepatobiliary lesions. The amount of toxic bacterial byproduct absorbed correlated directly with the degree of mucosal injury. While gentamicin and polymyxin did not prevent the development of the hepatobiliary lesions, tetracycline and metronidazole were effective, perhaps by reversing the *intestinal* mucosal injury, thereby preventing absorption of toxins[84]. The investigators specifically postulated that peptido-glycan–polysaccharide (PG-PS) polymers, which are present in the cell wall of many bacteria, were involved in the pathogenesis of hepatobiliary injury. Targeted disruption of the PG-PS polymer by mutanolysin, an enzyme which degrades PG-PS, prevented hepatobiliary injury[85,86]. It is possible that PG-PS, arising from enteric bacteria, activate Kupffer cell production of soluble inflammatory mediators such as TNF (tumour necrosis factor), which in turn initiates or perpetuates hepatic injury[86]. In rats with sepsis TPN augments the deleterious effects of TNF on vascular and endothelial cell function, as well as on liver function[87,88]. TNF and other cytokines may mediate cholestasis via inhibition of hepatic NaK-ATPase, thereby decreasing bile acid uptake by the liver[89].

Our observations (Table 1) indicate that infants who require TPN and develop cholestasis often have had serious antecedent intestinal disease such as meconium peritonitis, necrotizing enterocolitis, atresia, or malrotation

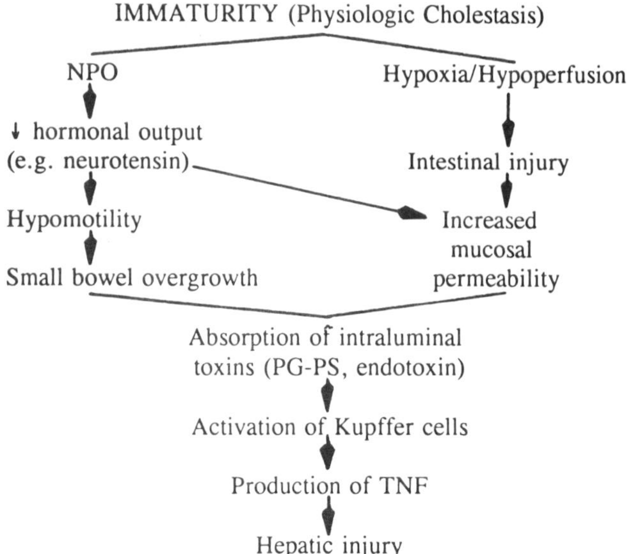

Fig. 1 *Unifying hypothesis*, interrelating several potential factors in the pathogenesis of TPN-associated hepatobiliary injury in low birth weight infants. Attendant to the multi-organ effects of premature birth, including a cholestatic tendency and a relative antioxidant deficiency, the immature infant is often unable to be fed via the enteral route (NPO) and must receive total parenteral nutrition (TPN). The absence of trophic hormones, such as neurotensin, leads to hypomotility with bacterial overgrowth and increased mucosal permeability. The latter may be abetted by *direct* intestinal injury due to hypoxia/hypoperfusion or reperfusion injury. The net result is an increased production and/or absorption of bacterial byproducts such as cell wall polysaccharides (peptidoglycan–polysaccharide; PG–PS), endotoxin, or secondary bile acids which may activate Kupffer cells, leading to an increased production of tumour necrosis factor (TNF), which mediates injury to a uniquely susceptible liver

with volvulus. In fact, at present in our institution, infants with documented TPN-AC most likely emerge from this subset. Massive loss of intestine is also associated with end-stage liver disease in adults receiving long-term TPN[90,91].

A unifying hypothesis of the pathogenesis to TPN-AC, interrelating sepsis and intestinal injury can therefore be generated (Fig. 1). This hypothesis also offers a conceptual framework to explain the apparent decline in the incidence of TPN-AC. For example, incremental improvement in the techniques of neonatal supportive care and the aggressive and early amelioration of hypoxaemia and hypotension might avoid initiation of the cascade leading to hepatobiliary injury (Fig. 1). The recent trend of early introduction of enteral feeding may allow stimulation of hormone release and thereby increase gut motility and bile flow. Alterations in gastrointestinal flora and a decrease in the incidence of necrotizing enterocolitis must also be incorporated into this concept. Whether the altered composition (qualitative or quantitative) of TPN solutions or a decrease in administered protein content contributes to the diminishing incidence remains to be proven. This unifying hypothesis also offers a rationale for management and perhaps prevention of TPN-AC.

MANAGEMENT

What is the optimal management of the infant who requires continual, optimal nutritional input yet has developed cholestasis during hyperalimentation? After other causes of cholestasis have been excluded, oral alimentation (continuous or bolus) should be initiated, even if only small volumes (1–2 ml/h) are tolerated. This should be the goal for *all* infants as the duration of TPN reaches 10–14 days. In patients in whom oral feedings are able to be administered, a slow, gradual resolution of hepatobiliary injury will occur[1,2,32]; portal fibrosis may persist[1]. The mechanism by which oral intake aids in aborting the development of cholestasis or decreasing the severity of hepatobiliary complications is presumably related to the tremendous surge in trophic and choleretic enteric hormones which occurs in response to early feeding[64,67]. Preliminary data support the hypothesis that early, even hypocaloric enteral feedings, will reduce the incidence of TPN-AC[92,93]; however, further studies are needed.

Certain infants are afflicted with severe gastrointestinal disease (e.g. short bowel syndrome) which precludes the administration of enteral nutrition in sufficient quantities to assure continued optimal growth. In these infants TPN-associated hepatic dysfunction may progress as long as the infusion continues[1,2,90,91,94–96]. For these patients there are several theoretical possibilities which may help ameliorate TPN-AC; however, there is very little supportive data: (1) alter the composition of the alimentation solution; e.g. use a taurine-containing parenteral amino acid mixture designed to maintain normal plasma amino acid concentrations[97,98]; (2) avoid 'oxidant–antioxidant imbalance' via restriction of the amount of copper and iron[99] and perhaps by provision of antioxidants (vitamin E, glutathione)[55,56,100,101]; (3) protect the TPN bottle from light, thereby reducing the potential for photo-oxidation and the resultant creation of toxic photo-products[102–104]; (4) stimulate bile flow via intermittent injections of CCK, phenobarbital[105], ceruletide, an analogue of CCK[106], or ursodeoxycholic acid (UDCA)[107,108].

UDCA, which has reported benefit in a wide variety of cholestatic disorders in adults and children, may be a safe and useful therapeutic agent for TPN-associated hepatobiliary dysfunction[107]. Lindor and Burnes have recently reported that UDCA administration was associated with a prompt and sustained decline in serum bilirubin levels in a patient who had developed TPN-AC[108]. The jaundice returned when UDCA was discontinued and once again abated with reinstitution. This ameliorative effect of UDCA may be related to: (1) the choleretic properties of this agent, (2) the displacement of toxic endogenous bile acids, (3) a specific cytoprotective effect on liver cell membranes, or (4) an effect on the intestinal mucosa[107]. For the patient who, despite all efforts, develops end-stage liver disease while receiving long-term TPN in the management of the short bowel syndrome, combined liver/small bowel transplantation might be a consideration[109].

SUMMARY

The routine practice of exclusive parenteral nutrient infusion (TPN) in efforts to promote growth and sustain nutrient homeostasis carries the risk of hepatobiliary injury. These reproducible abnormalities remain enigmatic, and despite a decline in the incidence of TPN-AC further detailed studies are needed. Precise prospective assessment of the relationship of all potential confounding factors is needed to further clarify the elements involved in progressive TPN-associated liver disease. In addition, basic research addressing the potential injurious factors is needed. For example, in order to test the unifying hypothesis (Figure 1), it may be fruitful to study the effect of intragastric neurotensin[69] or anti-TNF antibodies[109] in an experimental model. Regardless of the pathogenesis of TPN-AC, the possible risk of further hepatic injury by continued administration of the infusate must be weighed against the known risk of malnutrition in patients who cannot receive adequate oral nutrition.

Acknowledgements

The authors are grateful to Ms. Judy Dyrud for manuscript preparation, and Dr Steven Lichtman for his helpful comments.

References

1. Balistreri WF, Bove KE. Hepatobiliary consequences of parenteral nutrition. In: Progress in liver disease. New York: Grune and Stratton; 1989: IX:567–601.
2. Balistreri WF, Novak DA, Farrell MK. Bile acid metabolism, total parenteral nutrition and cholestasis. In: Lebenthal E, editor. Total parenteral nutrition – indications, complications and pathophysiological considerations in total parenteral nutrition and home total parenteral nutrition. New York: Raven Press; 1986:319–34.
3. Bernstein J, Chang C-H, Brough AJ, Heidelberger KP. Conjugated hyperbilirubinemia in infancy associated with parenteral alimentation. J Pediatr. 1977;90:361–7.
4. Postuma R, Trevenen CL. Liver disease in infants receiving total parenteral nutrition. Pediatrics. 1979;63:110–15.
5. Sondheimer JM, Bryan H, Andrews W, Forstner GG. Cholestatic tendencies in premature infants on and off parenteral nutrition. Pediatrics. 1978;62:984–9.
6. Bove KE, Kosmetatos N, Wedig KE et al. Vasculopathic hepatotoxicity associated with E-Ferol syndrome in low birthweight infants. J Am Med Assoc. 1985;254:2422–30.
7. Peden VH, Witzleben CL, Skelton MA. Total parenteral nutrition. J Pediatr. 1971;78:180–1.
8. Touloukian RJ, Seashore JH. Hepatic secretory obstruction with total parenteral nutrition in the infant. J Pediatr Surg. 19975;10:353–60.
9. Schwartz MZ, Maeda K. Short bowel syndrome in infants and children. Pediatr Clin N Am. 1985;32:1265–79.
10. Manginello FP, Javitt NB. Parenteral nutrition and neonatal cholestasis. J Pediatr. 1979;94:296–8.
11. Beale EF, Nelson RM, Bucciarelli RL et al. Intrahepatic cholestasis associated with parenteral nutrition in premature infants. Pediatrics. 1979;64:342–7.
12. Farrell MK, Balistreri WF, Suchy FJ. Serum sulfated lithocholate as an indicator of cholestasis during parenteral nutrition in infants and children. J Parent Ent Nutr. 1982;6:30–3.

13. Pereira GR, Sherman MS, DiGiacomo J *et al.* Hyperalimentation-induced cholestasis: Increased incidence and severity in premature infants. Am J Dis Child. 1981;135:842–5.
14. Seashore JH. Metabolic complications of parenteral nutrition in infants and children. Surg Clin N Am. 1980;60:1239–52.
15. Touloukian RJ, Downing SE. Cholestasis associated with long-term parenteral hyperalimentation. Arch Surg. 1973;106:58–62.
16. Zarif MA, Pildes RS, Szanto PB *et al.* Cholestasis associated with administration of L-amino acids and dextrose solutions. Biol Neonate. 1976;29:66–76.
17. Vileisis RA, Inwood RJ, Hunt CE. Prospective controlled study of parenteral nutrition-associated cholestatic jaundice: effect of protein intake. J Pediatr. 1980;96:893–7.
18. Cannon RA, Byrne WJ, Ament ME *et al.* Home parenteral nutrition. J Pediatr. 1980;96:1098–104.
19. Bell RL, Ferry GD, Smith EO *et al.* Total parenteral nutrition-related cholestasis in infants. J Parent Ent Nutr. 1986;10:356–9.
20. Black DD, Suttle EA, Whitington PF *et al.* The effect of short term total parenteral nutrition on hepatic function in the human neonate: a prospective randomized study demonstrating alteration of hepatic canalicular function. J Pediatr. 1981;99:445–9.
21. Balistreri WF, Heubi JE, Suchy FJ. Immaturity of the enterohepatic circulation in early life: factors predisposing to 'physiologic' maldigestion and cholestasis. J Pediatr Gastroenterol Nutr. 1983;2:346–54.
22. Balistreri WF. Fetal and bile acid synthesis and metabolism – clinical implications. J Inher Metab Dis. 1991;14:459–77.
23. Farrell MK, Gilster S, Balistreri WF. Serum bile acids: an early indicator of parenteral nutrition-associated liver disease. Gastroenterology. 1984;86:1074.
24. Farrell MK, Schilling S, Gorgone PA *et al.* All parenteral nutrition associated cholestasis is not solely to parenteral nutrition. Pediatr Res. 1980;20:239A.
25. Baker AL, Rosenberg IH. Hepatic complications of total parenteral nutrition. Am J Med. 1987;82:489–97.
26. Bowyer BA, Fleming CR, Ludwig J *et al.* Does long-term home parenteral nutrition in adult patients cause chronic liver disease. J Parent Ent Nutr. 1985;9:11–17.
27. Merritt RJ. Cholestasis associated with total parenteral nutrition. J Pediatr Gastroenterol Nutr. 1986;5:9–22.
28. Lindor KD, Fleming CR, Abrams A, Hirschkorn MA. Liver function values in adults receiving total parenteral nutrition. J Am Med Assoc. 1979;241:2398–400.
29. Bower RH. Hepatic complications of parenteral nutrition. Semin Liver Dis. 1983;3:216–24.
30. Jeejeebhoy KN, Langer B, Tsallas G *et al.* Total parenteral nutrition at home: studies in patients surviving 4 months to 5 years. Gastroenterology. 1976;71:943–53.
31. Kibort PM, Ulich TR, Berquist WE *et al.* Hepatic fibrosis and cirrhosis in children on long-term total parenteral nutrition. Gastroenterology. 1982;82:1099.
32. Pallares R, Sitges-Serra A, Fuentes J *et al.* Cholestasis associated with total parenteral nutrition. Lancet. 1983;1:758–9.
33. Robertson JFR, Garden OJ, Shenkin A. Intravenous nutrition and hepatic dysfunction. J Parent Ent Nutr. 1986;10:172–6.
34. Nanji AA, Anderson FH. Sensitivity and specificity of liver function tests in the detection of parenteral nutrition-associated cholestasis. J Parent Ent Nutr. 1985;9:307–8.
35. Bengoa JM, Hanauer SB, Sitrin MD *et al.* Pattern and prognosis of liver function test abnormalities during parenteral nutrition in inflammatory bowel disease. Hepatology. 1985;5:79–84.
36. Wagman LD, Burt ME, Brennan MF. The impact of total parenteral nutrition on liver function tests in patients with cancer. Cancer. 1982;49:1249–57.
37. Grant JP, Cox CE, Kleiman LM *et al.* Serum hepatic enzyme and bilirubin elevations during parenteral nutrition. Surg Gynecol Obstet. 1977;145:573–80.
38. Sheldon GF, Peterson SR, Sanders R. Hepatic dysfunction during hyperalimentation. Arch Surg. 1978;113:504–8.
39. Mashima Y. Effect of caloric overload on puppy livers during parenteral nutrition. J Parent Ent Nutr. 1979;3:139–45
40. Benjamin DR. Cholelithiasis in infants: the role of total parenteral nutrition and

gastrointestinal dysfunction. J Pediatr Surg. 1982;17:386–9.
41. Callahan J, Haller JO, Cacciarelli AA *et al.* Cholelithiasis in infants in association with total parenteral nutrition and furosemide. Radiology. 1982;143:437–9.
42. King DR, Ginn-Pease ME, Lloyd TV *et al.* Parenteral nutrition with associated cholelithiasis: Another iatrogenic disease of infants and children. J Pediatr Surg. 1987;22:593–6.
43. Whitington PF, Black DD. Cholelithiasis in premature infants treated with parenteral nutrition and furosemide. J Pediatr. 1980;97:647–9.
44. Roslyn JJ, Berquist WE, Pitt HA *et al.* Increased risk of gallstones in children receiving total parenteral nutrition. Pediatrics. 1983;71:784–9.
45. Roslyn JJ, Pitt HA, Mann LL *et al.* Gallbladder disease in patients on long-term parenteral nutrition. Gastroenterology. 1983;84:148–54.
46. Dahms BB, Halpin Jr. TC. Serial liver biopsies in parenteral nutrition-associated cholestasis of early infancy. Gastroenterology. 1981;81:136–44.
47. Cohen C, Olsen MM. Pediatric total parenteral nutrition: liver histopathology. Arch Pathol Lab Med. 1981;105:152–6.
48. Body JJ, Bleiberg H, Bron D *et al.* Total parenteral nutrition-induced cholestasis mimicking large bile duct obstruction. Histopathology. 1982;6:787–92.
49. Benjamin D. Hepatobiliary dysfunction in infants and children associated with long-term total parenteral nutrition: a clinico-pathologic study. Am J Clin Pathol. 1981;76:276–83.
50. Lowry SF, Benjamin MF. Abnormal liver function during parenteral nutrition: relation to infusion excess. J Surg Res. 1979;26:300–7.
51. Wolfe RR, O'Donnell TF, Stone MD *et al.* Investigation of factors determining the optimal glucose infusion rate in total parenteral nutrition. Metabolism. 1980;29:892–900.
52. Hall RI, Grant JP, Ross LH *et al.* Pathogenesis of hepatic steatosis in the parenterally fed rat. J Clin Invest. 1984;74:1658–68.
53. Roy CC, Belli DC. Hepatobiliary complications associated with TPN: an enigma. J Am Coll Nutr. 1985;4:651–60.
54. Whitington PF. Cholestasis associated with total parenteral nutrition in infants. Hepatology. 1985;5:693–6.
55. Pittschieler K, Lebenthal E, Bujanover Y, Petell JK. Levels of Cu-Zn and Mn superoxide dismutases in rat liver during development. Gastroenterology. 1991;100:1062–8.
56. Taylor SF, Devereaux MW, Khandwala RJ, Sokol RJ. Hepatic glutathione depletion precedes oxidative injury in weanling rats on total parenteral nutrition. Hepatology. 1900;12:935.
57. Nathanson MH, Boyer JL. Mechanisms and regulation of bile secretion. Hepatology. 1991;14:551–66.
58. Senger H, Boehm G, Beyreiss K. *et al.* Evidence for amino acid induced cholestasis in very low birthweight infants with increasing enteral protein intake. Acta Paediatr Scand. 1986;75:724–8.
59. Suchy FJ, Bucavalas JC, Novak DA. Determinants of bile formation during development: Ontogeny of hepatic bile acid metabolism and transport. Semin Liver Dis. 1987;7:77–84.
60. Bucuvalas JC, Goodrich AL, Blitzer BL, Suchy FJ. Amino acids are potent inhibitors of bile acid uptake by liver plasma membrane vesicles isolated from suckling rats. Pediatr Res. 1985;19:1298–364.
61. Graham M. Inhibition of bile flow in the perfused rat liver by a synthetic parenteral amino acid mixture. Hepatology. 1984;4:69–72.
62. Back P, Walter K. Developmental pattern of bile acid metabolism as revealed by bile acid analysis of meconium. Gastroenterology. 1980;78:671–6.
63. Shoda J, Mahara R, Osuga T *et al.* Similarity of unusual bile acids in human umbilical cord blood and amniotic fluid from newborns and in sera and urine from adult patients with cholestatic liver diseases. J Lipid Res. 1988;29:847–58.
64. Aynsley-Green A. Plasma hormone concentrations during enteral and parenteral nutrition in the human newborn. J Pediatr Gastroenterol Nutr. 1983;2(Suppl. 1):S108–12.
65. Greenberg G, Wolman S, Christofides N *et al.* Effect of total parenteral nutrition on gut hormone release in humans. Gastroenterology. 1981;80:988–93.
66. Hughes CA, Talbot IC, Ducker DA, Harran MJ. Total parenteral nutrition in infancy: Effect on the liver and suggested pathogenesis. Gut. 1981;24:241–8.

67. Lucas A, Bloom SR, Aynsley-Green A. Gut hormones and minimal enteral feeding. Acta Paediatr Scand. 1986;75:719–23.
68. Nakai H, Landing BH. Factors in the genesis of bile stasis in infancy. Pediatrics. 1961;27:300–7.
69. Helton WS, Scheltinga MR, Hong RW, Wilmore DW, Smith RJ. Neurotensin attenuates increased intestinal permeability during intravenous feeding in rats. Gastroenterology. 1991;100:A525.
70. Tomomasa T, Itoh K, Kourome T. Intragastric neurotensin stimulates gastrointestinal transit in suckling rats. Pediatr Res. 1990;27:118A.
71. Jirsova V, Janovsky M. Hyperbilirubinemia connected with parenteral administration of higher amounts of fluids in premature infants. Biol Neonate. 1978;33:132–4.
72. Pessayre D, Dolder A, Artigou J-V et al. Effect of fasting on metabolite-mediated hepatotoxicity in the rat. Gastroenterology. 1979;77:264–71.
73. Bernstein J, Brown AK. Sepsis and jaundice in early infancy. Pediatrics. 1962;29:873–82.
74. Lefkowitch JH. Bile ductular cholestasis: an ominous histopathologic sign related to sepsis and 'cholangitis lenta'. Human Pathol. 1981;13:19–24.
75. Alverdy JC, Aoys E, Moss GS. Total parenteral nutrition promotes bacterial translocation from the gut. Surgery. 1988;104:185–90.
76. Rooney JC, Hill DJ, Danks DM. Jaundice associated with bacterial infection in the newborn. Am J Dis Child. 1971;122:39–42.
77. Utili R, Abernathy C, Zimmerman H. Inhibition of Na^+,K^+-ATPase by endotoxin: A possible mechanism for endotoxin-induced cholestasis. J Infect Dis. 1977;136:583–7.
78. Zimmerman HJ, Fang M, Utili R et al. Jaundice due to bacterial infection. Gastroenterology. 1979;77:367–74.
79. Latham PS, Menkes E, Phillips MJ et al. Hyperalimentation-associated jaundice: an example of a serum factor inducing cholestasis in rats. Am J Clin Nutr. 1985;41:61–5.
80. Lichtman SN, Sartor RB. Hepatobiliary injury associated with experimental small-bowel bacterial overgrowth in rats. Infect Immun. 1991;59:555–62.
81. Lichtman SN, Sartor RB, Keku J, Schwab JH. Hepatic inflammation in rats with experimental small bowel bacterial overgrowth. Gastroenterology. 1990;98:414–23.
82. Lichtman SN, Keku J, Clark RL, Schwab JH, Sartor RB. Biliary tract disease in rats with experimental bacterial overgrowth. Hepatology. 1991;13:766–72.
83. Lichtman SN, Keku J, Schwab JH, Sartor RB. Evidence for peptidoglycan absorption in rats with experimental small bowel bacterial overgrowth. Infect Immun. (In press).
84. Lichtman SN, Keku J, Schwab JH, Sartor RB. Metronidazole and tetracycline prevent hepatic injury associated with small bowel bacterial overgrowth in rats. Gastroenterology. 1991;100:513–19.
85. Lichtman SN, Sartor RB, Keku J, Schwab JH. Mutanolysin prevents hepatic injury in rats with small bowel bacterial overgrowth. Hepatology. 1990;12:840 (abstr.).
86. Lichtman SN, Okoruwa E, Currin RT, Lemasters JJ. Kupffer cells have a role in hepatic injury associated with small bowel bacterial overgrowth. Hepatology. 1991 (In press).
87. Matsui J, Cameron RG, Kuo GC, Jeejeebhoy KN. Liver enlargement and proliferation of bile ductular cells during cachectin/TNF-alpha infusion with total parenteral nutrition. Gastroenterology. 1991;100:A536 (abstr.).
88. Tracey KJ, Vlassara H, Cerami A. Cachectin/tumour necrosis factor. Lancet. 1989;1:1122–6.
89. Whiting JF, Rosenbluth AB, Narciso JP, Gollan JL. Tumor necrosis factor-α inhibits taurocholate uptake by hepatocytes: implications for the pathogenesis of endotoxin-induced cholestasis. Gastroenterology. 1991;100:A811 (abstr.).
90. Stanko RT, Nathan G, Mendelow H et al. Development of hepatic cholestasis and fibrosis in patients with massive loss of intestine supported by prolonged parenteral nutrition. Gastroenterology. 1987;92:197–202.
91. Craig RM, Neumann T, Jeejeebhoy KN et al. Severe hepatocellular reaction resembling alcoholic hepatitis with cirrhosis after massive small bowel resection and prolonged total parenteral nutrition. Gastroenterology. 1980;79:131–7.
92. Dunn L, Hulman S, Weiner J, Kliegman R. Beneficial effects of early hypocaloric enteral feeding on neonatal gastrointestinal function: preliminary report of a randomized trial. J Pediatr. 1988;112:622–9.

93. Slagle TA, Gross SJ. Effect of early low-volume enteral substrate on subsequent feeding tolerance in very low birth weight infants. J Pediatr. 1988;113:526–31.
94. Hodes JE, Grosfeld JL, Weber TR *et al.* Hepatic failure in infants on total parenteral nutrition: Clinical and histopathologic observations. J Pediatr Surg. 1982;17:463–8.
95. Patterson K, Kapur SP, Chandra RS. Hepatocellular carcinoma in a non-cirrhotic infant after prolonged parenteral nutrition. J Pediatr. 1985;106:797–800.
96. Vileisis RA, Sorensen K, Gonzalez-Crussi F *et al.* Liver malignancy after parenteral nutrition. J Pediatr. 1982;100:88–90.
97. Buzby GP, Mullen JL, Stein TP *et al.* Manipulation of TPN caloric substrate and fatty infiltration of the liver. J Surg Res. 1981;31:46.
98. Heird WC, Dell RB, Helms RA *et al.* Amino acid mixture designed to maintain normal plasma amino acid patterns in infants and children requiring parenteral nutrition. Pediatrics. 1987;80:401–8.
99. Zlotkin S, Blosmanis E. Iron overload in patients on TPN. Ped Res. 1991;29:117A (abstr.).
100. Kennedy KA. Lung glutathione stores in newborn rats exposed to hyperoxia. Ped Res. 1990;27:309A (abstr.).
101. Hansen TN, Smith CV, Martin NE, Smith HW, Elliott SJ. Oxidant stress responses in ventilated newborn infants. Ped Res. 1990;27:208A (abstr.).
102. Bhatia J, Rassin DK. Photosensitized oxidation of tryptophan and hepatic dysfunction in neonatal gerbils. J Parent Ent Nutr. 1985;9:491–5.
103. Merritt RJ, Sinatra FR, Henton DH, Neustein H. Cholestatic effect of intraperitoneal administration of tryptophan to suckling rat pups. Pediatr Res. 1984;18:904–7.
104. Bhatia J, Moslen M, Haque A, McCleery R, Rassin D. Parenteral nutrition and hepatobiliary system: effects of nutrient-light interactions during hypocaloric alimentation. Ped Res. 1990;27:101A (abstr.).
105. Gleghorn EE, Merritt RJ, Subramanian N *et al.* Phenobarbital does not prevent total parenteral nutrition-associated cholestasis in noninfected neonates. J Parent Ent Nutr. 1986;10:282–3.
106. Schwartz JB, Merritt RJ, Rosenthal P *et al.* Ceruletide to treat neonatal cholestasis. Lancet. 1988;1:1219–20.
107. Balistreri WF, A-Kader HH, Ryckman FC, Whitington PF, Heubi JE, Setchell KDR. Biochemical and clinical response to ursodeoxycholic acid administration in pediatric patients with chronic cholestasis. In: Paumgartner G, Stiehl A, Gerok W, editors. Bile acids as therapeutic agents. Lancaster: Kluwer; 1991:323–33.
108. Lindor DL, Burnes J. Ursodeoxycholic acid for the treatment of home parenteral nutrition-associated cholestasis. Gastroenterology. 1991;101:250–3.
109. Langrehr JM, Reilly MJ, Banner B, Warty VJ, Lee KKW, Schraut WH. Hepatic steatosis due to total parenteral nutrition: the influence of short-gut syndrome, refeeding, and small bowel transplantation. J Surg Res. 1991;50:335–43.
110. Tracey KJ, Fong Y, Hesse DG *et al.* Anti-cachectin/TNF monoclonal antibodies prevent septic shock during lethal bacteraemia. Nature. 1987;330:662–4.

Section 4
Diagnostic Procedures in the Assessment of Cholestatic Liver Diseases

21
Imaging diagnosis of cholestasis in children

H. TSCHÄPPELER

INTRODUCTION

Cholestasis in children, and especially in neonates, is a common clinical problem[1]. The urine is dark and the stools are discoloured; the critical and important task is to establish the various causes of the cholestasis. They include lesions of the extrahepatic bile ducts (EHBD), intrahepatic bile ducts (IHBD) or of both. These sites correspond to the eventual treatment, as there are 'surgical' and 'medical' causes. EHBD disease accounts for about 5%, IHBD disease for about 55%, whereas the most important group of extra- and intrahepatic bile duct pathology, including biliary atresia (BA), represents 40%.

IMAGING MODALITIES

Imaging diagnosis is based on modalities, which demonstrate anatomy and morphology as well as function (Table 1). As there is no single and simple method providing both features, diagnostic evaluation of cholestasis has to be performed step by step.

Ultrasonography

High-resolution and colour Doppler ultrasonography is usually the first modality, which may also be applied for antenatal imaging.

Table 1 Imaging modalities

Ultrasonography	
CT	Anatomy
MR	Morphology
Cholangiography (PTC, POC, etc.)	
Scintigraphy	Function

PTC = percutaneous transhepatic cholangio-/cholecystography;
POC = peroperative cholangiography

The size of the gallbladder and its morphological appearance is well appreciated; the presence of dilated IHBD and EHBD is easily established. Parenchymal changes of the liver, as well as portal and hepatic venous or hepatic arterial flow, are assessed by colour Doppler sonography. Mass lesions at the porta hepatis or the adjacent areas are defined (cystic–solid). As ultrasonography is readily available (also as a bedside method) it is widely used as a screening modality, which can be repeated without any harm to the child. In order to avoid pitfalls the findings need careful interpretation.

Similar information concerning anatomy and morphology of the biliary tract is provided by computed tomography; however CT has several disadvantages including radiation exposure, need for intravenous contrast material, only cross-sectional display available and cost. It may be very useful in selected cases, whenever special information (e.g. before surgery) is mandatory.

Cholangiography

Cholangiography means visualization of the biliary system by positive contrast material. Before the sonographic era it was performed by intravenous injection of a iodinated water-soluble compound, which is preferentially eliminated by the liver and opacified the bile. One of the major disadvantages, however, was the failure of the examination in the presence of hyperbilirubin-aemia.

This disadvantage was overcome by percutaneous transhepatic cholangiography (PTC). This technique became possible only after appropriate puncture material was available and the biliary tract could be previously monitored by sonography demonstrating dilated ducts. Today PTC is a routine technique, applied both in adults and in children[2]. An alternative approach is percutaneous, transhepatic puncture of the gallbladder under sonographic guidance[3]. In both techniques the successful puncture is followed by injection of water-soluble contrast material directly into the biliary tract. Spot radiography is performed after appropriate opacification. Both procedures are invasive; in children either a good, controlled sedation and local anaesthesia or general anaesthesia is necessary. Opacification of the bile ducts may also be obtained during surgery by direct puncture of the gallbladder (peroperative cholangiography). Cholangiography visualizes even small intraluminal lesions and clearly demonstrates ductal patency. This latter feature facilitates separating obstructive from non-obstructive disease. In this regard cholangiography represents the 'gold standard'.

Retrograde cholangio- (and pancreato)graphy by endoscopic catheterization of the ampulla Vateri (ERCP) is another means to opacify the biliary and pancreatic ductal system; it is preferentially performed in combination with a therapeutic manoeuvre (e.g. removal of a gallstone).

Hepatobiliary scintigraphy

A large number of radiopharmaceuticals is available for hepatobiliary scintigraphy[4]. Both the function of the liver, i.e. extraction of the radionuclide (e.g. Tc-iminodiacetic acid = IDA) and its free excretion through the bile ducts into the intestinal tract can be appreciated. However accuracy of the latter depends on normal hepatic extraction, i.e. uptake by the liver could be increased by enzyme induction with phenobarbital prior to the test. This manoeuvre appears especially promising in infants with neonatal hepatitis. The major drawback is the lack of accurate information, since anatomical spatial resolution of scintigraphy is poor.

BILIARY ATRESIA

In neonates biliary atresia is the most common cause of cholestasis; among the congenital biliary malformations biliary atresia is the most frequent serious condition. Correct diagnosis as soon as possible is mandatory, since early treatment before the age of about 2 months improves prognosis and can delay or even avoid liver transplantation.

Biliary atresia, i.e. interruption of the EHBD, has a wide spectrum: usually there are no hepatic ducts, a small gallbladder may be present, associated atresia of the common bile duct occurs. In about 10% a solitary cyst at the porta hepatis represents the only finding of biliary atresia.

Though in up to 80% of all infants with biliary atresia the clinical presentation is typical (persistent acholic stools since birth, conjugated hyperbilirubinaemia with dark urine, enlarged liver) there are patients in whom a further investigation is indicated in order to exclude a 'medical' cause of cholestasis.

The initial imaging method – sonography – has two pitfalls: (1) unfortunately normal-sized common hepatic and bile ducts are not visible at this age, which means non-visualization of the ducts is of no diagnostic value; (2) the sonographic presence of a small gallbladder or its complete absence are not reliable; however a gallbladder longer than 3 cm suggests neonatal hepatitis rather than biliary atresia[5]. Sonography is diagnostic for biliary atresia, if a cystic structure at the porta hepatis without communication with any bile ducts is present[6], or if elements of the non-cardiac polysplenic syndrome are demonstrated (polysplenia, abdominal situs inversus, preduodenal portal vein, azygos continuation of the vena cava)[7].

Often non-invasive evaluation of neonatal jaundice also includes radionuclide studies. Interpretation of their findings has to take into consideration the age of the infant as well as liver function. Normal uptake in an infant younger than 3 months but without intestinal excretion favours the diagnosis of biliary atresia (Fig. 1a), whereas poor hepatic extraction in the same age group (with or without intestinal excretion) indicates neonatal hepatitis rather than biliary atresia. On the other hand in infants older than 3 months poor hepatic uptake with or without intestinal excretion is equivocal.

Patients in whom biliary atresia is strongly suspected should have operative

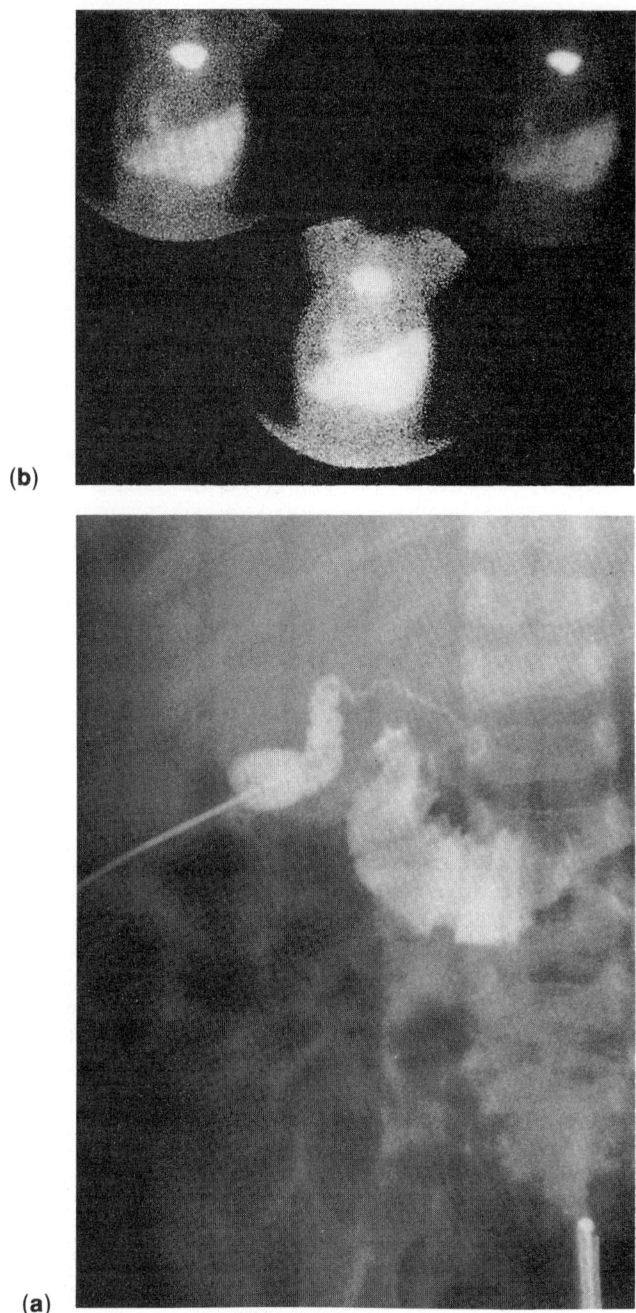

Fig. 1 Extrahepatic biliary atresia. (a) Hepatobiliary scintigraphy; adequate uptake of the tracer by the liver; no intestinal excretion. (b) Peroperative cholangiography. Opacification of the small gallbladder, cystic and common bile duct, duodenum; no common hepatic duct

cholangiography (Fig. 1b) and liver biopsy, usually followed by surgical therapy (e.g. Kasai procedure), whereas infants in whom neonatal hepatitis appears more likely should undergo closed or guided liver biopsy. The 'gold standard', however, to differentiate extrahepatic biliary atresia from neonatal hepatitis, remains cholangiography.

A large gallbladder allows sonographically guided percutaneous puncture, and direct biliary opacification can be performed in order to demonstrate patency of the common hepatic and/or common bile duct.

CHOLEDOCHAL CYST (CYSTIC DILATATION OF THE EHBD AND/OR IHBD)

Cystic dilatation of the bile ducts can present many different anatomical variants. Most often (80–90%) the common bile duct is dilated with a variety of appearances (segmental dilatation between the cystic duct and the duodenum is the most common type; diverticulum of the common bile duct is very rare; segmental dilatation of the intraduodenal duct is choledochocele; segmental dilatation with involvement of the hepatic, cystic and common bile ducts). Caroli's disease consists of multiple, mostly intrahepatic cysts.

Choledochal cyst is discovered in 25% of cases within the first year of life; more and more often antenatal diagnosis is established. The classical triad suggesting the diagnosis includes abdominal pain, right upper quadrant mass and intermittent cholestasis; this topical presentation is quite rare, especially in the younger child.

Confirmation of the diagnosis is primarily based on the sonographic findings (Fig. 2a): the most common type is characterized by a cystic mass within the hepatic pedicle; there is communication with bile ducts, their intra- and extrahepatic size being quite variable. Furthermore the gallbladder is easily identified. However, before surgery definition of the precise anatomy may be required, and pre- or peroperative cholangiography is necessary (Fig. 2b). Differential diagnosis of a cystic mass in a patient with cholestasis (apart from a choledochal cyst in biliary atresia) is a duodenal duplication which compresses the distal portion of the common bile duct.

LITHIASIS

Due to the high sensitivity and specificity of ultrasound, sludge and/or gallstones within the gallbladder are easily detected (Fig. 3a); quite often it is an incidental finding in an asymptomatic child. There are well-known causes of calculi, which are most often pigment stones without or with incorporation of calcium: haemolytic disorders, cystic fibrosis, gastrointestinal dysfunction, parenteral nutrition or furosemide therapy, especially if applied in prematures.

On the other hand, in a cholestatic child sonography detects biliary obstruction without difficulty by demonstrating mild to moderate, even dilatation of the biliary tree (Fig. 3b); however, direct identification of the

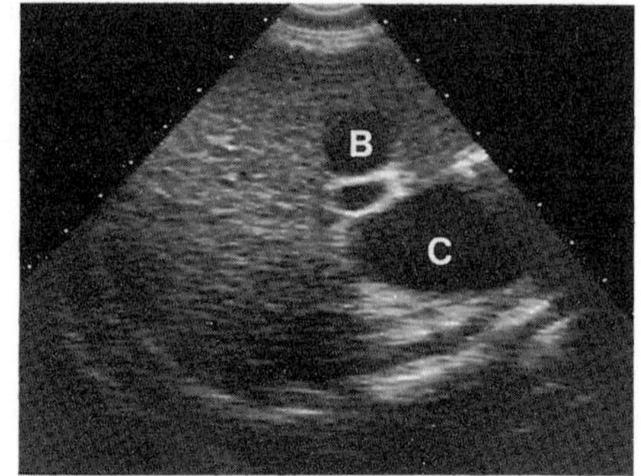

(a)

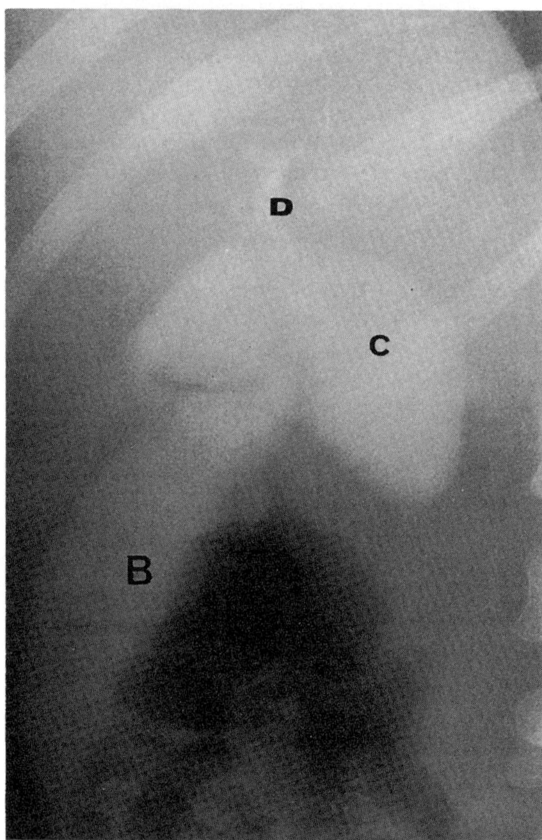

(b)

Fig. 2   Choledochal cyst. (**a**) Ultrasonography; cystic structure (C) at the porta hepatis, dilated bile duct, gallbladder (B). (**b**) (Intravenous) cholangiogram. Considerable cystic dilatation (C) of the common bile duct, dilated hepatic ducts (D), gallbladder (B)

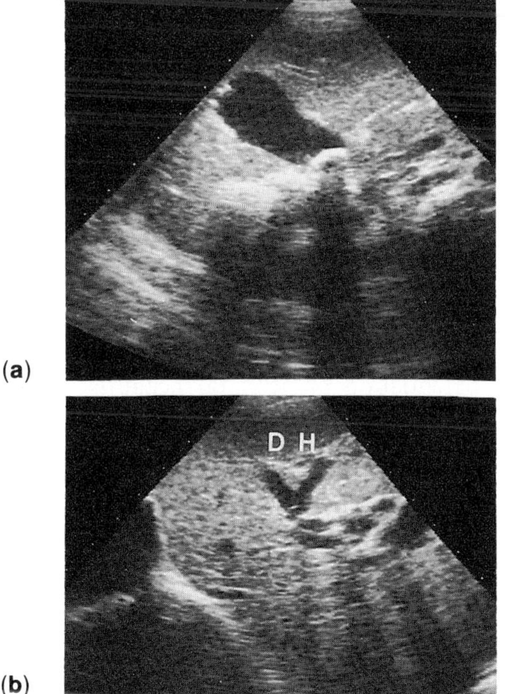

Fig. 3 Obstructing cholelithiasis. (a) Cholecystolithiasis. (b) Dilatation of common bile duct (with small intraluminal calculus) and hepatic ducts (DH)

responsible calculus fails in some patients[8]. Though spontaneous resolution occurs, and can be documented sonographically, cholangitis and even liver abscesses may complicate obstructing choledocholiathasis. Its treatment may include flushing of the biliary tree by (percutaneous) cholangio- or cholecystography in order to push the calculus into the duodenum[9] or direct removal by ERCP, thus avoiding surgery.

EXTRINSIC COMPRESSION

Cholestasis due to external compression of the common bile duct is a rare condition in children. Duodenal duplication and enlarged lymph nodes at the porta hepatis are possible causes. Together with the accompanying ductal dilatation they are detected by sonography and/or complementary CT examination.

Fortunately, and in contrast to the adult patient, in children obstructing primary neoplastic biliary disease – a very challenging diagnostic and therapeutic task – is very rare.

Among the 'medical' causes sclerosing cholangitis is an infrequent entity characterized by an inflammatory obliterative fibrosis of the intra- and extrahepatic biliary system. It results in chronic progressive liver disease.

Association with various diseases (e.g. chronic inflammatory bowel disease) is known. Imaging diagnosis is possible by cholangiography: rarefaction of segmental branches, stenosis and focal dilatation of the ducts are present[10].

For diagnosis of intrahepatic cholestasis imaging methods have a minor role, as diagnosis is mainly based on the combination of biochemical and histological findings. Demonstration of 'butterfly'-shaped vertebrae may suggest Alagille syndrome[11].

CONCLUSION

In paediatric cholestasis ultrasonography is the initial and often definitively diagnostic imaging modality. Being aware of the sonographic pitfalls in the most important differentiation of neonatal hepatitis from biliary atresia hepatobiliary scintigraphy may add crucial findings. However, cholangiography remains the gold standard modality before surgical treatment. Sonography and cholangiography play a major role in the diagnosis (and treatment) of the other extrahepatic diseases causing cholestasis.

References

1. Gates GF, Sinatra FR, Thomas DW. Cholestatic syndromes in infancy and childhood. Am J Roentgenol. 1980;134:1141–8.
2. Franken EA, Smith WL, Smith JA *et al*. Percutaneous cholangiography in infants. Am J Roentgenol. 1978;130:1057–8.
3. Garel LA, Belli D, Grignon A *et al*. Percutaneous cholecystography in children. Radiology. 1987;165:639–41.
4. Gerhold JP, Klingensmith WC, Kuni CC *et al*. Diagnosis of biliary atresia with radionuclide hepatobiliary imaging. Radiology. 1983;146:499–504.
5. Kirks DR, Coleman RE, Filston HC *et al*. An imaging approach to persistent neonatal jaundice. Am J Roentgenol. 1984;142:461–5.
6. Torrisi JM, Haller JO, Velcek FT. Choledochal cyst and biliary atresia in the neonate: Imaging findings in five cases. Am J Roentgenol. 1990;155:1273–6.
7. Abramson SA, Berdon WE, Altman RP *et al*. Biliary atresia and non-cardiac polysplenic syndrome: US and surgical considerations. Radiology. 1987;163:377–80.
8. Brunelle F, Descos B, Bernard O *et al*. Common bile duct calculi in infants. Ann Radiol. 1983;26:147–54.
9. Pariente D, Bernard O, Gauthier F *et al*. Radiological treatment of common bile duct lithiasis in infancy. Pediatr Radiol. 1989;9:104–8.
10. Sisto A, Feldman P, Garel L *et al*. Primary sclerosing cholangitis in children: study of five cases and review of the literature. Pediatrics. 1987;24:918–21.
11. Alagille D, Estrada A, Hadchouel M *et al*. Syndromic paucity of interlobular bile ducts: review of 80 cases. J Pediatr. 1987;110:195–200.

22
The role of dynamic liver function tests in liver transplantation

M. BURDELSKI, M. OELLERICH, B. RODECK, A. LATTA and
J. DÜWEL

INTRODUCTION

After more than 20 years of clinical experience liver transplantation has
come of age. There is a remarkable increase of liver transplantations especially
in the United States and in Europe during the past decade[1], indicating that
this surgical therapy of otherwise fatal liver diseases is accepted as a routine
method. This is outstanding progress, but this progress has created the need
for new methods in hepatology, i.e. the need for liver function tests with
reliable prognostic information. This new quality of tests is essential in donor
rating, choosing the next patient for transplantation and in monitoring liver
function after transplantation.

The need for donor organ quality assessment arises from the fact that
between 6% and 8% of all transplanted organs show primary non-function[2],
organs with severely impaired primary function not taken into account.
Static conventional liver function tests have been shown to be unreliable
predictors of this most critical complication in the early postoperative
course[3]. Avoiding primary non-function by better selection of donor organs
would also lead to an improvement in survival after liver transplantation.

As far as choosing the candidate for the next transplantation is concerned,
this problem depends very much on the local donor situation. If there is no
lack of donor organs the waiting time from presentation of the patient to
realization of his transplantation is so short that choosing the candidate for
the next transplantation is possible without ethical, medical or social
problems[4–7]. However, in centres with long waiting lists due to relative
or absolute lack of donors the situation is completely different. Many
transplantation candidates die on the waiting list[5]. Under such conditions
choosing the candidate for the next transplantation is extremely difficult.
The aim should be to select a candidate by objective methods, for instance
by means of prognostic criteria which allow allocation of the risk of a patient
surviving the next year without transplantation.

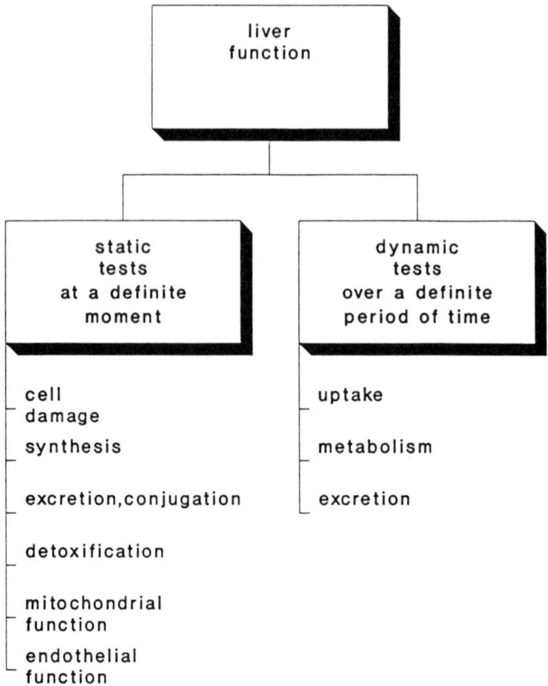

Fig. 1 Static and dynamic liver function tests

It is justified to offer liver transplantation as a therapeutic option only if there is evidence that the patient will benefit from the procedure, and not for only a few years. Long-term survival after liver transplantation has been reported[8,9], but information about quality of liver function in these long-term survivors is poor.

Since conventional static liver function tests seem to lack specificity in predicting disease severity[10], dynamic liver function tests based on drug disposition were proposed as an attractive alternative to these conventional parameters[10–13] (Fig. 1). These dynamic liver function tests have been used extensively in our centre[13–18] in order to obtain answers to the questions mentioned above. The results of some of these studies will be reported. The tests used have been described in detail elsewhere[13–18].

DONOR ORGAN QUALITY ASSESSMENT

In our pilot study from 1986 to 1987 a comparison of static and dynamic liver function tests showed that out of all tests performed only monoethylglycinexylidide (MEGX) formation after i.v. lidocaine injection in the donor before explantation was able to predict primary function or non-function of the graft in the corresponding recipient with satisfactory prognostic value (Fig. 2)[14]. Based on these results the study was continued until December

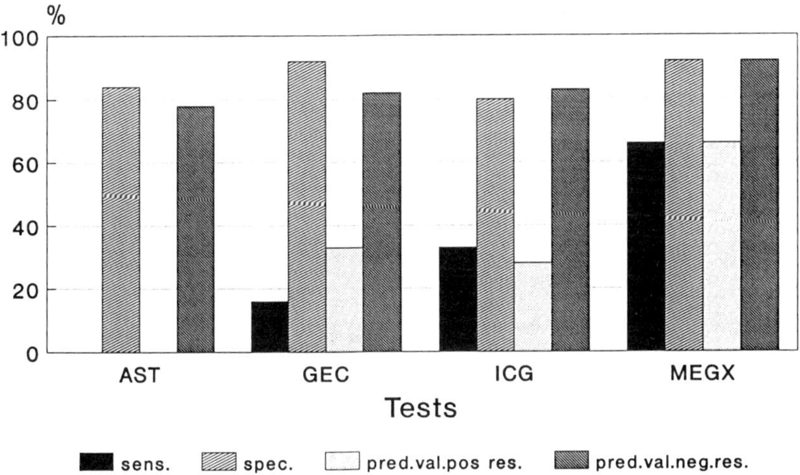

Fig. 2 Prognostic sensitivity, specificity, predictive value of a positive and predictive value of a negative result of static (AST) and dynamic (glucose-elimination capacity (GEC), ICG clearance (ICG) and MEGX formation, 15 min value (MEGX)) liver function tests in the donor, predicting primary non-function in the recipient ($n = 36$). Modified from ref. 14

1989[18,19]. At the end of this prospective study 171 donor–recipient pairs, corresponding to 52% of all transplantations performed in this time, were analysed. The Kaplan Meier curves of graft survival from those organs which were tested in the donor showed a highly significant relationship between surival and good MEGX results in the donor (Fig. 3) and vice-versa ($p < 0.00005$). These data show that there is a relationship between lidocaine metabolism and the functional state of the liver.

Intact cytochrome P-450 activity, bound to intact structures of the endoplasmic reticulum, is indicated by good MEGX formation. Thus, useful information is provided by this dynamic liver function test with regard to graft survival in the corresponding recipient. In clinical practice test results should be interpreted in the context of all available data from donor and recipient only. In general, donor MEGX findings $< 50\,\mu g/l$ indicate a 70% risk of primary non-function. On the other hand, those organs from donors with test results $> 90\,\mu g/l$ have a 70% chance of surviving the initial post-transplant period[18,19]. If used in a rational way this dynamic liver function test will contribute to a better and more efficient use of the limited donor pool.

TRANSPLANT CANDIDATE SELECTION

In accord with our experience other centres report that, for every three paediatric patients transplanted, one died waiting[20]. This situation slightly improved after the technique of partial liver transplantation had been developed[21-23]. Small children at about 1 year of age may now be transplanted using this technique; otherwise these children would not have survived

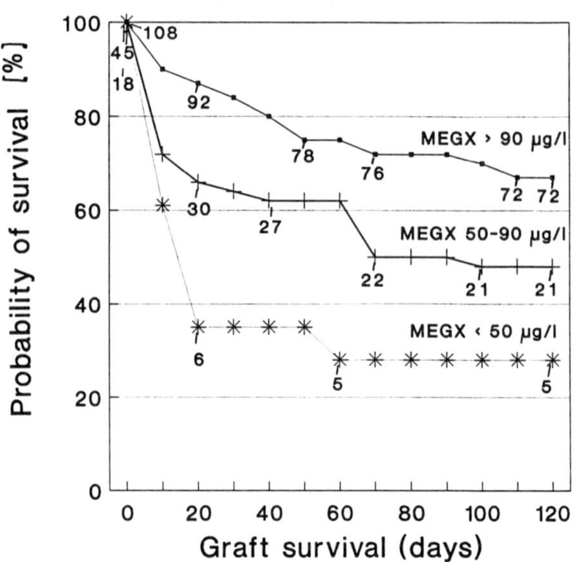

Fig. 3 Life-table showing probability of graft survival in relation to MEGX test results presented as 15 min values in donors ($n = 171$). The differences between favourable ($> 90\,\mu g/l$), intermediate ($50–90\,\mu g/l$) and unfavourable ($< 50\,\mu g/l$) test results are highly significant ($p < 0.00005$). Modified from ref. 19

because whole organs of appropriate size are extremely rare. In many centres, however, the waiting lists still cover more patients than can be transplanted in time. Under these circumstances objective criteria are needed to decide which patient from the waiting list should receive the next organ.

Proposals for such objective criteria in children differ from those in adults. A retrospective study has been performed in Pittsburgh[20] showing, by means of multivariate analysis, that cholesterol below 100 mg/dl, history of ascites, concentrations of indirect bilirubin above 6 mg/dl and a prolongation of prothrombin time above 20 s had been significantly related with death of the patient within 120 days. The only prospective study in children so far has been performed in our institution[24]. From November 1986 to April 1989 all patients referred to our hospital for evaluation of liver transplantation entered the study. At the time of inclusion, presence or absence of ascites was recorded and the following liver function tess have been performed: indocyanine green (ICG) $t_{1/2}$, MEGX formation, serum concentration of albumin, bilirubin, total bile acids, creatinine and tyrosine, serum catalytic concentrations of alkaline phosphatase and cholinesterase with butyryl-thiocholine as substrate and prothrombin time. After entering the study 10 children out of 51 were transplanted during the observation period of 365 days. The baseline characteristics of the remaining 41 patients are shown in Table 1. MEGX test and ICG were performed as described elsewhere[13,15,16].

The results of all static and dynamic liver function tests were examined with regard to 365-day survival. In addition, results were cross-tabulated at different cut-off points with transplant candidate survival and analysed by

Table 1 Characteristics of the study: biochemical and pharmacokinetic data of paediatric patients ($n = 41$) with chronic end-stage liver disease expressed as median and 16–84 percentile

Parameter	Median	16%	84%
Albumin (g/l)	38	30	42
Alkaline phosphatase (U/l)	578	223	1269
Bile acids (μmol/l)	93	23	212
Bilirubin (μmol/l)	77	18	292
Cholinesterase (kU/l)	2.1	1.2	5.4
Creatinine (μmol/l)	35	18	54
ICG $t_{1/2}$ (min)	11	5.5	22.3
MEGX (30 min value, μg/l)	26	2	66
Prothrombin time (percentage of normal)	67	52	92
Tyrosine (μmol/l)	94	68	145

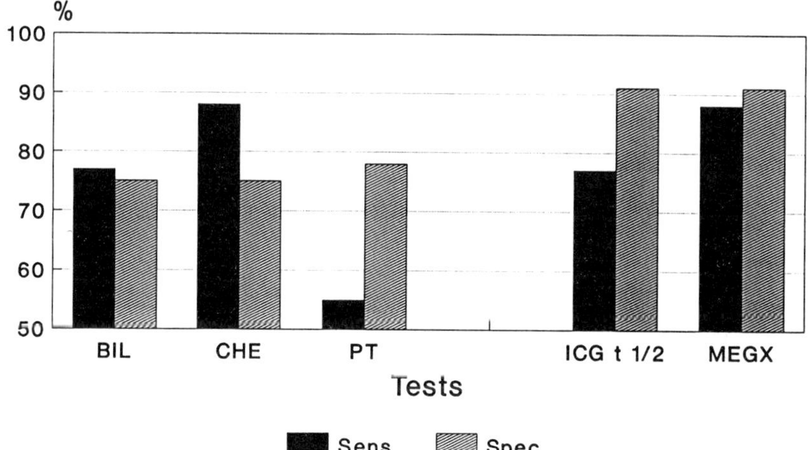

Fig. 4 Prognostic sensitivity and specificity of conventional static (Bil = bilirubin, CHE = cholinesterase, PT = prothrombin time) and dynamic (ICT $t_{1/2}$ = indocyanine green half-life and MEGX = MEGX test, 30 min value) liver function tests as predictors of 1-year survival of transplantation candidates without transplantation ($n = 41$)

the chi-square method using the Statistical Package of Social Sciences. Prognostic sensitivity and specificity of bilirubin, cholinesterase, prothrombin time, ICG $t_{1/2}$ and MEGX test were calculated as described elsewhere[25]. Finally, a stepwise survival analysis was performed by means of the Cox proportional hazards model (BMDP program 2L) in order to find the best prognostic indicators for 1-year survival of these patients.

Out of 41 patients entering the study nine died within 365 days, before liver transplantation could be performed. The prognostic sensitivity and specificity of static and dynamic liver function tests differed greatly (Fig. 4). The best prognostic sensitivity was observed in both dynamic tests, reaching 91%. None of the static tests achieved this prognostic quality. As far as prognostic specificity is concerned, the best results were obtained with cholinesterase (88%) and MEGX formation (89%). The combination of

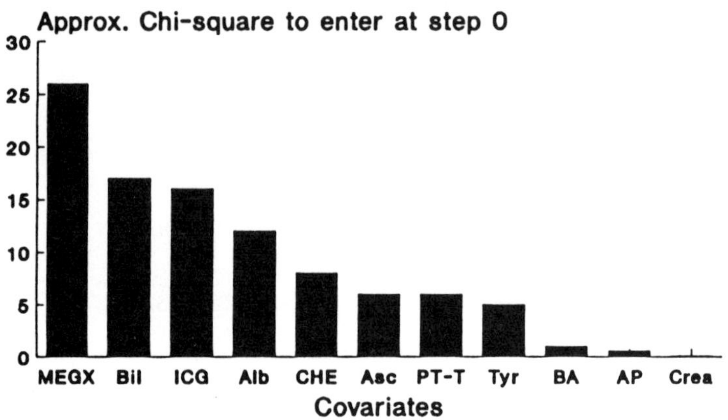

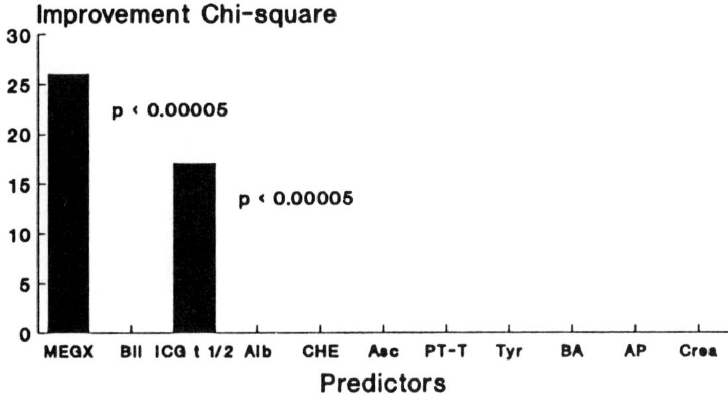

Fig. 5 Influence of transplant candidate variables as covariates on the hazard function in the Cox model in 41 paediatric patients with cirrhosis with regard to 1-year survival (top). MEGX (30 min value) Bil = bilirubin; ICG: $t_{1/2}$; Alb = albumin; CHE = cholinesterase; Asc = ascites; PT-T = prothrombin time; Tyr = tyrosine; AP = alkaline phosphatase' BA = bile acids; Crea - = creatinine. The lower part shows the summary of stepwise results from the Cox proportional-hazards regression analysis indicating significant predictors of 365-day survival in these patients

bilirubin, cholinesterase, prothrombin time, weight percentile[26] and MEGX formation did not improve the prognostic sensitivity and specificity if compared with the results of MEGX formation alone (sensitivity 77% vs 88%; specificity 91% vs 91%).

The influence of all parameters as covariates on the hazard function in the Cox model is shown in Fig. 5. At step zero, MEGX showed the highest chi-square values to enter the stepwise analysis followed by bilirubin, ICG, albumin, cholinesterase, ascites, prothrombin time, tyrosine, alkaline phosphatase, and creatinine. At the final step only the MEGX and ICG test had entered the model and could not be removed. Ascites and the conventional static liver function tests studied did not remain as independent and significant predictors of 1-year survival of these patients.

These findings suggest that dynamic liver function tests based on drug disposition are indeed an attractive alternative to conventional liver function tests if prognostic information is needed. The prognostic value of the MEGX test depends on both liver blood flow and metabolic capacity of the liver, whereas ICG depends merely on liver blood flow[16,19]. The results of a prospective study in adult liver transplantation candidates performed at the same time showed similar results[16]. The highest chi-square to enter the stepwise analysis in the Cox model in this study was also reached by dynamic liver function tests. At the first rank there was ICG, followed by MEGX, bilirubin and cholinesterase. At the final step, ICG, MEGX and cholinesterase had entered the model and could not be removed. The differences between the studies, though small, might be explained either by the different nature of the underlying diseases in both age groups – biliary atresia and Byler's disease in children and biliary and posthepatic cirrhosis in adults – or by the fact that the statistical basis in the paediatric series might still be too small to allow final conclusions. Nevertheless, the available evidence favours the primarily flow-dependent dynamic liver function tests. This supports the contention that the implications of intra- and prehepatic shunting are of great importance with regard to 1-year survival in chronic end-stage liver disease.

In clinical practice the MEGX test is much easier to perform than the ICG test because the needed blood volume is much smaller (two specimens of 1 ml vs four of 3 ml), blood samples for MEGX determination may be stored without problems, ICG samples have to be analysed immediately because of the instability of the compound. We therefore recommend only performing the MEGX test. However, if there are contradictory findings with regard to clinical findings and clinical chemical results the additional performance of the ICG test will give further prognostic support.

EVALUATION OF LONG-TERM EFFECT OF LIVER TRANSPLANTATION ON LIVER FUNCTION

There are few reports on long-term survival after liver transplantation[9,27-30]. In these reports there is little information with regard to liver function. Normal static liver function tests are reported in some studies[9], leaving the question open to what extent immunosuppressive therapy, including cyclosporin and steroids, may affect the functional state of the liver[31].

In a cross-sectional study we investigated our liver-transplanted children on the occasion of the yearly clinical control examination. As shown in Fig. 6 there was no significant difference between normals[32] and our patients 1– 3 years after transplantation. These findings suggest that medical therapy does not alter liver function measured with a dynamic liver function test. However, prospective studies are needed to answer this question properly.

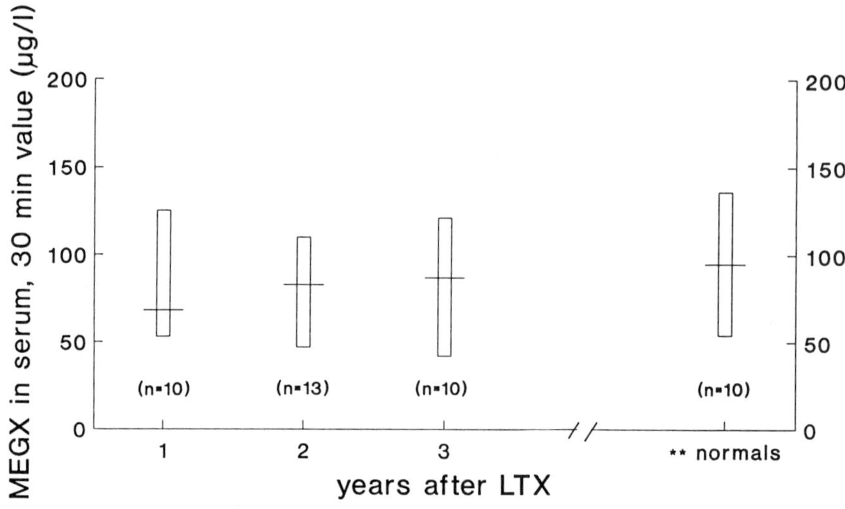

Fig. 6 Results of MEGX tests expressed as median and 16–84 percentile in patients 1–3 years after liver transplantation on the left. Values from normal children are shown as mean ± SD on the right part. From ref. 19

CONCLUSIONS

In conclusion, the data presented give good evidence that dynamic liver function tests such as MEGX formation after lidocaine injection and determination of indocyanine green half-life are effective tools as far as donor organ quality assessment, survival probability of transplant candidates and liver function of successfully transplanted patients are concerned. Conventional static liver function tests are less effective with regard to this concern.

References

1. Gordon RD, Bismuth H. Liver Transplant Registry Report. Transplant Proc. 1991;23:58–60.
2. Bismuth H. European Liver Transplant Registry. Personal communication; 1990.
3. Makowka L, Gordon RD, Todo, S, Ohkohchi N, Marsh JW, Tzakis AG, Yokvi H, Legash J, Esquivel CO, Satake M, Iwatsuki S, Starzl TE. Analysis of donor criteria for the prediction of outcome in clinical liver transplantation. Transplant Proc. 1987;19:2378–82.
4. Busuttil RW. Living-related liver donor (Con). Transplant Proc. 1991;23:43–5.
5. Samuel D, Benkamou JP, Bismuth H, Gugenheim J, Ciardello M, Saliba F. Criteria for selection for liver transplantation. Transplant Proc. 1987;19:2383–6.
6. Asher N, Evans RW. Designation of liver transplant centers in the United States. Transplant Proc. 1987;19:205.
7. Shaw BM Jr. Exclusion criteria for liver transplant recipients. Transplant Proc. 1989;21:3484–6.
8. Starzl TF, Demetris AJ, van Thiel D. Liver transplantation (first of two parts). N Engl J Med. 1989;321:1014–22.
9. Burdelski M, Pichlmayr R, Ringe B, Rodeck B, Brodehl J. Pediatric liver transplantation – ten years experience in Hanover. In: Terasaki PJ, editor. Clinical Transplants. Los Angeles:

UCLA Tissue Typing Laboratory; 1987;55–62.

10. Howden CW, Birnie GG, Brodie MJ. Drug metabolism in liver disease. Pharmacol Ther. 1989;40:439.

11. Branch RA. Drugs as indicators of hepatic function. Hepatology. 1982;2:97–105.

12. Huet PM, Villeneuve JP. Determinants of drug disposition in patients with cirrhosis. Hepatology. 1983;3:913.

13. Oellerich M, Burdelski M, Lautz HU, Rodeck B, Düwel J, Schulz M, Schmidt FW, Brodehl J, Pichlmayr R. Assessment of pretransplant prognosis in patients with cirrhosis. Transplantation. 1991;51:801–6.

14. Burdelski M, Oellerich M, Lamesch P, Raude E, Ringe B, Neuhaus P, Bortfeld S, Kämmerling C, Raith H, Scheruhn M, Westphal C, Worm M, Pichlmayr R. Evaluation of quantitative liver function tests in liver donors. Transplant Proc. 1987;19:3838–9.

15. Oellerich M, Raude E, Burdelski M, Schulz M, Schmidt FW, Ringe B, Lamesch P, Pichlmayr R, Raith H, Scheruhn H, Wrenger M, Wittekind Ch. Monoethylglycinexylidide formation kinetics: a novel approach to assessment of liver function. J Clin Chem Clin Biochem. 1987;25:845–53.

16. Oellerich M, Burdelski M, Lautz HU, Binder L, Pichlmayr R. Predictors of one-year pretransplant survival in patients with cirrhosis. Hepatology. 14 (In press).

17. Burdelski M, Oellerich M, Raude E, Lamesch P, Ringe B, Raith H, Scheruhn M, Westphal C, Worm S, Bortfeld C, Schulz M, Wittekind Ch, Hoyer PF, Pichlmayr R. A novel approach to assessment of liver function in donors. Transplant Proc. 1988;20(Suppl 1):591–3.

18. Oellerich M, Burdelski M, Ringe B, Lamesch P, Gubernatis G, Bunzendahl H, Pichlmayr R, Hermann H. Lignocaine metabolite formation as a measure of pre-transplant liver function. Lancet. 1989;1:640–2.

19. Oellerich M, Burdelski M, Ringe B, Wittekind Ch, Lamesch P, Lautz HU, Gubernatis G, Beyrau R, Pichlmayr R. Functional state of the donor liver and early outcome of transplantation. Transplant Proc. 1991;23:1575–8.

20. Malatack JJ, Schaid DJ, Urbach AH, Gartner JC, Zitelli BJ, Rockette H, Fischer J, Starzl TE, Iwatsuki S, Shaw BW Jr. Choosing a pediatric recipient for orthotopic liver transplantation. J Pediatr. 1987;111:479–89.

21. de Hemptinne B, de Ville de Goyet J, Kestens PJ, Otte JB. Volume reduction of the liver graft before orthotopic transplantation: report of a clinical experience of 11 cases. Transplant Proc. 1987;19.3317–22.

22. Brölsch Ch, Emond JC, Thistlethwaite JR, Bonch DA, Whitington PF, Lichtor JL. Liver transplantation with reduced size donor organs. Transplantation. 1988;45:519–24.

23. Ringe B, Pichlmayr R, Burdelski M. A new technique of hepatic vein reconstruction in partial liver transplantation. Transplant Int. 1988;1:30–5.

24. Burdelski M, Oellerich M, Düwel J, Rodeck R, Brodehl J. Predictors of one-year survival in pediatric liver cirrhosis. Hepatology. 1990;12:858.

25. Oellerich M, Burdelskki M, Lautz HU. Prognostic sensitivity and specificity of the monoethylglycinexylidide liver function test in transplant candidates. J Clin Chem Clin Biochem. 1989;27:757.

26. Burdelski M, Schmidt K, Hoyr PF, Galaske R, Brodehl J, Pichlmayr R. Indications for liver transplantation in pediatric patients. Transplant Proc. 1986;18(Suppl. 3):89–91.

27. Iwatsuki S, Starzl TE, Todo S, Gordon RD, Esquivel CO, Tzakis AG, Makowka L, Marsh JW, Koncru B, Stieber A, Klintmalm G, Henberg B. Experience in 1000 liver transplants under cyclosporine–steroid therapy: a survival report. Transplant Proc. 1988;20(Suppl. 1)98–504.

28. Colonna JO, Brems JJ, Hiatt JR, Millis JM, Ament ME, Baldrich-Quinones WJ, Berquist WE, Besbris D, Brill JE, Goldstein LI, Nuesse BJ, Ramming KP, Saleh S, Vargas JH, Busutttil RW. The quality of survival after liver transplantation. Transplant Proc. 1988;20(Suppl. 1):594–7.

29. Urbach AH, Gartner JC Jr, Malatack JJ. Linear growth following liver transplantation. Am J Dis Child. 1987;141:547–9.

30. Spolidoro JVN, Berquist WE, Pekivanoglu E, Busuttil RW. Growth acceleration in children after orthotopic liver transplantation. J Pediatr. 1988;112.41–4.

31. Stiller CR, Opelz G. Should cyclosporine be continued indefinitely? Transplant Proc. 1991;23:36–40.

32. Gremse DA, A-Kader HH, Schroeder TJ, Balistieri WF. Assessment of lidocaine metabolite formation as a quantitative liver function test in children. Hepatology. 1990;12:565–9.

23
Diagnosis of liver allograft rejection

J. NEUBERGER and D. ADAMS

INTRODUCTION

One of the major challenges facing those involved with organ transplantation is prevention of rejection. Conventional treatments for the prevention and treatment of rejection affects the immune system in a broad way, so that the price of prevention of rejection is that of increased susceptibility to infection. Techniques to treat the graft to induce tolerance are promising, but are not yet applicable for general clinical use[1,2]. Because of the trade-off between acceptance of the graft and increased susceptibility to infection, accurate and reliable diagnosis of liver allograft rejection is of clinical importance.

CLINICAL PATTERNS OF LIVER ALLOGRAFT REJECTION

Broadly, there are three clinical patterns of liver allograft rejection: hyper-acute/fulminant rejection, acute reversible rejection and chronic irreversible or ductopenic rejection[3-6]. There is not, as yet, universal agreement over terminology, and certainly this classification has a number of deficiencies.

Fulminant/hyperacute rejection

Fulminant/hyperacute rejection may occur within a few hours of transplantation but more commonly occurs after several days of normal graft function[7,8]. Initially the patient is well but rapidly develops liver failure with hepatic encephalopathy[9,10]. The only treatment is liver replacement. Although the diagnosis can usually be made on the basis of liver biopsy (see below), in practice, because of the impaired coagulation, it is usually not possible to obtain tissue for diagnosis.

The underlying mechanisms are uncertain; immune involvement is suggested by the increased deposition of immunoglobulins on sinusoidal lining cells and vascular endothelium[9,11]. It has been suggested that hyper-acute rejection occurs more commonly in those receiving ABO-incompatible grafts[9,11,12], and some centres report ABO mismatch in all cases of fulminant rejection. However, in our own series ABO mismatch was seen in only 18% of cases of hyperacute rejection[10].

Acute/reversible rejection

Acute rejection is usually apparent between 4 and 14 days after liver transplantation and clinically presents with fever, malaise and jaundice. Liver tests show characteristic changes with an early increase in the serum bilirubin followed by the liver enzymes. These changes are non-specific. The diagnosis is confirmed on liver biopsy, which shows the characteristic features, which are discussed below. The majority of cases of acute rejection respond well to treatment with increased immunosuppression. The conventional treatment is with either high-dose corticosteroids or anti-T-lymphocyte immunoglobulin such as monoclonal antibody to the CD3 receptor, OKT3. There is increasing interest in newer immunosuppressive agents, FK506, rapamycin, deoxyspergualin, mycophenolic acid ester and monoclonal antibodies such as anti-CD4, anti-CD7, anti ICAM-1, anti LFA-1 and anti-CD54. These are being evaluated in animal models and the clinical situation, with encouraging results[13].

Chronic/irreversible rejection

This form of rejection is characterized clinically by increasing progressive cholestasis, and histologically by the progressive loss of bile ducts; hence the term vanishing bile duct syndrome (VBDS). Although the onset may be within the first 2–4 weeks following liver transplantation, it is more commonly apparent 4–8 months after transplantation when good graft function has been established. Characteristically the first signs are those of biochemical evidence of cholestasis with a progressive rise in serum alkaline phosphatase followed by serum bilirubin. The patient complains of symptoms of cholestasis; jaundice, pruritus, pale stools and dark urine. Although more recently some instances of the vanishing bile duct syndrome have been shown to be reversible[14], most fail to respond to all forms of immunosuppression, and unless treated by re-transplantation, death from cholestasis appears inevitable. Recurrence is more common in those regrafted for irreversible rejection[15].

FREQUENCY OF DIFFERENT PATTERNS OF REJECTION

A recent analysis of patterns of clinical rejection was undertaken at the Liver Unit at the Queen Elizabeth Hospital, Birmingham (Dousset, personal communication). A total of 172 consecutive adult patients who received liver grafts were retrospectively assessed. Hyperacute rejection occurred in three patients and the onset was between day 7 and 9 post-transplant. All patients had received ABO identical grafts. Two patients died waiting for an emergency graft; the third was re-grafted.

Acute rejection occurred in 70% of the patients. While the majority had only one episode, 9% of the patients with rejection had two episodes and at least 6% had three episodes of rejection. The rejection episode usually occurred 12 days after transplant but five patients had their first episode of rejection between 20 and 116 days after transplantation. Only 7% of patients failed to respond to a 3-day course of high-dose corticosteroids and were subsequently treated with the monoclonal antibody OKT3.

Chronic rejection occurred in nine of the 172 patients and was diagnosed between 42 and 720 days post-transplant (median 122 days). Of these, three patients had undergone recurrent episodes of acute rejection and two had required OKT3 to control corticosteroid-resistant acute rejection. Of the nine patients, seven were re-transplanted. The occurrence of chronic rejection in those re-grafted for chronic rejection was 43% compared with 5% in the original graft. In none of these cases was there any clinical, serological or histological evidence of cytomegalovirus (CMV) infection, which has been implicated with the development of rejection by some series. Three patients had acute 'vanishing bile duct syndrome'. This was apparent between 14 and 28 days following transplantation. All had an episode of severe acute rejection and three of them required additional OKT3 therapy. In all cases patients received ABO identical livers. Transplantation was required in all cases.

Thus, while acute rejection is common after liver transplantation, it is hyperacute rejection and irreversible ductopenic rejection that are the major causes of graft loss.

HISTOLOGY OF LIVER ALLOGRAFT REJECTION

The diagnostic gold standard of allograft rejection is that of liver histology[3,4,6,7]. Liver can be obtained either by needle biopsy or by fine-needle aspiration.

Histological features of hyperacute rejection

The histological features of hyperacute rejection are those of extensive graft infarction, often with a widespread haemorrhagic element; there are clusters of hepatocytes undergoing necrosis with sinusoidal congestion and haemorrhage. As the process continues, the conventional features of acute rejection may become apparent (Fig. 1).

Acute rejection

The characteristic histological features of acute rejection are seen in the portal tracts, and the triad of rejection was initially described by Snover and colleagues[6]. The triad consists of a mixed portal tract infiltrate, bile duct damage and a venous endothelialitis (Fig. 2). It must be remembered that the histological picture may be modified by the current immunosuppressive drugs. The mixed portal inflammatory infiltrate consists of lymphocytes,

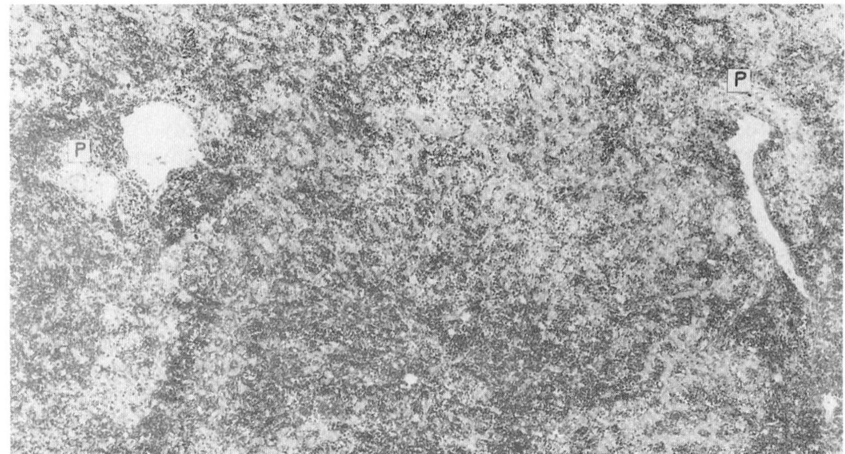

Fig. 1 Histology of end-stage liver with fulminant rejection showing panacinar haemorrhage and hepatic necrosis. Surviving portal tracts are seen (P)

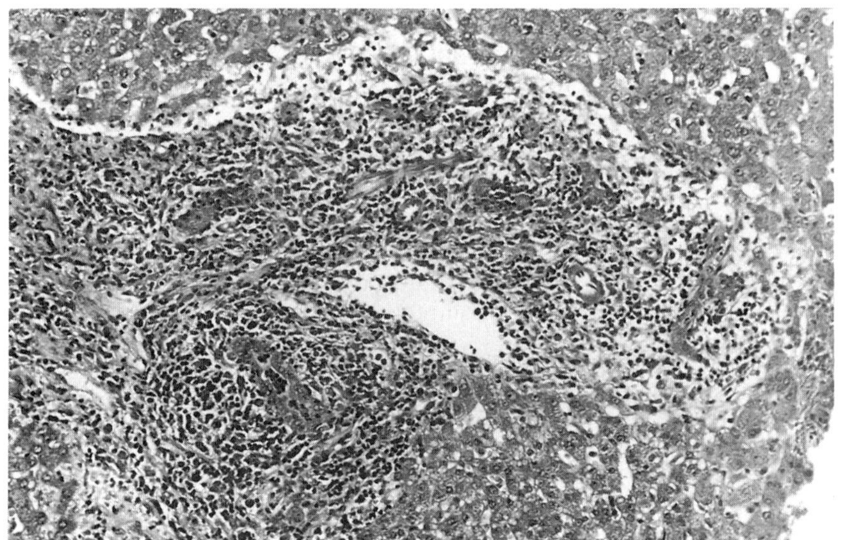

Fig. 2 Section of liver allograft 7 days post-transplant showing a portal tract infiltrate, inflammatory infiltration of bile ducts and venous endothelial cell inflammation

monocytes, plasma cells, neutrophils and eosinophils. Foster has suggested that neutrophils and eosinophils are specific for acute rejection[16]. The small and medium-sized bile ducts are infiltrated by neutrophils and mononuclear cells. In our experience the presence in the bile of neutrophils in the absence of bacteria is characteristic of rejection rather than cholangitis. The biliary epithelium itself shows features of degeneration with pyknosis and cytoplasmic eosinophilia. In more severe cases the bile ducts themselves are damaged and disrupted. Venous endothelial inflammation is characterized by, in mild cases, lymphoid cells attached to the lymphoid surface of the endothelium which, in more severe cases, progresses to subendothelial infiltration with lifting of the endothelium.

Parenchymal lesions are less marked but consist of lymphocytic infiltration, cholestasis, hepatocyte necrosis and ballooning which are mainly located in the perivenular region. Lymphocytic infiltration is, however, typical of acute allograft rejection.

Fine-needle aspiration biopsy

Fine-needle aspiration biopsy was originally developed for use in renal transplants as a reliable and atraumatic method of monitoring rejection. The technique is safe with few side-effects, and can be performed even when the platelet count is below 20 000/l and the coagulation factor V below 15%[17]. A drop of blood has to be taken simultaneously. Additional studies can be performed on activation markers on the cells. Although bacterial infection does not give rise to diagnostic problems, viral hepatitis and other inflammatory processes can make the diagnosis of rejection more difficult.

The sample is taken from the liver, the specimen is put through the cytocentrifuge and stained. The cell types are counted and a weighting factor is given for the different types of inflammatory cells. Thus, lymphoblast cells, plasma cells, monoblasts and macrophages have the highest correction factor (1.0) whereas lymphocytes carry a low correction factor (0.1), activated lymphocytes (0.5), large granulomatous lymphocytes (0.2), polymorphs (0.1) and monocytes (0.2) carry intermediate correction factors. The overall intensity of inflammation is expressed numerically in corrected increment units (CIU), and this finally corrected after subtracting the blood background. A CIU of 3 or more, and the presence of lymphoblastoid cells in the biopsy, is considered evidence of the onset of immune activation and rejection[18,19] (Fig. 3). A high macrophage count is said to predict progression to ductopenic rejection.

Fine-needle aspiration biopsy can achieve a predictive value of 86%, sensitivity 77% and specificity 90%[20]. Fine-needle aspiration biopsy, while safe and effective for the diagnosis of acute rejection, is less helpful in cases of chronic rejection and for assessing some of the complications occurring later[21].

Chronic rejection

There are two characteristic features of chronic rejection: bile duct damage and a vasculopathy. The bile duct damage is typically a destruction and subsequent absence of the small and medium-sized intrahepatic bile ducts, leading to the term 'vanishing bile duct syndrome'. The vasculopathy is an obliterative process involving large and medium-sized arteries (Fig. 4).

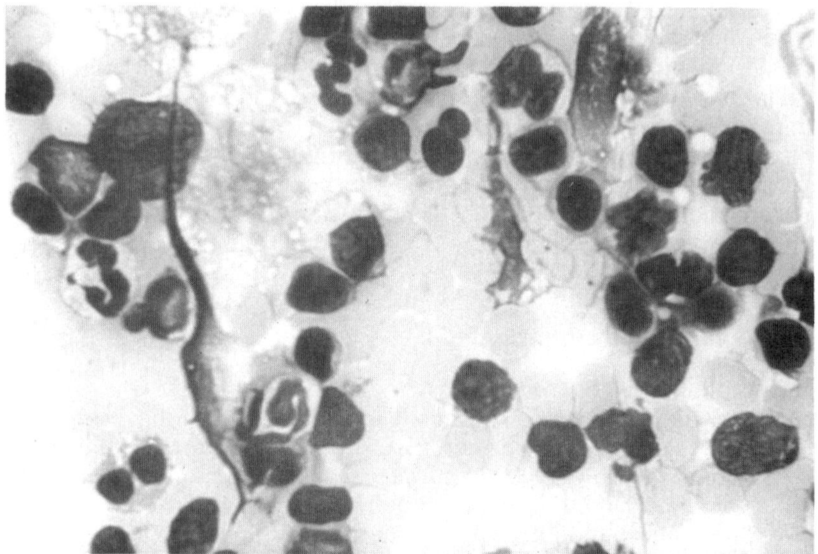

Fig. 3 Fine-needle aspirate from liver taken during acute graft rejection, showing neutrophils, lymphocytes and activated macrophages (courtesy of Dr J Young)

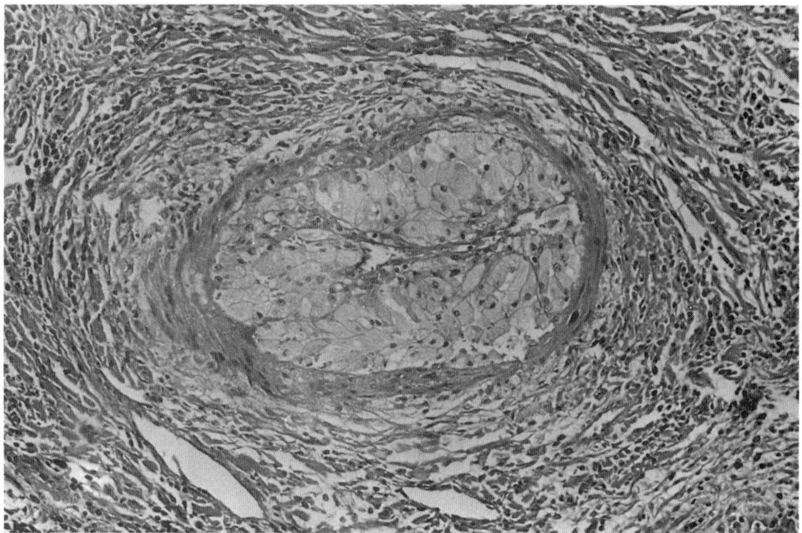

Fig. 4 Medium-sized artery from a hepatectomy specimen showing foamy cell infiltrate of the intima, typical of chronic rejection

Perivenular cholestasis and hepatocyte necrosis are present in the parenchyma. Although in the early stages of chronic rejection there is a prominent portal inflammatory infiltrate centred around bile ducts, as the disease progresses these inflammatory infiltrates are seen less clearly and the number

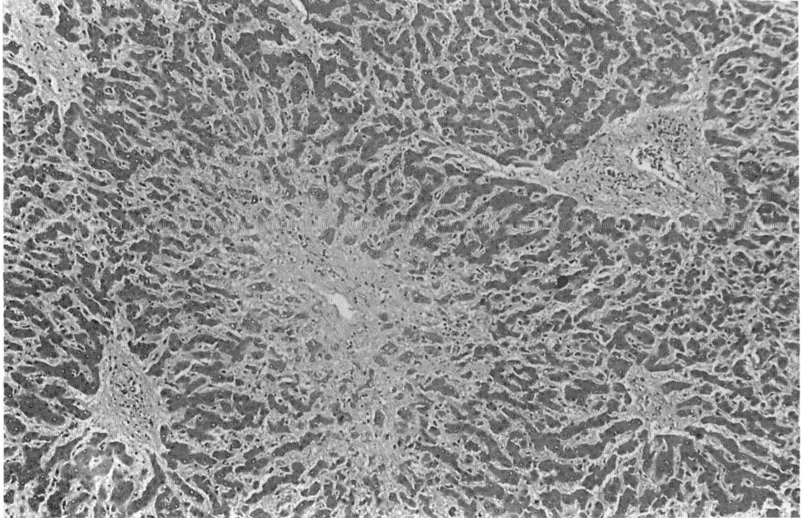

Fig. 5 End-stage chronic rejection (liver obtained at post-mortem) showing four portal tracts with a 'burnt-out' appearance and no evidence of inflammation. The liver parenchyma shows a characteristic lesion of perivenular hepatocyte drop-out and fibrosis

of bile ducts within the portal tracts progressively falls (Fig. 5). This condition contrasts with other vanishing bile duct syndromes such as primary biliary cirrhosis in that there is virtually no ductular proliferation in chronic rejection. The arterial lesions of chronic rejection consist of deposition of foam cells in the intima of large and medium-sized vessels. The foam cells may infiltrate the liver parenchyma but are not usually seen on needle biopsies.

Serological markers of acute rejection

Standard liver tests are not specific for acute rejection. Serum guanase and F-protein may be more sensitive than serum transaminases, but are not specific[21,22]. It has been suggested that a rise in sugar-conjugated bilirubin and fall in protein-bound bilirubin is helpful in diagnosing rejection[23]. Acute phase proteins such as orosomucoid, α-anti-chymotrypsin and amyloid A all show a rise but are not specific[24,25]. Abnormalities of coagulation and of bile acids occur during rejection but neither is specific for rejection[26,27].

The lack of specificity of the standard liver tests for the diagnosis of allograft rejection has led to the investigation of other markers of greater specificity. The rejection process is a manifestation of the inflammatory cascade[28] which starts with the presentation of allograft antigens to the host immune system resulting in immune activation, recruitment and ultimately progressive graft damage.

Markers of lymphocyte activation and recruitment

Lymphocyte activation is accompanied by both phenotypic and functional changes, including expression of activation markers on the cell membrane and secretion of cytokines which are involved in amplification of the immune response. Accurate measurement of cytokines in serum is difficult. The group of Tilg[29] have measured a number of different markers of immune activation and cytokines after organ transplantation and found detectable levels in serum of γ-interferon, β_2-microglobulin and neopterin, changes were not specific for rejection[30,31]. Interleukin-2 could not be detected. Others have confirmed the lack of specificity of β_2-microglobulin and neopterin for rejection. Assays for the soluble products of activation markers have shown, for example, that the soluble form of the interleukin-2 receptor (SIL-2R) is increased during rejection, this is not specific enough for routine clinical use[32,33]. In chronic rejection, serum levels tend to fall with time.

Assessment of the effector response has also been used to assess acute rejection. Effector cells include eosinophils, neutrophils, monocytes and perhaps most importantly cytotoxic T cells. Although T-cell numbers in peripheral blood change during rejection, most workers agree that these are not specific for the diagnosis of rejection[34–36]. However, unpublished observations from our unit (Hathaway and Adams) suggest that soluble CD-8 levels start to rise before episodes of acute rejection. It is not yet established whether similar changes are seen during infection. In peripheral blood, neutrophils are activated during episodes of rejection and, *in vitro*, increased responses to chemotactic stimuli and enhanced secretion of superoxide radicals and proteolytic enzymes can be shown[37]. These changes occur also during infection. Eosinophils are also seen in the portal tract infiltrate during episodes of rejection, and Foster and colleagues have shown that the peripheral blood eosinophil count starts to rise before rejection is apparent and this is, in their experience, both sensitive and specific[38]. Monocytes and macrophages are also present in inflammatory infiltrate of rejection. Levels of tumour necrosis factor (TNF), a product of activated macrophages and lymphocytes, rise during episodes of acute rejection, but again the specificity of increased TNF for rejection is inadequate for diagnostic use[39,40].

The third approach has been to look for evidence of target cell damage. With respect to the biliary epithelial cell, two proteins which are confined to the biliary epithelial cell in the liver are the epithelial cell membrane antigen EMA and secretory component. EMA is detected in bile following transplantation but levels do not rise during episodes of rejection. Secretory component is shed into bile during rejection, but similar amounts are found in bacterial cholangitis[41]. Biliary epithelial cells express HLA molecules and it is the class I molecules which may be the target of the lymphocyte-mediated attack[42]. As indicated above, serum levels of β_2-microglobulin are non-specifically elevated during rejection, but one study reported that biliary levels are more specific for rejection[29,43]. Pollard has shown that soluble class I antigens are released into serum and bile during rejection, and this may be of potential diagnostic value[44]. Biliary levels of the soluble form of ICAM-1 are also more specific for acute rejection than serum levels[45].

Table 1 Sensitivity and specificity of immunological markers of rejection (percentages)

Variable (and reference)	Sensitivity	Specificity
Blood eosinophilia[16]	83	100
Bile B2M[43]	96	87
Bile SIL2R[32]	94	84
Serum TNF[42]	89	88
Bile cICAM-1[45]	93	96

B2M, β_2-microglobulin; SIL2R, soluble interleukin 2 receptor; TNF, tumour necrosis factor; cICAM-1, circulating ICAM-1

Lymphocyte infiltration of the graft occurs by recruitment and local proliferation. Recruitment occurs in response to locally secreted chemotactic factors and these can be studied *in vitro*. In the 1–2 days preceding the clinical diagnosis of acute allograft rejection, factors chemotactic for lymphocytes can be detected in bile. These factors, which are probably secreted by CD-4 helper T cells, show preferential activity for recruitment of CD-8$^+$ T cells[46]. Although a chemotaxis assay to detect these factors can be performed within 6 h, this approach is more helpful in understanding the mechanism of allograft rejection rather than providing a test for the diagnosis of allograft rejection.

Immune damage to endothelial cells may be important in both acute and chronic rejection. Hepatic endothelial cell damage can be assessed by serum levels of hyaluronic acid, a proteoglycan which is specifically removed from the circulation by the hepatic endothelial cells. Other markers of endothelial cell dysfunction, such as the factor VIII-related antigen, reflect not only hepatic but also vascular endothelial cell damage. Circulating hyaluronic acid levels are increased 24 h before clinical rejection becomes apparent, and tend to be higher during rejection than other complications[47]. Again, the lack of specificity does not allow use of this measurement for the diagnosis of allograft rejection.

For serological markers to be of clinical value, both a high specificity and sensitivity are required. Of those series where such data are given (Table 1) it appears that serum levels are of little value. In contrast, measurements of factors in bile are of greater specificity.

PHYSICAL TESTS

Coulden and colleagues[47] suggested that Doppler ultrasound examination of hepatic veins could be of benefit in the diagnosis of acute rejection. Of 23 patients with biopsy-proven rejection, Doppler ultrasound showed an abrupt damping of pulsatile blood flow. Reduced pulsation was seen in cholangitis. However, in our experience this is not specific for acute rejection.

CONCLUSIONS

At present there is little doubt that hepatic allograft rejection remains a major problem following liver transplantation. The basis of diagnosing allograft rejection remains that of examining liver material. For acute rejection, both fine-needle aspiration and liver biopsy are of great sensitivity and specificity, while liver biopsy is of greater value in the diagnosis of chronic rejection. Serological markers of rejection are as yet of insufficient specificity for introduction into routine clinical use.

References

1. Platt JL, Vercellotti GM, Dalmasso A *et al.* Transplantation of discordant xenograft: a review of progress. Immunol Today. 1990;ii:450–6.
2. Bach FH, Sachs DH. Transplantation immunology. N Engl J Med. 1987;317:489–92.
3. Demetris AJ, Lasky S, Van Thiel D, Starzl TE, Dekker A. Pathology of hepatic transplantation. Am J Pathol. 1985;118:151–61.
4. Adams D, Neuberger JM. Patterns of graft rejection following liver transplantation. J Hepatol. 1990;10:113–19.
5. Hubscher SG. Histological findings in liver allograft rejection. Histopathology. 1990;18:377–83.
6. Snover DC, Sibley RK, Freese DK *et al.* Orthotopic liver transplantation: a pathological study of 63 serial liver biopsies from 17 patients. Hepatology. 1984;4:1212–23.
7. Starzl TE, Demetris AJ, Todo S *et al.* Evidence for hyperacute rejection of human liver grafts. Clin Transplant. 1989;3:37–45.
8. Bird G, Friend P, Donaldson P *et al.* Hyperacute rejection in liver transplantation. Transplant Proc. 1989;21:3742–4.
9. Gugenheim J, Samuel D, Reynes M, Bismuth H. Liver transplantation across ABO blood group barriers. Lancet 1990;336:519–23.
10. Hubscher SG, Adams DH, Neuberger J *et al.* Massive haemorrhagic necrosis of the liver after transplantation. J Clin Pathol. 1989;42:360–70.
11. Gugenheim J, Samuel D, Fabiani B *et al.* Rejection of ABO incompatible liver allografts in man. Transplant Proc. 1989;21:2223–4.
12. Demetris AJ, Jaffe R, Tzakis A *et al.* Antibody mediated rejection in human orthotopic liver allograft. Am J Pathol. 1988;132:489–502.
13. Adams D, Neuberger J. Treatment of acute allograft rejection. Sem Liver Dis. 1991 (In press).
14. Hubscher SG, Buckels JAC, Elias E, McMaster P, Neuberger J. Vanishing bile duct syndrome after liver transplantation: is it reversible? Transplantation. 1991;51:1004–10.
15. Wiesner RH, Van Hoek B, Ludwig J, Paya L. Recurrence of ductopenic rejection in liver allograft after transplantation for the vanishing bile duct syndrome. Transplant Proc. 1991 (In press).
16. Foster PF, Sankary HN, Hart M, Ashmann M, Williams J. Blood and graft eosinophilia as prediction of rejection in human liver transplantation. Transplantation. 1989;47:72–4.
17. Lautenschlager I, Hockerstedt K, Hayry P. Fine needle aspiration biopsy in the monitoring of liver allograft. Transplant Int. 1991;4:54–61.
18. Vogel W, Margreiter R, Schmalzl F, Judmaier G. Preliminary results with fine needle aspiration biopsy in liver graft. Transplant Proc. 1984;16:1240–2.
19. Lautenschlager I, Hockerstedt K, Ahonen J *et al.* Cellular characteristics of liver allograft rejection. Transplant Proc. 1987;19:2485–6.
20. Kirby RM, Young JA, Hubscher SG *et al.* Aspiration cytology in the diagnosis of rejection after orthotopic liver transplantation. Transplant Proc. 1989;19:3808–9.
21. Crary GS, Yasminek WG, Snover DC, Vine W. Serum guanase: a biochemical indicator of rejection in liver transplant recipients. Transplant Proc. 1989;21:2315–16.
22. Forbes GM, Oliviera D, Hughes R, O'Grady J, Calne R, Williams R. Serum F-protein in liver allograft recipients with graft dysfunction. Transplantation. 1989;118:995–7.
23. Cox CJ, Valdiserri RD, Zerbe TR, Genter JL. Ektachem bilirubin fraction BC as a predictor of liver transplant rejection. Transplantation. 1987;44:536–9.
24. Maury CPS, Teppo AM, Hockerstedt K. Acute phase proteins and liver allograft rejection. Liver. 1988;8:75–9.

25. Maury CPH, Hockerstedt K, Lautenschlager I, Scheinin TM. Monitoring of high density lipoprotein associated amyloid A protein after liver transplantation. Transplant Proc. 1987;19:3825–6.
26. Forster J, Greig PD, Glynn MF et al. Coagulation factors as indication of early graft function following liver transplantation. Transplant Proc. 1989;21:2308–9.
27. Herrera J, Coddceo R, Mora NP et al. Bile acid as an early indicator of allograft function during orthotopic liver transplantation. Transplant Proc. 1989;21:2313–14.
28. Adams DH. Mechanisms of human allograft rejection. Clin Sci. 1990;78:343–50.
29. Tilg H, Vogel W, Aulitsky WE et al. Evaluation of cytokines and cytokine induced secondary messages in sera of patients after liver transplantation. Transplantation. 1990;49:1074–84.
30. Maury CPS, Hockerstedt K, Tepo AM, Lautenschlager I, Ischeinin TM. Changes in serum amyloid A protein and beta-2-microglobulin in association with liver allograft rejection. Transplantation. 1984;38:551–5.
31. Oldhafer KS, Schaefer O, Wonigeit K, Ringe B, Pichlmayr R. Monitoring of serum neopterin levels after liver transplantation. Transplant Proc. 1988;20:671–7.
32. Adams DH, Wang L, Hubscher S, Elias E, Neuberger J. Soluble interleukin-2 receptors in serum and bile of liver transplant recipient. Lancet. 1989;1:469–72.
33. Perkins JD, Belson DL, Rakela J, Grambsch PM, Krom R. Soluble interleukin 2 receptor level as an indicator of liver allograft rejection. Transplantation. 1989;47:77–87.
34. Herron HG, Williams JW, Dean PJ. Alteration in immunologic measurements in patients experiencing early hepatic allograft rejection. Transplantation. 1988;45:923–5.
35. Munn SR, Tominaga S, Perkins SB, Hayes DH, Weisner RH, Krom RAF. Increasing peripheral T-lymphocytes count predict rejection in human liver allograft. Transplant Proc. 1988;20:674–5.
36. Hathaway M, Adams DH, Burnett D, Elias E. Recruitment of lymphocytes in human liver allograft during rejection. Transplant Proc. 1990;22:2306–7.
37. Adams DH, Wang LF, Burnett D, Stockley R, Neuberger J. Neutrophil activation: an important cause of tissue damage during allograft rejection. Transplantation. 1990;50:86–91.
38. Sankary H, Foster P, Hart M, Ashmann M, Schwartz D, Williams J. An analysis of the determinant of hepatic allograft rejection using stepwise logistic regression. Transplantation. 1989;47:77–81.
39. Adams DH, Garner C, Neuberger J. Serum tumour necrosis factor in liver transplantation. Transplant Proc. 1990;22:2310.
40. Adams DH, Burnett D, Stockley R, McMaster P, Elias E. Markers of biliary epithelial damage in liver allograft rejection. Transplant Proc. 1989;19:3820–1.
41. Steinhoff G. Major histocompatibility antigens in human liver transplantation. J Hepatol. 1990;11:9–15.
42. Imagawa DK, Millis JM, Olthoff KM et al. The role of tumour necrosis factor in allograft rejection. Transplantation. 1990;50:219–25.
43. Adams DH, Burnett D, Hubscher SG, McMaster P, Elias E. Biliary beta-2-microglobulins in liver allograft rejection. Hepatology. 1988;8:1565–70.
44. Pollard SG, Davies I, Calne RY. Soluble class I antigen in human bile. Transplantation. 1989;48:712–14.
45. Adams DH, Mainolfi E, Neuberger J, Elias E, Rothlein R. Secretion of circulating ICAM-1 into bile ducts during liver allograft rejection. Gut. 1991;32:A576.
46. Hathaway M, Adams DH, Burnett D, Elias E. Secretion into bile of chemotactic factor for CD$^+$ lymphocytes during rejection of human liver allograft. Transplant Proc. 1991;23:1424–33.
47. Coulden RA, Britton PD, Farman P, Nobile-Jamieson G, Wight D. Preliminary report: hepatic vein Doppler in the early diagnosis of acute liver transplant rejection. Lancet. 1990;336:273–5.

24
Value of bile acid determination and hepatic scintigraphy for the diagnosis of neonatal jaundice

J. PAWŁOWSKA, Z. BOGONIOWSKA, M. SZCZYGIELSKA-KOZAK, Z. WRÓBLEWSKA and J. SOCHA

INTRODUCTION

Cholestatic jaundice in early infancy requires early determination of the cause and appropriate treatment. A variety of causative factors and necessity to differentiate intra and extrahepatic cholestasis make numerous diagnostic tests mandatory. The differentiation of cholestasis has considerable practical implication since extrahepatic biliary tract atresia, which is the main cause of extrahepatic cholestasis, demands surgical treatment as soon as possible[1-5].

In spite of new diagnostic tests the differentiation of cholestasis is difficult in this early period. Liver biopsy is considered to be the most valuable test, and in expert hands has a diagnostic accuracy of over 95%[6].

In 1958 Carey[7] drew attention to serum bile acids in diseases of the liver and biliary tract. Serum bile acids concentration is known to increase manifold with the complete cessation of the enterohepatic circulation in biliary tract obstruction. Bile acid levels also increase in intrahepatic cholestasis due to, among other factors, 'leakage' from the damaged hepatocytes into the circulatory system. Cholestyramine administration may effect changes in bile acid metabolism[8-15].

In the search for methods permitting the differential diagnosis of cholestasis in infancy an attempt was made to assess the value of hepatic scintigraphy and bile acid determination in the serum and duodenal contents.

MATERIALS AND METHODS

The study included 90 infants aged 1–44 weeks admitted to hospital for prolonged jaundice after serological incompatibility had been excluded.

In all infants serum conjugated bile acid concentration, total and direct bilirubin, as well as alkaline phosphatase and alanine transferase, were determined prior to and following 3-day oral administration of 1 g/kg per 24 h cholestyramine in four daily doses. The duodenal contents were collected after a fast, and bile acid concentrations determined. In 35 infants functional hepatobiliary scintigraphy was performed.

The infants were subdivided into two groups:

Group I – 60 infants with intrahepatic cholestasis (34 infants aged 2–10 weeks and 26 infants aged 10–40 weeks);

Group II – 30 infants with extrahepatic cholestasis (15 infants aged 1–10 weeks and 15 infants aged 10–44 weeks).

In group I the diagnosis was confirmed by laparotomy in eight cases, autopsy in five cases and long-term (12–36 months) clinical observation in 47 cases. In group II the final diagnosis was established at operation on 28 infants and in two cases at autopsy.

Serum concentrations of conjugated bile acids were determined by radioimmunoassay[16] using a commercially available kit (Becton Dickinson, New York, USA). Serum bile acid concentration in a control group of children[17] was ($x \pm$ SEM) $2.61 \pm 0.37 \,\mu$mol/l.

Free and conjugated bile acids in duodenal contents were qualitatively and quantitatively determined by thin-layer chromatography and spectrophotometry. Bile acid concentration in duodenal contents in the control group of children[18] averaged 4.88 ± 2.01 mmol/l.

Functional hepatobiliary scintigraphy was performed with a Nuclear Ohio Sigma 410 camera using ^{99m}Tc-Hida (Sorin) as a radiotracer in a dose of $30–50 \,\mu$Ci/kg. In children with bilirubin concentration exceeding 5 mg/dl the radiotracer dose was increased to $200 \,\mu$Ci/kg.

The findings were analysed statistically using Student's t-test and the nonparametric Wilcoxon test.

The study was conducted in full compliance with the principles of the 'Declaration of Helsinki', and with the laws and regulations of Poland.

RESULTS

Serum bile acid concentrations were markedly elevated in all patients with cholestasis. Concentrations were higher in older infants; this presumably reflects increasing hepatocellular injury. Serum bile acid concentrations were statistically significantly higher in the extrahepatic cholestasis group compared with the intrahepatic disease group (Fig. 1). Similarly, total and direct bilirubin were also more elevated in group II.

Oral administration of cholestyramine produced a decrease in absolute values of serum bile acids (and bilirubin) concentrations in infants with intrahepatic but not extrahepatic cholestasis under 10 weeks of age (Fig. 2).

The mean bile acid concentrations in duodenal juice in groups I and II were 2.81 ± 4.10 mmol/l and 0.17 ± 0.18 mmol/l, respectively ($p < 0.001$). Complete absence of bile acids in the duodenal contents was established in 24 infants with extrahepatic cholestasis (Table 1). In the intrahepatic group

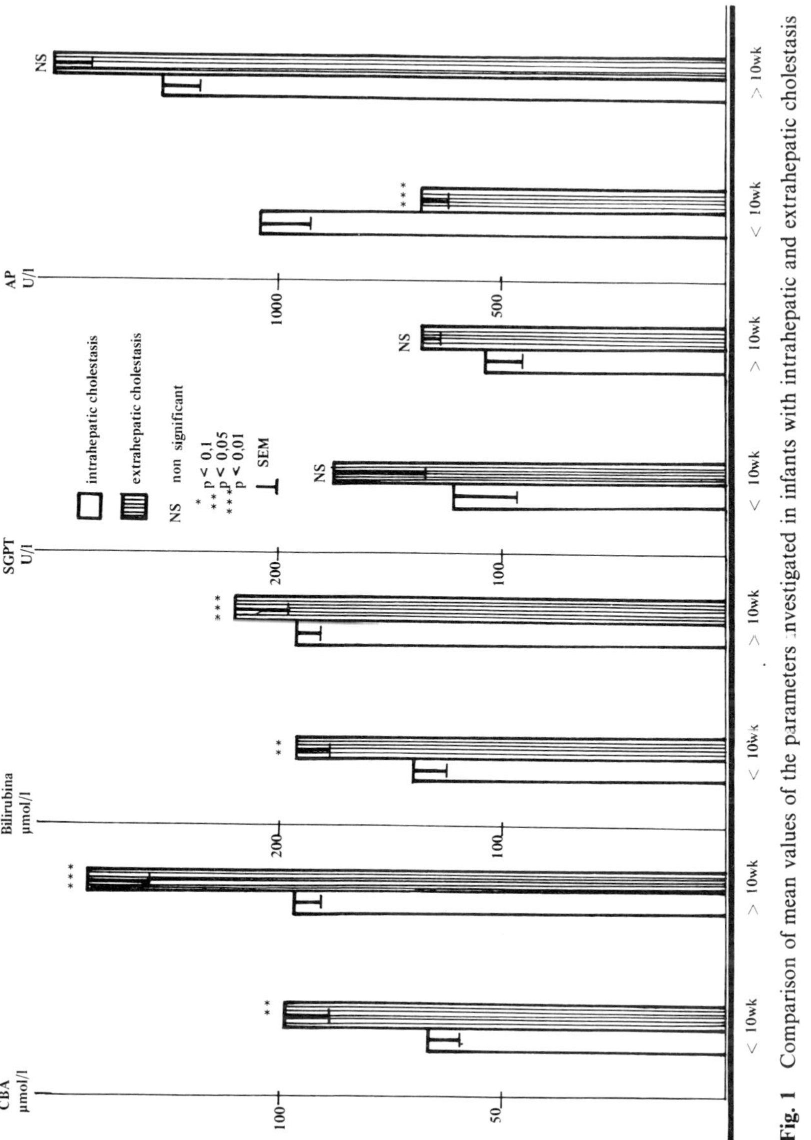

Fig. 1 Comparison of mean values of the parameters investigated in infants with intrahepatic and extrahepatic cholestasis

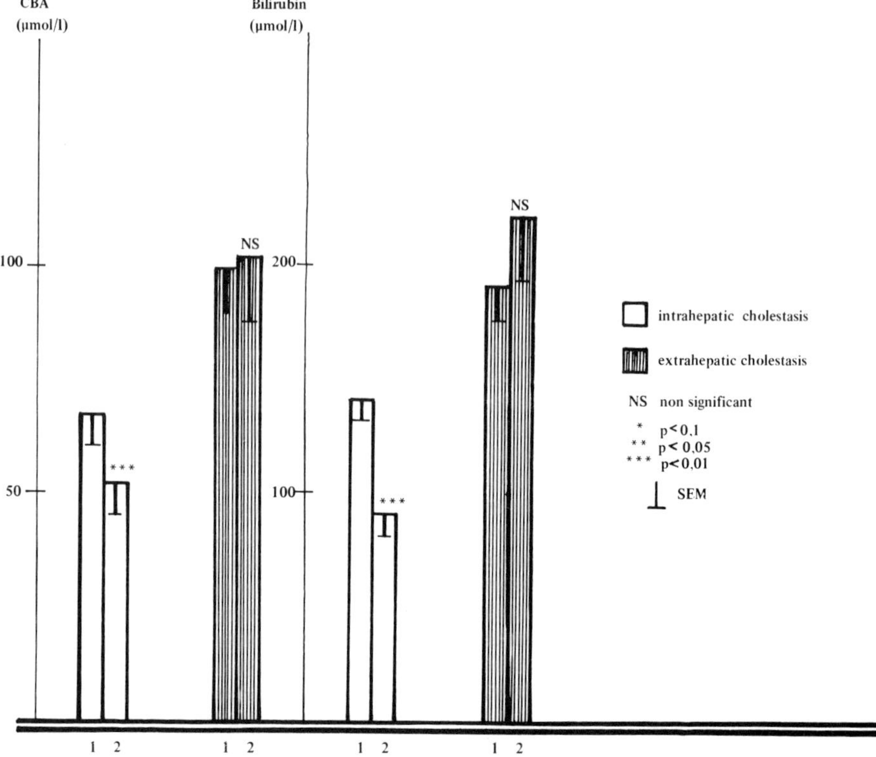

Fig. 2 Mean values of the parameters investigated before (1) and after (2) cholestyramine administration in infants aged 10 weeks

Table 1 Bile acid in the duodenal contents in children with cholestasis (percentages in parentheses)

	BA in duodenal fluid		Total
	Absent	Present	no. of cases
Group I: Extrahepatic cholestasis	24 (26.7)	6* (6.7)	30
Group II: Intrahepatic cholestasis	8 (8.9)	52** (57.7)	60
Total no. of cases	32	58	90

$\chi^2 = 2163.4$ *$X = 0.17 \pm 0.18$ mmol/l
$p \ll 0.001$ **$X = 2.81 \pm 4.10$ mmol/l

bile acids were present in the duodenal contents in 52 patients. The method had 84.4% sensitivity.

In 76.3% of the infants from group I who underwent hepatic scintigraphy the findings were in agreement with the bile acid assessment (Table 2). In two cases both studies yielded false-positive results.

Table 2 Correlation between bile acids in duodenal fluid and ^{99m}Tc-IDA scintigraphy in patients with intrahepatic cholestasis (percentages in parentheses)

| | ^{99m}Tc-IDA scintigraphy | | Total |
	+	−	no. of cases
Bile acids in duodenal fluid			
+	16 (66.7)	3	19
−	2	2 (9.6)	4
Total no. of cases	18	5	23

Table 3 Relative values of bile acids (percentages in parentheses)

CBA after cholestyramine administration	Group I		Group II	
	< 10 weeks	> 10 weeks	< 10 weeks	> 10 weeks
Elevated	4 (11.8)	3 (11.5)	4 (26.7)	7 (46.7)
Unchanged	10 (29.4)	2 (7.7)	5 (33.3)	1 (6.6)
Declined	20 (58.8)	21 (80.8)	6 (40.0)	7 (46.7)
Total no. of cases	34 (100)	26 (100)	15 (100)	15 (100)

DISCUSSION

Early differential diagnosis of cholestatic jaundice in infancy has for years constituted an important clinical problem. Considering the necessity of selecting the appropriate therapeutic approach the diagnosis should be established prior to 10 weeks of age. Clinical signs alone do not allow distinguishing between intrahepatic and extrahepatic cholestasis. In both syndromes jaundice appears in the first days or weeks of life, accompanied by hypocholic or acholic stools and dark urine. Occasionally the infant looks exceptionally well, although in some cases, especially in intrahepatic cholestasis, the patient may be seriously ill. Numerous studies have demonstrated that intrahepatic cholestasis in the course of neonatal hepatitis is more common in boys, prematurely born and low birth weight infants[19–22]. Familial occurrence is observed in 15–20% of cases.

In our material a significant decrease in absolute values of bile acids following cholestyramine administration was observed in the intrahepatic cholestasis group in younger infants. This probably reflected the still-efficient liver with preserved patency of the biliary tract, as severe injury to the hepatocyte is thought to be associated with the absence of response to cholestyramine.

Our study did not prove the superiority of serum bile acid determinations to bilirubin assessment in the diagnosis of biliary tract patency. It seems, however, that, particularly in the cases of intrahepatic cholestasis, serial determinations of serum bile acid concentration may provide additional information on liver cell function.

In children with intrahepatic cholestasis cholestyramine also has therapeutic effect since bile acids can cause injury to the hepatocyte.

Duodenal intubation with appraisal of the collected contents is employed in a few centres only[23-26]. These authors based their diagnoses on the presence of bilirubin in duodenal contents. Since bilirubin constitutes only 10% of organic anions in bile, while bile salts are the main component (60%), we thought that determination of bile acids in duodenal contents could more accurately reflect disturbances in bile secretion.

The absence of bile acids in the duodenal contents of infants with intrahepatic cholestasis could be due to several causes. Thus, bile flow into the duodenum is not constant, being affected by several factors, including food, enterohormonal stimulation and duodenal intubation itself. Therefore, extending the sampling over a longer period of time could improve the sensitivity of this test. Marked injury to the hepatocyte may be another cause for failure to excrete bile salts.

Bile acids were found in the duodenal contents of six infants with extrahepatic cholestasis. In two of them histology of an excised fragment of extrahepatic bile ducts revealed single spaces lined with columnar epithelium. This confirms the reports by Chandra[27] and Lea et al.[28], who are of the opinion that the presence of bile acids in the duodenal contents of infants with biliary obstruction may be caused by the flow of bile into the gallbladder before complete atresia has occurred.

It seems that the method of bile acid determination may become established as a reliable screening test allowing prompt differentiation between intrahepatic and extrahepatic cholestasis. It is a simple, not too invasive and cheap method. Additionally, bile acid determination in the duodenal contents after surgery may serve as one of the criteria of its effectiveness. The investigation is also less expensive and may be performed more frequently than e.g. scintigraphy.

References

1. Alagille D. Clinical aspects of neonatal hepatitis. Am J Dis Child. 1972;123:287–93.
2. Hays DM. Biliary atresia: the current state of confusion. Surg Clin N Am. 1973;53:1257–73.
3. Hitch DC, Shikes RH, Lilly JR. Determinants of survival after Kasai's operation for biliary atresia using actuarial analysis. J Pediatr Surg. 1979;14:310–13.
4. Kaliciński P, Cedro A, Kamiński W. Niedrożność dróg żołciowych: patogeneza, rozpoznanie, leczenie operacyjne i rokowanie. Przegl Ped. 1986;1:39–46.
5. Kobayashi A, Utsunomiya T, Kowai S, Ohbe Y. Congenital biliary atresia. Analysis of 97 cases with reference to prognosis after hepatic portoenterostomy. Am J Dis Child. 1976;130:830–3.
6. Brough AJ, Bernstein J. Morphologic approach to the evaluation of infantile conjugated hyperbilirubinemia. In: Javitt NB, editor. Neonatal hepatitis and biliary atresia. International workshop sponsored by NIH, DHEW Publication (NIH), 1979:381–96.
7. Carey JB, Jr. Serum trihydroxy–dehydroxy bile acid ratio in liver and biliary tract disease. J Clin Invest. 1958;37:1494–503.
8. Cox KL, Stadalnik RC, McGbahan JP, Sanders K, Cannon RA, Ruebner BH. Hepatobiliary scintigraphy with technetium-99m disofenin in the evaluation of neonatal cholestasis. J Pediatr Gastroenterol Nutr. 1987;6:885–91.
9. Iwańczak F, Prandota J, Iwańczak B. Diagnostyka różnicowa żołtaczek w wieku noworodkowym i niemowlécym. Ped Pol. 1981;2:209–14.
10. Javitt NB. Cholestasis in infancy – status report and conceptual approach. Gastroenterology. 1976;70:1172–84.

11. Javitt NB, Morrissey KP, Siegel E, Goldberg H, Gartner LM, Hollander M. Cholestatic syndromes in infancy. Diagnostic value of serum bile acid pattern and cholestyramine administration. Pediatr Res. 1973;7:119–25.
12. Deleze G, Paumgartner G. Bile acids in serum and bile of infants with cholestatic syndromes. Helv Paediatr Acta. 1970;32:29–32.
13. Morrisey KP, Javitt NB. Extrahepatic biliary atresia: diagnosis by serum bile acid patterns and response to cholestyramine. Surgery. 1973;74:116–21.
14. Poley JR, Caplan DB, Magnani HN, Alaupovic P, Smith EJ, Campbell DP, Bhatia M, Burdelski M, Bojanowski D. Quantitative changes of serum lipoprotein-x after cholestyramine administration in infants with cholestatic biliary tract and liver disease. Eur J Clin Invest. 1978;8:397–405.
15. Poley JR, Magnani HN. Cholestatic jaundice in infancy: diagnosis, differential diagnosis and treatment. Aust Pediatr J. 1976;12:134–53.
16. Spenny JG. An ^{125}I radioimmunoassay for primary conjugated bile salts. Gastroenterology. 1977;72:305–12.
17. Socha J, Bogoniowska Z, Szymański W, Pawłowska J, Woźniewicz B. Kwasy żółciowe w surowicy w przewlekłych zapaleniach watroby. Ped Pol. 1983;3:263–9.
18. Szymański W. Kwasy żółciowe w soku dwunastniczym w zespołach złego wchłaniania u dzieci. Ph. thesis, Child Health Center, Warszawa; 1981.
19. Altman RP. Biliary atresia. Pediatrics 1981;68:896–8.
20. Balistreri WE. Neonatal cholestasis. J Pediatr. 1985;106:171–84.
21. Javitt NB. Bile salts and liver diseases in childhood. Postgrad Med J. 1974;50:354–61.
22. Norris WJ, Hays DM. Problems in diagnosis associated with obstructive neonatal jaundice. Am J Surg. 1957;94:321–33.
23. Green HL, Helinek GL, Maran R, O'Neil J. Diagnosis of prolonged obstructive jaundice. J Pediatr. 1979;95:412–14.
24. Harada T. Differential diagnosis of congenital biliary atresia and neonatal hepatitis by 25-hour collection of duodenal fluid. Jpn J Pediatr Surg. 1981;13:759–65.
25. Hashimoto S, Tsugawa C, Kimura K, Matsumoto T, Morihana U, Araki M, Takamine H, Nishiyama S. Naso-duodenal tube technique for rapid diagnosis of congenital biliary atresia. J Jpn Soc Pediatr Surg. 1978;11:889–92.
26. Yamada R, Tsunoda A, Nishi T, Gamatoto H, Oohama Y. Differential diagnosis between biliary atresia and neonatal hepatitis by examination of duodenal fluid. In: Kasai M, editor. Biliary atresia and its related disorders. Amsterdam-Oxford-Princeton: Excerpta Medica; 1987:133–6.
27. Chandra RS. Histopathology of the liver and the fibrous remnant in biliary atresia. Proceedings of the 4th International Symposium on Biliary Atresia, 1986; Sendai.
28. Lea E, Penna FJ, Ferreira RA, Roquete MLV, Carvalho AST, Moto JAC. Obstructive jaundice of the infant. Diagnostic value of the duodenal intubation. Proceedings of the International Forum of Pediatric Gastroenterology and 2nd Annual Meeting of the Latin American Society for Pediatric Gastrology and Nutrition; 1976; São Paulo.

25
Procollagen type III peptide in evaluation of hepatic fibrosis in children with α_1-antitrypsin deficiency

J. RUJNER, J. SOCHA, R. JANAS and B. WOŹNIEWICZ

Diagnosis of hepatic fibrosis is established mainly on the grounds of histological examination. For many years attempts have been made to develop non-invasive techniques of assessment of hepatic fibrosis. Markers of collagen synthesis (prolyl-hydroxylase, PIIIP) and of degradation (collagenase, prolinase), or non-collagen glycoproteins (fibronectin, laminin, hepatonectin) and glycosaminoglycans have been considered[1]. Since 1974 numerous reports have studied the value of PIIIP levels to assess hepatic fibrosis. However, the majority of the reports deal with adult populations[3-7].

Cholestasis in infants with inborn α_1-antitrypsin deficiency (ATD) usually progresses to liver cirrhosis or fibrosis. The process develops at a different rate in different individuals[8,9].

In our study we make an attempt to assess the value of serum PIIIP in children with ATD estimating the degree of hepatic fibrosis and monitoring its progression.

MATERIALS AND METHODS

Investigations were carried out in 31 children with ATD (23 PiZZ, 6 PiMZ, 1 PiSS, 1 PiFZ). The patients were seven girls and 24 boys, aged 9 weeks to 14 years.

PIIIP concentration was measured using the RIA kit supplied by Hoechst, Germany.

In order to evaluate liver function and cholestasis the following parameters were determined: conjugated bile acid level — CBA (Abbott CG-RIA Diagnostic Kit), total bilirubin (Jędrasik's method), ALAT activity (enzymatic method with reagents by Boehringer Mannheim, and display on the Centrifichen apparatus by Union Carbide), alkaline phosphatase (optimal standard method at 30°C using centrifugation analysis with the Centrifichen 400

Table 1 Correlation between serum PIIIP concentration expressed as SDS depending and the degree of the liver fibrosis

Cholestasis present		Fibrosis degree			
		$III°$	$II°$	$I°$	0
Yes	$\bar{x}$	4.04	2.52	2.30	3.61
		23.08–(−)2.41	6.60–0.17	3.6–(−)0.1	—
	No	11	4	3	1
No	$\bar{x}$	0.55	0.15	0.90	−0.32
		3.1–(−)0.48	2.45–(−)2.69	4.09–(−)2.32	4.09–(−)1.18
	No	3	13	7	12
Total	$\bar{x}$	3.29 ± 1.78	0.71 ± 0.54	1.32 ± 0.61	−0.06 ± 0.34
		23.08–(−)2.41	6.60–(−)2.69	4.09–(−)2.32	3.61–(−)1.88
	No	14	17	10	13

apparatus and reagents by Boehringer Mannheim), and prothrombin index. None of the children had renal failure.

The investigations were carried out at certain time intervals, being done three times in seven children, twice in nine children, and once in the remaining children.

Examination of liver specimens obtained by percutaneous needly biopsy included, among others, severity of hepatic fibrosis, which was graded as follows: 0 = absent, I = mild, II = moderate, III = severe.

In children normal PIIIP values vary with age. When analysing our results we used the criteria established by Trivedi et al.[10] for children up to 200 weeks of age, Eriksson and Sveger[11] criteria for children between 8 and 12 years, and the criteria of Danne et al.[12] for pubertal children. Individual values were converted to standard deviation scores (PIIIP SDS) according to the following formula:

$$\text{SDS} = \frac{\text{Observed value} - \text{mean value for age-matched controls}}{\text{SD for age-matched controls}}$$

or presented as the ratio of the observed value to the mean value for the given age.

RESULTS

The results of all the determinations presented as PIIIP SDS are listed in Table 1 as a function of the degree of hepatic fibrosis and the presence or absence of cholestasis. No correlation was found between the degree of hepatic fibrosis and serum PIIIP concentration. However, the mean concentration value was raised in all the patient groups with coexisting cholestasis.

Table 2 shows the results presented as the ratio of the observed value to the mean value for age in accordance with the degree of hepatic fibrosis and coexisting pneumonia, sepsis, or urinary infection. Analysis of the above data showed no correlation between the degree of hepatic fibrosis and the observed values. However, increased values were noted in groups 0, II and III with

Table 2   Correlation between serum PIIIP concentration expressed as SDS depending on the cholestasis or infection (pneumonia, urinary infection, sepsis) coexistent with liver fibrosis

Infection present		Fibrosis degree			
		$III°$	$II°$	$I°$	0
Yes	$\bar{x}$	2.75	1.46	1.42	1.89
		6.25–0.56	2.11–1.05	1.57–0.98	—
	No	6	3	4	1
No	$\bar{x}$	1.10	1.06	1.60	0.89
		2.02–0.39	1.82–0.04	2.42–0.71	1.55–0.56
	No	8	4	6	12

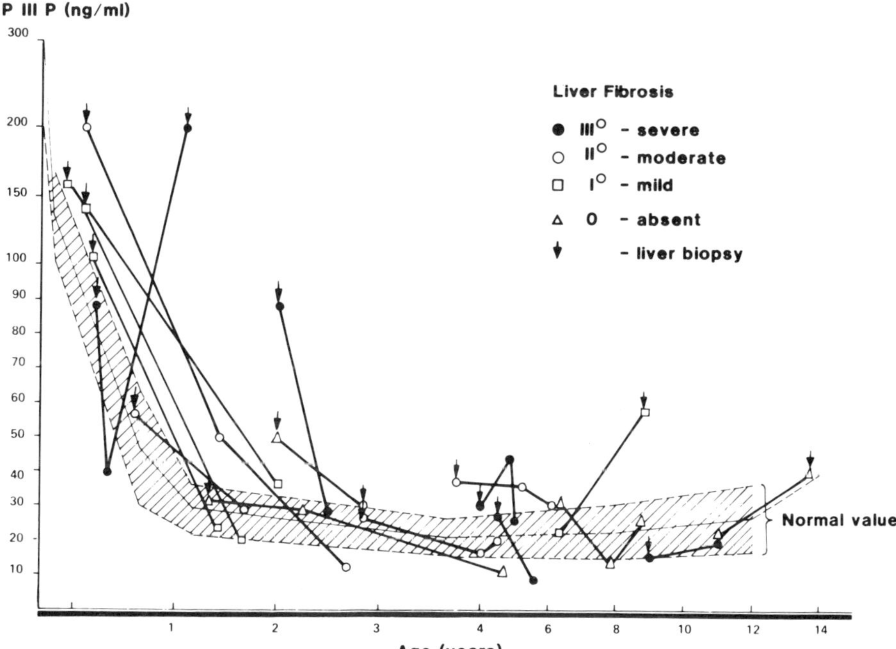

Figure 1   Serum PIIIP concentration in relation to liver fibrosis and age in each patient in repeated examinations. Serum PIIIP concentration increased in each patient with ongoing infection (mostly sepsis)

coexisting extrahepatic inflammation. In severe liver cirrhosis and non-inflammatory hepatic fibrosis the values were lower in cirrhosis ($\bar{x}$ 1.29) and fibrosis (1.13) than in progressive inflammatory cirrhosis ($\bar{x}$ 2.59).

Patterns of PIIIP concentration in repeated investigations in 16 children are presented in Fig. 1. Follow-up examinations showed raised values in 31.2% (5 out of 16 patients) as compared with the initial 50% (8 out of 16 patients).

Figure 2 shows the relationships between PIIIP levels and the different conventional liver tests.

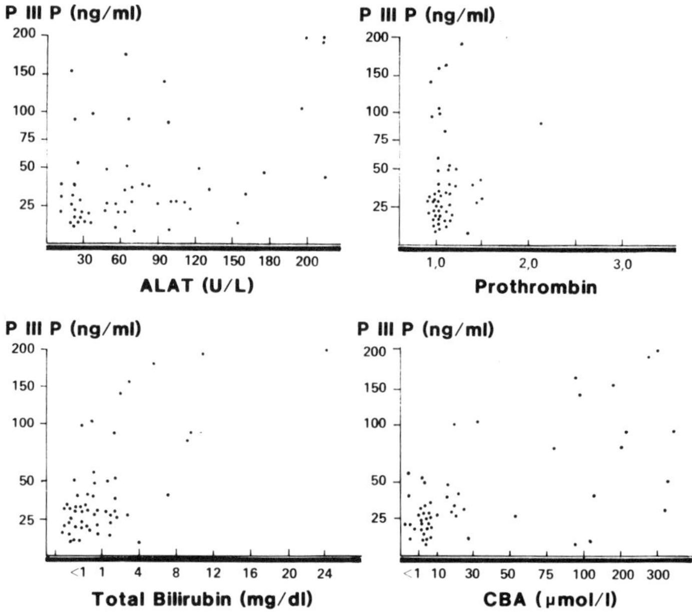

Figure 2 Correlation between serum PIIIP concentration expressed as SDS depending on the serum concentration of ALAT, prothrombin index, total bilirubin and CBA. Serum PIIIP concentration showed no significant correlation with ALAT ($y = 0.0059x + 0.6511, r = 0.1217$), prothrombin index ($y = 0.0120x + 1.0259, r = 0.0046$) and weak correlation with bilirubin ($y = 0.3167x + 0.5439, r = 0.2684$) and with CBA ($y = 0.001x + 0.4209, r = 0.3936$)

DISCUSSION

The level of serum procollagen type III peptide depends on synthesis and degradation of tissue collagen (liver, bones, lungs, etc.) as well as on its excretion by the kidneys and biliary tract[13]. High serum PIIIP levels were found in healthy children during their rapid growth and in children with dwarfism treated with HGH, as well as in adults with Paget's disease, myelofibrosis, scleroderma, fibrotic pulmonary diseases, and rheumatoid arthritis[12,14–17]. In inflammatory processes a high activity of macrophages, which, among others, produce fibronectin, results in increased collagen formation[18]. Surrenti *et al.* found increased PIIIP levels in as many as 73.4% of patients with chronic active hepatitis and only 36.3% of those with chronic persistent hepatitis[19]. Similar results were reported by Rhode *et al.*[20]. Surrenti demonstrated a positive correlation between serum PIIIP levels and presence of inflammatory infiltrates in the portal space, necrosis and degenerative processes[19]. Our results confirm these data. We observed that the mean PIIIP concentration was twice as high in patients with liver cirrhosis and an accompanying inflammatory process than that in patients with inactive cirrhosis and non-inflammatory hepatic fibrosis. PIIIP concentration was also raised in children with coexisting extrahepatic inflammation (pneumonia, sepsis, urinary infection) as compared with those without any infections, regardless of the degree of hepatic fibrosis. This finding implies involvement of PIIIP resulting from extrahepatic collagen metabolism. It is especially significant in monitoring progression of hepatic fibrosis in children with ATD who have a higher incidence of pneumonia and bronchitis.

In the liver itself the ratio of particular collagen fractions to one another varies with the degree of hepatic fibrosis. At the initial stage, when the amount of newly produced collagen is not significant, the ratio between type I and type III is 1:1. With an increased amount of collagen the level of collagen type I markedly rises and the ratio changes[21] to 2:1. This should account for our findings of low PIIIP levels in severe inactive liver cirrhosis. Similar evidence was also reported by other authors[4,5,10]. Trivedi *et al.* assessed serum PIIIP levels in children with ATD and cirrhosis, and found normal PIIIP levels in three out of seven children with liver cirrhosis without jaundice[10].

We did not observe any correlation between serum PIIIP and the degree of hepatic fibrosis on histological examination. Raised levels observed in all the degrees of fibrosis were noted when cholestasis developed. This may be associated with a delayed PIIIP excretion by the biliary tract since renal failure had been excluded in all the children.

The influence of a great number of extrahepatic factors on serum PIIIP levels including different growth rate results in the lack of specificity of PIIIP determination in the assessment of hepatic fibrosis in ATP. Thus, diagnosis of hepatic fibrosis or liver cirrhosis in children will still require liver biopsy.

References

1. Myara I, Cosson C. Fibrose hepatique: modifications du collagene et marqueurs seriques lies a son metabolisme. Gastroenterol Clin Biol. 1988;12:99–106.
2. Hahn EG, Schuppan D. Collagen metabolism in liver disease. In Bianchi L *et al.*, editors. Liver in metabolic diseases. Lancaster: MTP Press; 1983:309–23.
3. Bell H, Raknerud N, Orjasaeter H, Hang E. Serum procollagen III peptide in alcoholic and other chronic liver disease. Scand J Gastroenterol. 1989;24:1217–22.
4. McCullough A, Stassen WN, Wiesner RH, Czaja A. Serum type III procollagen peptide concentrations in severe chronic active hepatitis: Relationship to cirrhosis and disease activity. Hepatology. 1987;7:49–54.
5. Schneider M, Voss B, Hogemann B, Eberhardt G, Gerlach U. Evaluation of serum laminin P_1, procollagen III peptides, and *N*-acetyl-beta-glucosaminidase for monitoring the activity of liver fibrosis. Hepato-Gastroenterol. 1989;36:506–10.
6. Torres-Salinas M, Pares A, Caballeria J, Jimenez W, Heredia D, Bruguera M, Rodes J. Serum procollagen type III peptide as a marker of hepatic fibrogenesis in alcoholic hepatitis. Gastroenterology. 1986;90:1241–6.
7. Weigand K, Zaugg PY, Frei A, Zimmermann A. Long-term follow-up of serum N-terminal propeptide of collagen type III levels in patients with chronic liver disease. Hepatology. 1984;4:835–8.
8. Dick MC, Mowat AP. Hepatitis syndrome in infancy – an epidemiological survey with 10 year follow up. Arch Dis Child. 1985;60:512–16.
9. Latimer JS, Sharp HL. Alpha-1-antitrypsin deficiency in childhood. Curr Probl Pediatr. 1980;11:4–30.
10. Trivedi P, Cheeseman P, Portmann B, Mowart AP. Serum type III procollagen peptide as a non-invasive marker of liver damage during infancy and childhood in extrahepatic biliary atresia, idiopathic hepatitis of infancy and alpha-1-antritrypsin deficiency. Clin Chim Acta.

1986;161:137–46.
11. Eriksson S, Sveger T. Procollagen type III peptide in asymptomatic children with alpha-1-antitrypsin deficiency. J Pediatr Gastroenterol Nutr. 1988;7:938–9.
12. Danne T, Gruters A, Schnabel K, Burger W, L'allermand D, Enders I, Helge H, Weber B. Long term monitoring of treatment with recombinant human growth hormone by serial determinations of type III procollagen-related antigen in serum. Pediatr Res. 1988;23:167–71.
13. Alcorn J, Chojkier M. Procollagen III peptide (PIIIP): can it reflect hepatic fibrosis? Hepatology. 1987;7:981–3.
14. Apaja-Sarkkinen M, Autio-Harmainen H, Alavaikko M, Risteli J, Risteli L. Immunohistochemical study of basement membrane proteins and type III procollagen in myelofibrosis. Br J Haematol. 1986;63:571–80.
15. Cavalleri A, Gobba F, Bacchella L, Luberto F, Ziccardi A. Serum type III procollagen peptide in asbestos workers: an early indicator of pulmonary fibrosis. Br J Indust Med. 1988;45:818–23.
16. Hasselbach H, Junker P, Horslev-Petersen K, Lisse I, Bentsen KD. Procollagen type III aminoterminal peptide in serum in idiopathic myelofibrosis and allied conditions: relation to disease activity and effect of chemotherapy. Am J Hematol. 1990;33:18–26.
17. Risteli J, Sogaard H, Oikarinen A, Risteli L, Karvonen J, Zachariae H. Aminoterminal propeptide of type III procollagen in methotrexate-induced liver fibrosis and cirrhosis. Br J Dermatol. 1988;119:321–5.
18. Rojkind M, Kershenobich D. In: Csomos G, Thoder H, editors. Clinical hepatology. Berlin: Springer-Verlag; 1983;126.
19. Surrenti C, Casini A, Milani S, Ambu S, Ceccatelli P, D'Agata A. Is determination of serum N-terminal procollagen type III peptide (sPIIIP) a marker of hepatic fibrosis? Digest Dis Sci. 1987;32:705–9.
20. Rohde H, Vargas L, Halm E, Kalbfleisch V, Burguera M, Timpl R. Radioimmunoassay for type III procollagen peptide and its application to human liver disease. Eur J Clin Invest. 1979;9:451–9.
21. Rojkind M. Fibrogenesis. In Arias IM *et al.*, editors. The liver, biology and pathobology. New York: Raven Press; 1982:801.

26
Gallbladder emptying in patients with cystic fibrosis compared with healthy controls

R.-D. STENGER and B. BEYER

INTRODUCTION

Cystic fibrosis (or mucoviscidosis) has an approximate prevalence of 1:2000, which makes it the most widespread inborn error of metabolism in Caucasian populations.

A generalized disorder of most exocrine glands is responsible for an abnormal composition of their secretory products. These contain abnormal mucoproteins and evidence pathological changes in the water and electrolyte content.

In addition to the lungs, paranasal sinuses, sweat glands, pancreas and male gonads, the liver is also affected in about 25% of cases. The disorders are already apparent in childhood and, when followed by cholestasis, can finally result in a focal biliary cirrhosis[1].

Ultrasonography of the liver and gallbladder makes it possible not only to identify morphological changes but also to examine the dynamics of gallbladder emptying[2-6].

The use of ultrasound to evaluate gallbladder function is reliable and has taken the place of radiological and nuclear medical techniques because it has no side-effects[7,8]. We therefore used this method to examine whether, in CF, gallbladder contraction is perhaps disturbed as a consequence of cholestasis, or whether there are other causes.

MATERIALS AND METHODS

The study comprised 10 children with cystic fibrosis (six males and four females, average age 10.6 ± 1.6 years) and 10 children as controls (six females and four males, average age 7.8 ± 1.8 years).

The serum bilirubin, ASAT and ALAT were within normal limits in all cases. The CF patients all had an alkaline phosphatase activity in excess of $5\,\mu$mol/s per litre.

The three major dimensions of the gallbladder – length, breadth, and anterior/posterior diameter (depth) – were measured by ultrasonography and the position of the transducer was marked on the skin of the abdomen so that repeated measurements were always performed at the same angles (Fig. 1).

The gallbladder volume (V) was calculated according to the following ellipsoid equation:

$$V = \frac{\pi}{6} \times \text{length} \times \text{breadth} \times \text{depth}$$

The size of the gallbladder was measured after at least 12 h of fasting. A gastric stimulant was given consisting of 130 ml water, 20 ml sorbitol in a 40% solution and an egg yolk, and then further measurements were taken after 5, 10, 15, 30, 45 and 60 min according to Krönert et al.[4].

The Mann–Whitney U-test was used to calculate the significance because the number of cases in both groups was small and could not guarantee a normal distribution.

RESULTS

After the gastric stimulant the gallbladder volume declined by $69.80 \pm 19.38\%$ in the CF patients (range of variation 28.27–90.03%) and by $95.64 \pm 2.06\%$ in the controls (range of variation 92.20–98.21%). This difference is statistically significant ($p < 0.01$) and was already evident after 15 min (Fig. 2). The gallbladder fasting volume increases with age but gallbladder contraction does not increase to the same extent (Fig. 3). In some of the older test subjects in both groups the contraction effect of the gastric stimulant had already declined by the 60th minute. In our CF patients we could detect no signs of liver cirrhosis, gallstones or microgallbladder.

DISCUSSION

Gallbladder motility has become a subject of scientific research thanks to the introduction of real-time ultrasonography. The contraction of the gallbladder can be disturbed in diabetes mellitus[4], cholelithiasis[9] and other diseases. Until now it has been unknown whether gallbladder motility is disturbed in cystic fibrosis. Our investigation indicated disturbances of gallbladder contraction in CF patients after a gastric stimulant. The effect was more marked in the older patients, although a decrease in gallbladder reaction with increasing age must be taken into account. The mean age of the CF group was slightly higher than that of the controls. These results need to be confirmed by further studies of larger groups of patients.

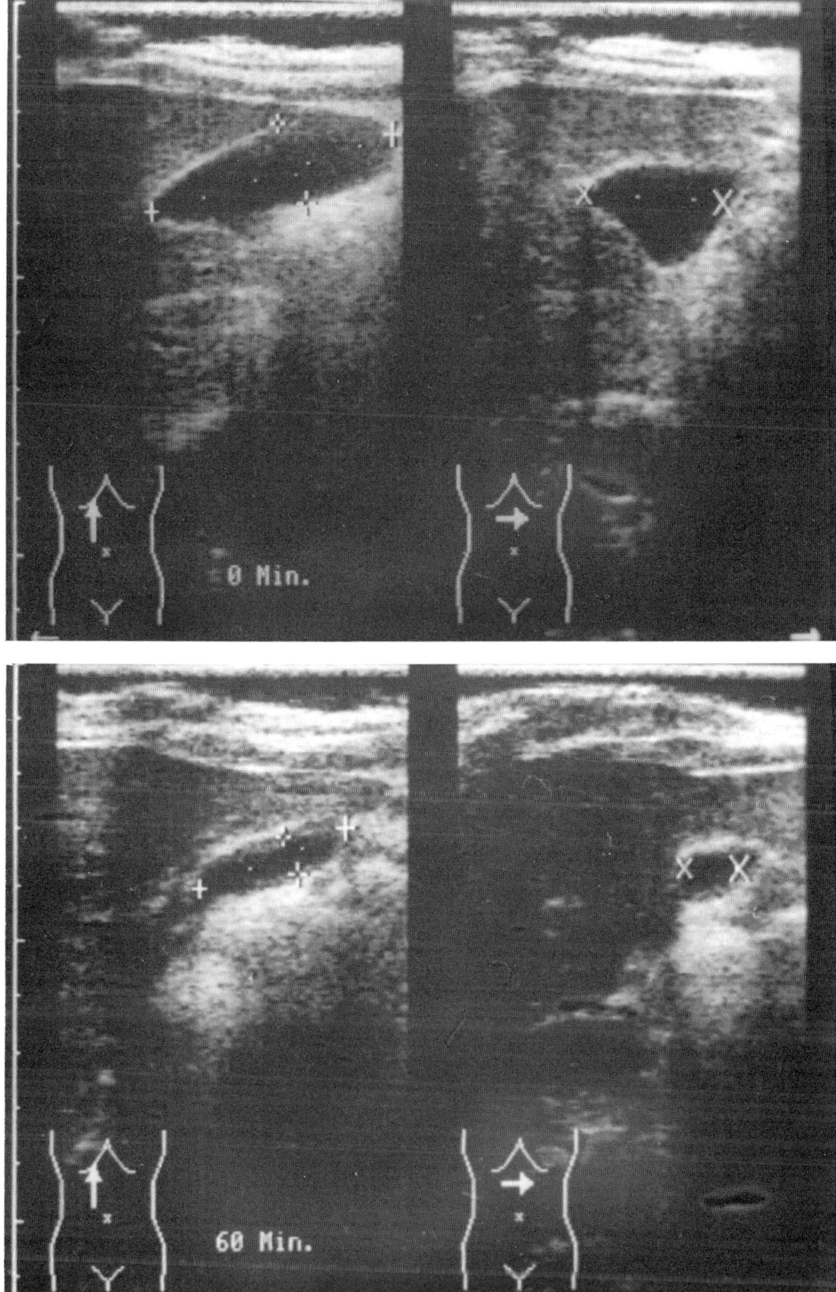

Fig. 1 Axial and transverse measurements of the gallbladder of a CF patient before (**a**) and 60 min after (**b**) gastric stimulant. The shape and contours of the gallbladder provide no indication of pathology. The measurement angles have been marked in each case

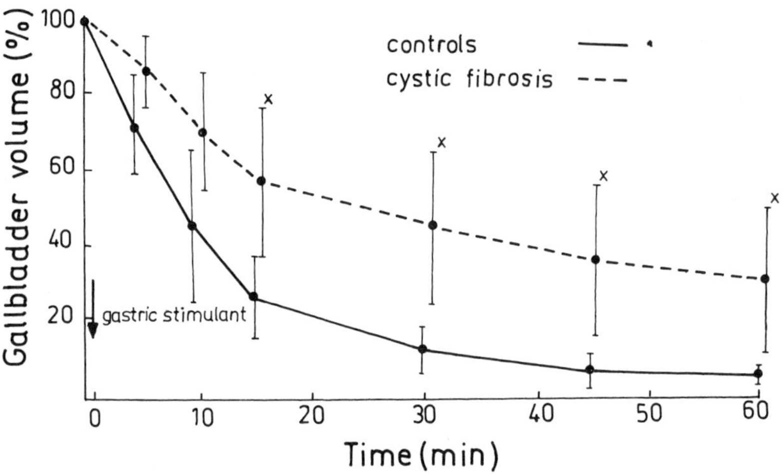

Fig. 2 Gallbladder emptying (mean $\pm$ SD in percentage of fasting volume) of CF patients ($n = 10$) and controls ($n = 10$) after a gastric stimulant; *$p < 0.01$

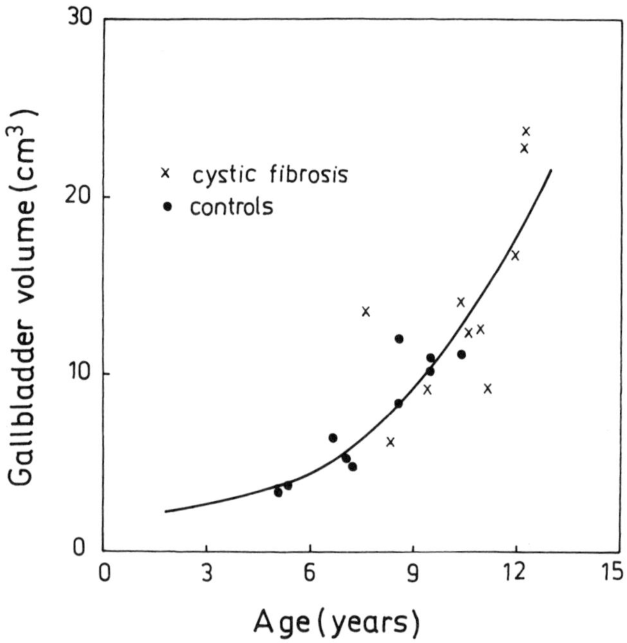

Fig. 3 Correlation between fasting gallbladder volume and age in children with CF ($n = 10$) and a control group ($n = 10$)

Acknowledgements

The authors wish to thank Mrs Holz, Mrs Sack, and Mrs Wettengel for technical assistance.

References

1. Lentze MJ. Mukoviszidose (zystische Fibrose), Leber und Gallenwege. In: Betke K, Künzer W, Schaub J, editors. Lehrbuch der Kinderheilkunde, 6. neubearbeitete und erweiterte Auflage. Stuttgart–New York: Georg Thième; 1991:820–1.
2. Arienti V, Magri F, Boriani L, Belotti M, Ugenti F, Gasbarrin G. Levosulpiride versus clebopride in gastric and gallbladder emptying in patients with functional dyspepsia: ultrasonographic evaluation. Curr Ther Res. 1991;49:575–87.
3. Janowitz P, Swobodnik W, Wechsler IG, Hagel S, Ditschuneit H. Sonographische Beurteilung der Gallenblasenfunktion mittels Planimetrie. Ultraschall Med. 1990;11:135–8.
4. Krönert K, Götz V, Reuland P, Luft D, Eggstein M. Gallbladder emptying in diabetic patients and control subjects assessed by real-time ultrasonography and cholescintigraphy: a methodological comparison. Ultrasound Med Biol. 1989;15:535–9.
5. Quvist N, Rafaelson S, Øster-Jørgensen E, Rasmussen L, Hovendal C, Pedersen SA. The simultaneous use of 99m-Tc-HIDA scintigraphy and ultrasound in the determination of gallbladder storage and emptying in the fasting state. Eur J Gastroenterol Hepatol. 1991;3:657–61.
6. Wedmann B, Schmidt G, Wegner M, Coenen C, Ricken D, Dröge C. Sonographic evaluation of gallbladder kinetics: *in vitro* and *in vivo* comparison of different methods to assess gallbladder emptying. J Clin Ultrasound. 1991;19:341–9.
7. Bellamy PR, Hicks A. Assessment of gallbladder function by ultrasound: implication for dissolution therapy. Clin Radiol. 1988;39:511–12.
8. Ereson GT, Johnson ML, Kern F. A critical evaluation of real-time ultrasonography for the study of gallbladder volume and contraction. Gastroenterology. 1980;83:773–6.
9. Schaffer EA, McOrmond P, Duggan H. Quantitative cholescintigraphy: assessment of gallbladder filling and emptying and duodenal–gastric reflux. Gastroenterology. 1980;79:899–906.

27
Ultrasound examination of the biliary system in children with acute viral hepatitis

V. USONIS, K. MOCISKIENE, V. DAUGELAVICIUS, A. CEKUOLIS,
S. KAROSIENE and R. MYKOLAITIENE

INTRODUCTION

In newborns and infants ultrasound is the most common means for diagnosing the absence of the biliary tree and the gallbladder[1,2]. It is also often used for discovering gallstones[3], severe inflammatory diseases of the gallbladder and biliary system[4-6]. The diagnoses of the disorders of the biliary system revealed by ultrasound have been usually confirmed using other techniques[7-9]. The most distinctive findings during acute viral hepatitis are: the increased overall echogenicity of the liver and in some cases the markedly thickened gallbladder wall[10,11]. Sometimes dilated intrahepatic bile tracts are visible[12].

An attempt has been made to reveal deformations of the biliary system in children with acute viral hepatitis. These disorders worsening the course of disease and prolonging rehabilitation may be considered as one of the reasons for cholestasis.

PATIENTS AND METHODS

Two hundred and thirty-three children with acute viral hepatitis were under investigation. The mean ($\pm$ SD) age was 7.9 $\pm$ 1.2 years, with 104 (44.6%) girls and 129 (55.4%) boys. Diagnosis of viral hepatitis was based on routine clinical, biochemical findings, and confirmed by detecting hepatitis virus markers – anti HAV/IgM for viral hepatitis A (215 or 92.3% of patients in our study) and HDsAg, HBcAg/IgM, HBeAg for viral hepatitis B (18 or 7.7% of patients). The patients were categorized as follows: (1) having no changes in the biliary system; (2) having anatomical defects without inflammatory changes and (3) having inflammatory changes such as cholecystitis or cholangitis.

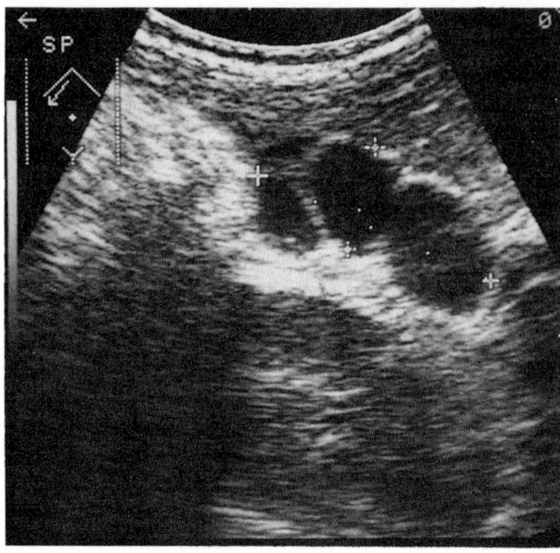

Fig. 1 A girl aged 9 years: congenital septae in fundal part of gallbladder

Ultrasonography of the hepatobiliary system was performed after an overnight fast, by means of ultrasound scanner Picker International LS-2700, using 5 and 3.5 MHz linear probes and Picker International LSC-7000 using 3.5 MHz convex probes.

RESULTS

Alterations of the biliary system have been registered in 58.4% (136) of all cases; they were not related to sex or age of the patients investigated. In five patients, defects in the development of the gallbladder (such as septum of the fundal region of the gallbladder) have been detected (Fig. 1). In 102 patients (43.8% of all under examination!), deformations of the gallbladder and/or intrahepatic biliary ducts have been found. The most common findings were the following: strictures of the gallbladder (Fig. 2), bendings of the caudal part of the gallbladder and multiple bendings of the cystic duct. Inflammatory changes of the biliary system such as cholecystitis (Fig. 3) and cholangitis (Fig. 4) were observed in 34 (14.6%) patients. The diagnoses of inflammatory changes of the biliary system were based on clinical symptoms, thickened walls of the gallbladder or bile ducts revealed by ultrasound, routine blood and bile tests.

The clinical course of acute viral hepatitis and biochemical changes in patients with disorders of the biliary tract were significantly longer and more severe compared with patients without these disorders (Table 1).

Clinical and biochemical data were identical in all three groups at the beginning of the disease while significant differences became evident after only 10 days. Hyperbilirubinaemia, hepatomegaly and elevated levels of alanine aminotransferase lasted significantly longer in patients with disorders

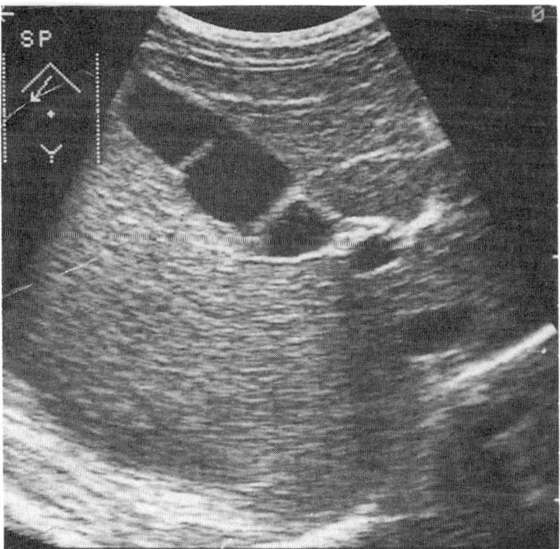

Fig. 2 A boy aged 6 years: deformations of the gallbladder

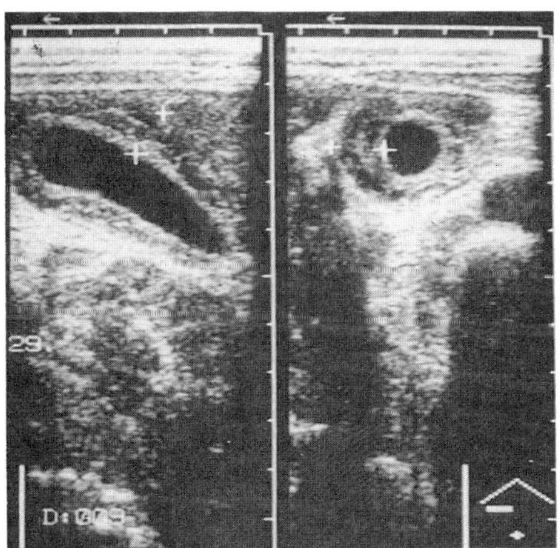

Fig. 3 A boy aged 8 years: cholecystitis

of the biliary tract, especially in those with inflammatory processes in the biliary tract.

DISCUSSION

Deformations of the biliary system detected in our patients are unlikely to be caused by hepatitis viruses and they were identified accidentally.

It seems that the disorders of the biliary tract revealed in our study could be explained by: (1) anatomical and functional peculiarities of the children's liver which disappear with age; (2) undiagnosed deformations of the children's

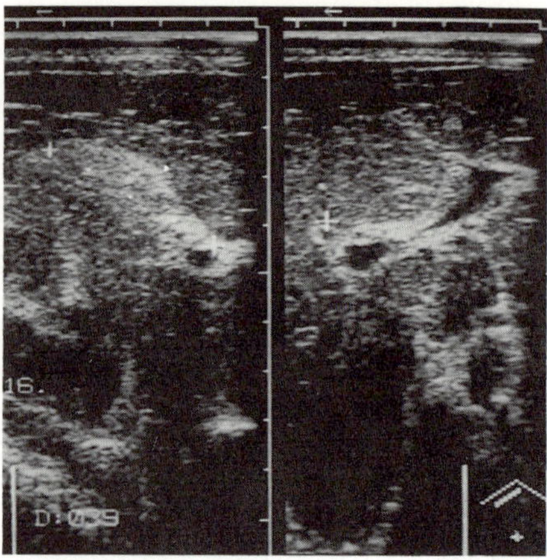

Fig. 4 A girl aged 7 years: intrahepatic cholangitis

Table 1 Parameters of the patients with acute viral hepatitis: number of patients (and percentage)

	Time scale from onset of disease				
	2–3 days	*10 days*	*1 month*	*3 months*	*6 months*
Viral hepatitis without changes in the biliary system (n = 97)					
Hyperbilirubinaemia	85	10	0	0	0
	(87.6)	(10.3)	(0)	(0)	(0)
Elevated level of alanine	97	57	4	1	0
aminotransferase	(100)	(58.8)	(4.1)	(1.0)	(0)
Hepatomegaly	86	31	0	0	0
	(88.7)	(32.0)	(0)	(0)	(0)
Anatomical defects without inflammation (n = 102)					
Hyperbilirubinaemia	89	76	26	2	1
	(87.2)	(74.5)	(25.5)	(2.0)	(1.0)
Elevated level of alanine	102	82	9	4	0
aminotransferase	(100)	(80.4)	(8.8)	(3.9)	(0)
Hepatomegaly	96	81	24	7	5
	(94.1)	(79.4)	(23.5)	(6.9)	(4.5)
Inflammations of the biliary tract (n = 34)					
Hyperbilirubinaemia	33	17	8	1	0
	(97.1)	(50.0)	(23.5)	(2.9)	(0)
Elevated level of alanine	34	28	22	1	0
aminotransferase	(100)	(82.3)	(64.7)	(2.9)	(0)
Hepatomegaly	32	28	26	4	3
	(94.1)	(82.3)	(76.5)	(11.8)	(8.8)

biliary tract may lead to severe diseases in adults.

The alterations of the intrahepatic biliary tract visualized by ultrasound should lead to detailed investigations of the reasons for these changes. Ultrasonography is one of the most suitable means for the identification of deformations of children's intrahepatic biliary tract.

References

1. Abramson SJ, Treves S, Teele RL. The infant with possible biliary atresia: evaluation by ultrasound and nuclear medicine. Pediatr Radiol. 1982;12:1–5.
2. Chandra RS. Biliary atresia and other structural anomalies in the congenital polysplenia syndrome. J Pediatr. 1974;85:649–53.
3. Reif S, Sloven DG, Lebenthal E. Gallstones in children. Am J Dis. Child. 1991;145:105–8.
4. Blankenberg F, Wirth R, Jeffrey RB, Mindelzun R, Francis I. Computed tomography as an adjunct to ultrasound in the diagnosis of acute acalculous cholecystitis. Gastrointest Radiol. 1991;16:149–53.
5. Engstrom C-F, Wiechel K-L. Endoluminal ultrasound of the bile ducts. Surg Endosc. 1990;4:187–90.
6. Stott MA, Farrands PA, Guyer PB, Dewbury KC, Browning JJ, Sutton R. Ultrasound of the common bile duct in patients undergoing cholecystectomy. J Clin Ultrasound. 1991;19:73–6.
7. Han BK, Babcock DS, Gelfand MH. Choledochal cyst with bile duct dilatation: sonography and 99mTc-IDA cholescintigraphy. Am J Roentgenol. 1981;136:1075–9.
8. Teefey SA, Baron RL, Bigler SA. Sonography of the gallbladder: significance of striated (layered) thickening of the gallbladder wall. Am J Roentgenol. 1991;156:945–7.
9. Urbain D, Jeanmart J, Lemone M, Kiromera A, Muls V, Arendt V, Dewit S. Cholestasis in a patient with the acquired immune deficiency syndrome: comparison between ultrasonographic and cholangiographic findings. Am J Gastroenterol 1991;86:574–6.
10. Garel L, Pariente D, Sauvergrain J. Ultrasound in infancy and childhood. Clin Gastroenterol. 1984;13:161–82.
11. Juttner HU, Ralls PW, Quiann MF, Jenney JM. Thickening of the gallbladder wall in acute hepatitis: ultrasound demonstration. Radiology. 1982;142:465–8.
12. Raskin M. Ultrasonography of the gallbladder and biliary system. In: Sarti DA, Sample WF, editors. Diagnostic ultrasound: text and cases. Boston, MA: G.K. Hall; 1980:116–67.

Section 5
Treatment of Cholestatic Disorders:

1: Surgical and Conservative

28
Place of liver transplantation in biliary atresia

J. DE VILLE DE GOYET and J. B. OTTE

INTRODUCTION

Biliary atresia is the most common cause of chronic cholestasis in children. Since its introduction the results of the Kasai portoenterostomy have improved[1], but a substantial proportion of those patients still develop progressive liver disease[2,3]. In a recent Japanese review of 251 patients, with an overall mortality of 59%, Ryoji Ohi demonstrates the relationships between survival rate and, on one hand, the experience of the team and, on the other hand, the age at the time of surgery[4]. Even with a positive bile flow rate higher than 90% in 96 patients operated between 1977 and 1988, only 56 (58%) are jaundice-free. Kimura and Akiyama have collected 325 long-term (> 10 years) survivals from 49 institutions in Japan and concluded that only 157 (48.3%) of them are healthy[5]. It is well established by now that even if Kasai portoenterostomy has dramatically improved the prognosis, long-term follow up demonstrates a poor prognosis, regarding survival, morbidity or quality of life.

INDICATION OF LIVER TRANSPLANTATION (Fig. 1)

Depending on the failure of a restitution of the bile flow and early cholangitis a substantial proportion of patients develop liver insufficiency in early childhood and most of them die before the age of 3[2,3] if liver replacement is not performed. Later in childhood, even with a good liver function, portal hypertension and haemorrhage from oesophageal or gastrointestinal tract varices can occur: in a series of 225 cases with a survival rate of 42%, oesophageal varices were endoscopically confirmed in 26 of 66 examined patients (39%), 52 of them being free of jaundice[6]. Portal hypertension is a major late complication, and controversy around the optimal treatment (conservative endoscopic sclerotherapy, decompressive shunting or liver transplantation) exists. Depending on the age of the patient and the estimated

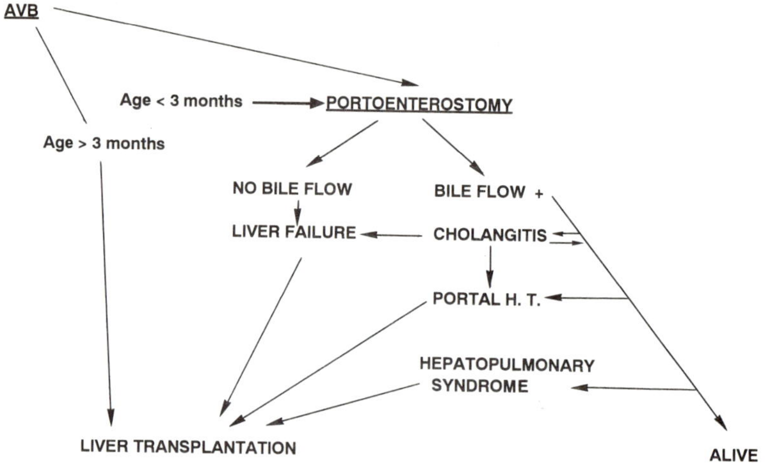

Fig. 1 Indication of liver transplantation in biliary atresia

evolution of the liver function, liver transplantation has to be taken into account[7]. Severe hypoxia due to a hepatopulmonary syndrome can be the only indication for replacement of the liver in older children or adolescents. For long-term survivors the risk of the development of a cancer probably exists, as in other fibrotic and cirrhotic livers: this is still not evaluated but liver transplantation could be indicatd.

KASAI VERSUS TRANSPLANTATION

Scarring from prior surgery and anatomical abnormalities are special difficulties which could reduce the success of transplantation in comparison to other indications. However, training and experience of the transplanting team (surgeons, anaesthetists and paediatricians) are the most important factors: previous abdominal operations enhance morbidity but do not affect mortality, even if most of the patients are less than 3 years and weigh less than 12 kg. Thus existence of a prior portoenterostomy does not appear to adversely affect the prognosis of the transplanted child.

To the contrary, avoiding primary portoenterostomy could reduce technical difficulties, but this strategy would lead to a dramatic increase of small candidates for liver transplantation, exactly the population where the greatest difficulty for locating suitable donors exists[8]. This increased demand would lead to high mortality on the waiting list.

The modern approach to the treatment of biliary atresia is a sequential strategy based on Kasai's portoenterostomy, performed under the best conditions and, in case of failure, followed by liver transplantation[8-15]. Regarding the possibility of later transplantation, surgical procedures should be performed with care being taken not to cause unnecessary adhesions and not to create stomas (which have been proved to be inefficient in preventing cholangitis). Reoperations have to be performed only in strictly limited

Table 1 Anatomic abnormalities in 166 consecutive transplantations for biliary atresia (1984–91)

Incidence: 61 abnormalities in 26 patients (15%)	
Findings:	
No inferior vena cava	13
Preduodenal portal vein	10
Hypoplastic portal vein	18
Aberrant hepatic artery	8
Situs inversus	3
Midgut malrotation	9

indications, such as cessation of bile flow after a successful initial operation. When the diagnosis is delayed (after the age of 3 months) the indication of a primary transplantation could be proposed, regarding the disappointing results of the Kasai.

EVALUATION OF CANDIDATES FOR LIVER TRANSPLANTATION

Criteria for contraindications have changed with increased experience[14-17]. Small size and young age of the patient cannot now be limits for transplantation, when most children with a failed Kasai procedure need a transplantation when less than 2 years of age and weighing less than 12 kg. Good results in children of less than 1 year are now achieved by various teams[18,19].

Size and permeability of the portal vein have been important criteria for technical acceptance[20], but if the portal vein is hypoplastic or absent, the splenomesenteric confluent and the superior mesenteric vein can be checked by real-time echo Doppler. Revascularization of the graft can be performed from both sites.

Anatomical abnormalities are frequent in the biliary atresia group (Table 1), usually concomitant in the so-called 'polysplenia syndrome': polysplenia, preduodenal hypoplastic portal vein, absent inferior vena cava, anomalous origin of the hepatic artery, liver symmetry, and occasionally intestinal malrotation and situs inversus[12,21]. In our series this syndrome is more frequent in children of less than 1 year at the time of transplantation. There is no significant difference in survival with or without anatomical abnormalities[22].

Pretransplant clinical evaluation includes exclusion of advanced disease of other systems. Neurological examination is critical, and more difficult because of the young age of the patients. In our experience lack of growth in the circumference of the head can be correlated with deficiency in weight and size. Severe disproportion suggests neurological defects. Critical malnutrition and severe hepatic dysfunction can be observed when children are referred late in their evolution, or when they have clinically deteriorated during the waiting time. Intensive 2–3-week medical care allows both evaluation and preoperative management. By clinical response to optimal therapy the perioperative prognosis can be estimated, and a transplantation can be proposed[23].

Table 2 Waiting time and death according to age

Registration		Delays (days) till transplantation			Death during waiting time	
Age (years)	n	n	Median	Range	n	Percentage
< 1	102	64	143	2–574	22	21.5
> 1 < 3	98	69	175	0–722	11	11.2
> 3 < 6	30	25	70	1–839	2	6.6
> 6 < 15	46	40	17	0–430		
	276				35	12.6

Experience (1984–90) at University of Louvain Medical School.

TIMING

Shortage of donor organs is critical in paediatric liver transplantation. Both in North America and in Europe, 15–30% of children on the transplant waiting list die before they can be operated[24–26] (Table 2). Lack of size-matched organs is the worst for infants and young children where the major part of the need for liver replacement exists. Use of reduced size transplant could increase the proportion of candidates transplanted and reduce overall mortality[25,26]. Paradoxically, despite the use of increasingly innovative surgical solutions the average waiting time[6] does not get shorter: the growing numbers of transplant centres, and the increasing variety of indications, dramatically increase overall need for liver replacement. Earlier referral is necessary in order to offer all candidates the chance of a liver transplantation. The children who do not have biliary drainage should be evaluated and listed as early as 6 months of age[27]. Early referral, optimal medical treatment during the waiting time and the recent use of adult donors (left lateral lobe graft) has decreased the death rate of the waiting children in our series during the past 2 years.

OPERATION PROCEDURE

Because of prior abdominal surgery and extensive adhesions in association with portal hypertension, and because mean age and weight are lower, the transplant procedure for biliary atresia patients tends to be more difficult. Vascular and biliary reconstruction are often more complex and anatomical abnormalities are found in 15%. Operation time and blood loss are increased, but not significantly[8,11]. Iatrogenic intestinal traumatism is more frequent: in our series of 245 children, peritonitis secondary to intestinal perforation occurred in 11 children out of 166 biliary atresia patients (6.6%) and two out of 79 non-biliary atresia children (2.5%). Despite those technical difficulties, liver transplantation can be successful. Standard orthotopic liver transplantation is performed, using innovative modifications for vascular (hepatic artery, portal vein and caval drainage) implantation of the graft, depending on the size of the vessel, the vascular abnormalities and/or the use of reduced and segmental grafts[21]. Biliary reconstruction is always performed using choledochojejunostomy on the previous Roux-Y limb.

Table 3 Liver transplantation for biliary atresia: age distribution

< 1 year	30	(18%)
> 1 and < 3 years	103	(62%)
> 3 and < 6 years	19	(11.5%)
> 6 and < 15 years	14	(8.5%)
	166	

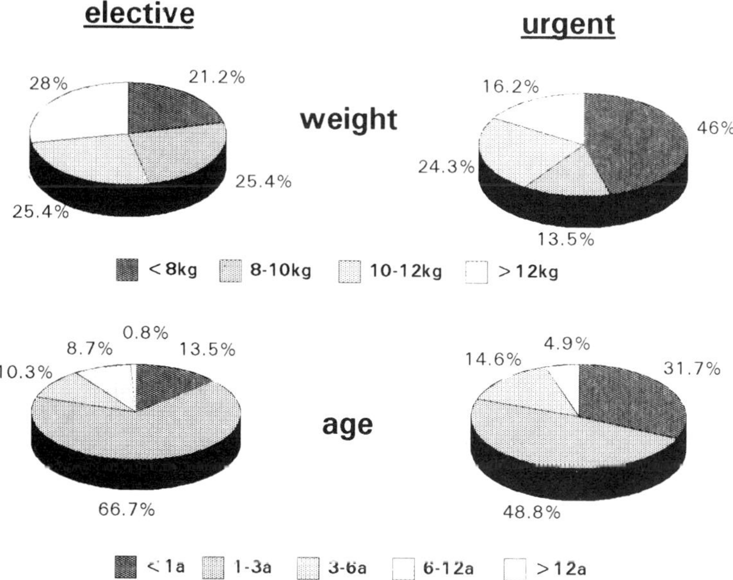

Fig. 2 Patient weight and age distribution according to urgent or elective transplantation ($n = 166$)

Prevention of ascendant cholangitis can be achieved either by a 60 cm loop length or a Tsuchida antireflux valve[28].

RESULTS

Between May 1984 and August 1991 we transplanted 245 children, 166 of them (68%) with biliary atresia. Of this latter group, 133 were less than 3 years old at the time of transplantation (including 30 less than 1 year) (Table 3). Seventy-seven weighed under 10 kg (46.4%) and 38 others between 10 and 12 kg (22.9%). The transplantation was urgent for 40 (24%) and elective for 126 children (76%). In the two groups the majority of the patients is between 1 and 3 years of age. In the urgent group most of the children weigh less than 10 kg (Fig. 2). Of the 166 first grafts used 88 were full-size grafts (53%), and innovative techniques were used for 78 transplantations (47%) (44 reduced grafts, 29 segmental grafts and five split-liver grafts).

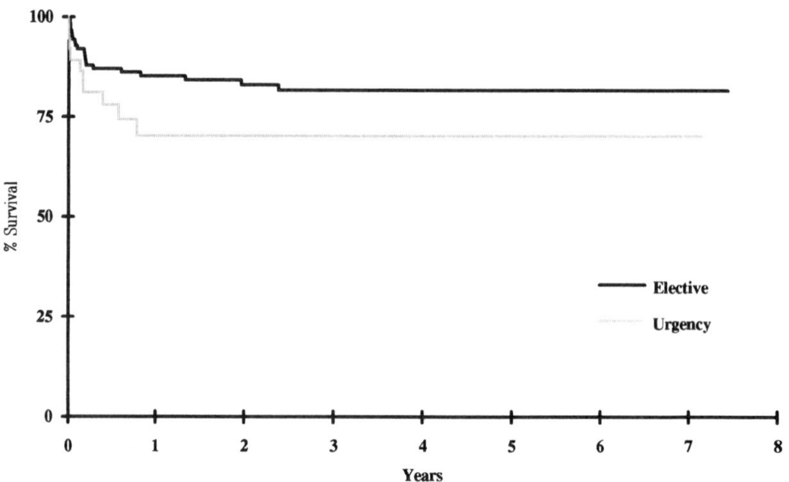

Fig. 3 Long-term survival after paediatric liver transplantation for biliary atresia ($n = 166$)

Table 4 Long-term survival according to pretransplant status

Clinical status	n	5 year survival[a]	Age (years)	Weight (kg)
Urgent	40	67.4 ± 7.9	2.10 ± 1.81	9.7 ± 4.4
Elective	126	82.9 ± 3.6	2.65 ± 2.39	11.4 ± 6.5
		$p = 0.029$[b]	$p = 0.058$[c]	$p = 0.061$[c]

[a]Kaplan–Meier. [b]Cox model with Wold test. [c]Wilcoxon rank sum test.

It has been well established that transplantations using reduced or segmental grafts have the same survival rate and the same quality of liver function as full-size grafts (FSG)[29,30]. This technique is now routinely used for elective cases. In our experience there is no difference between full-size and innovative techniques (IT), regarding primary non-function or retransplantation rates. Moreover, we found a significant lower incidence of hepatic artery thrombosis and biliary complications in the IT group. The proportions of urgent recipients transplanted with FSG or IT are 38% and 62% respectively (retransplantation excluded). The corresponding values for the elective cases are 57% and 43%. This indicates that more IT were used in high-risk recipients and consecutively, overall survival rate is lower for IT (74% versus 83% in FSG). But when transplantation is electively performed the values are 81.5% (IT) and 82% (FSG) respectively.

Long-term survivals (5 years) were achieved in 82.9% of the elective patients and in 67.4% when transplantation was very urgent (overall survival 79.3%) (Kaplan–Meier product limit estimate; Fig. 3). Light weight (< 10 kg) and low age (< 1 year) are not correlated with a lower success rate in a multifactorial analysis (Cox proportional hazards model). On the contrary, urgent transplantation is significantly ($p = 0.02$) associated with a high risk ($\times 2.2$) of deaths (Table 4).

CONCLUSIONS

The best management for biliary atresia is a sequential strategy, combining Kasai portoenterostomy and liver transplantation, when necessary. Most candidates for liver transplantation are small for weight and age, but these can no longer be limits for acceptance. Anatomical abnormalities and technical problems are now rare exclusion criteria. Because of extreme scarcity of small paediatric donors, innovative surgical techniques are necessary and the waiting time on the list for transplantation is long. Poor residual liver function and urgency of liver replacement are the most important bad prognostic factors. Early referral to transplantation centres is thus critical. When liver transplantation for biliary atresia is performed electively, long-term survival and good quality of life is now achieved in 81.7% of candidates.

References

1. Ohi R. A history of the Kasai operation: hepatic portoenterostomy for biliary atresia. World J Surg. 1988;12:871–4.
2. Schweizer P. Treatment of extrahepatic bile duct atresia: results and long-term prognosis after hepatic portoenterostomy. Pediatr Surg Int. 1986;1:30–6.
3. Houwen RJH, Zwierstra RP, Severijnen RSVM, Bouquet J, Madern G, Vos A, Bax NMA, Heymans HSA, Bijlveld CMA. Prognosis of extrahepatic biliary atresia. Arch Dis Child. 1989;64:214–18.
4. Ryoji O, Masaki N, Tsuneo C, Naobumi E, Makoto G, Mohamed I. Long-term follow-up after surgery for patients with biliary atresia. J Pediatr Surg. 1990;25:442–5.
5. Ohi R, Mochizuki I, Komatsu K *et al.* Portal hypertension after successful hepatic portoenterostomy in biliary atresia. J Pediatr Surg. 1986;21:271–4.
6. Ryoji O, Izumi M, Kazuhisa K, Morio K. Portal hypertension after successful hepatic portoenterostomy in biliary atresia. J Pediatr Surg. 1986;21:271–4.
7. Willis C, Van Thiel MDH. Liver transplantation: an overview. Hepatology. 1988;8:948–59.
8. Wood PR, Langnas AN, Stratta RJ, Pillen TJ, Williams L, Lindsay S, Meiergerd D, Shaw BW, Jr. Optimal therapy for patients with biliary atresia: portoenterostomy ('Kasai' procedures) versus primary transplantation. J Pediatr Surg. 1990;25:153–62.
9. Cavanti JP, Shambergerr RC, Eraklis A, Lillehei CW. The therapy of biliary atresia combining the Kasai portoenterostomy with liver transplantation: a single center experience. J Pediatr Surg. 1990;25:149–52.
10. Stewart BA, Hall RJ, Lilly JR. Liver transplantation and the Kasai operation in biliary atresia. J Pediatr Surg. 1988;23:623–26.
11. Cuervas-Mons V, Rimola A, Van Thiel DH, Gavaler JS, Schade RR, Starzl TE. Does previous abdominal surgery alter the outcome of pediatric patients subjected to orthotopic liver transplantation? Gastroenterology. 1986;90:853–7.
12. Lilly JR, Starzl TE. Liver transplantation in children with biliary atresia and vascular anomalies. J Pediatr Surg. 1974;9:707–14.
13. Otte JB. Pediatric transplantation. Cur Sc. ISSN 1040-8703 – Cur Opin Pediatr. 1991;3:471–7.
14. Otte JB, de Ville de Goyet J, Sokal E *et al.* Liver transplantation in children: indications and results in 167 patients (Part 1). Jap J Pediatr Surg. 1990;26:1050–6.
15. Shaw BW, Wood RP, Kaufman SS *et al.* Liver transplantation therapy for children (Part 1). J Pediatr Gastroenterol Nutr. 1988;7:157–66.
16. Kalayoglu M, Stratta RJ, Sollinger HW *et al.* Liver transplantation in infants and children. J Pediatr Surg. 1989;24:70–6.
17. Malatack JJ, Schaid DJ, Urbach AH *et al.* Choosing a pediatric recipient for orthotopic

liver transplantation. J Pediatr. 1987;111:479–89.
18. Sokal EM, Veyckemans F, de Ville de Goyet J, Moulin D, Van Hoorebeeck N, Alberti D, Buts JP, Rahier J, Van Obbergh L, Clapuyt P, Carlier M, Claus D, Latinne D, de Hemptinne B, Otte JB. Liver transplantation in children less than 1 year of age. J Pediatr 1990;117:205–9.
19. Esquivel CO, Koneru B, Karrer F *et al.* Liver transplantation before 1 year of age. J Pediatr. 1987;110:545–8.
20. Claus D, Clapuyt P. Liver transplantation in children: role of the radiologist in the preoperative assessment and the postoperative follow-up. Transplant Proc. 1987;19:3344–57.
21. Lerut J, Tzakis AG, Bron K, Gordon RB, Iwatsuki S, Esquivel CO, Makowka L, Toso S, Starzl TE. Complications of venous reconstruction in human orthotopic liver transplantation. Ann Surg. 1987;205:404–13.
22. Falchetti D, Brant de Carvalho F, Clapuyt P, de Ville de Goyet J, de Hemptinne B, Claus D, Otte JB. Liver transplantation in children with biliary atresia and polysplenia syndrome. Report of twelve cases. J Pediatr Surg. 1991;26:1–4.
23. de Ville de Goyet J, Sokal E, Otte JB. La transplantation hépatique chez l'enfant. In: Neuhaus P, editor. Leber transplantation. Berlin, Heidelberg, New York: Springer (In press).
24. Shaw BW, Wood RP, Kaufman SS, Williams L, Antonson DL, Kelly DA, Vanderhoof JA. Liver transplantation therapy for children (part 2). J Pediatr Gastroenterol Nutr. 1988;7:797–815.
25. Otte JB, de Ville de Goyet J, Sokal E, Alberti D, Moulin D, de Hemptinne B, Veyckemans F, Van Obbergh L, Carlier M, Clapuyt Ph, Claus D, Jamart J. Size reduction of the donor liver is a safe way to alleviate the shortage of size-matched organs in pediatric liver transplantation. Ann Surg. 1990;211:146–57.
26. Broelsch CE, Emond JC, Thistlethwaite JR, Rouch DA, Whittington PF, Lichtor JL. Liver transplantation with reduced-size donor organs. Transplantation. 1988;45:519–23.
27. Kalayoglu M, Stratta RJ, Sollinger HW, Hoffmann RM, D'Alessandro AM, Pirsch JD, Belze FO. Liver transplantation in infants and children. J Pediatr Surg. 1989;24:70–6.
28. Nakajo T, Hashizume K, Saeki M, Tsuchida Y. Intussusception-type antireflux valve in the Roux-en-Y loop to prevent ascending cholangitis after hepatic portojejunostomy. J Pediatr Surg. 1990;25:311–14.
29. Brant de Carvalho F, Falchetti D, de Ville de Goyet J *et al.* Analysis of liver graft loss in infants and children below 4 years. Transplantation Society, San Francisco, August 1990. Transplant Proc. 1991;23(1).
30. Otte JB, de Ville de Goyet J, Alberti D, de Hemptinne B, Sokal E, Moulin D, Veyckemans F, Carlier MA, Van Obbergh L, Rahier J, Clapuyt P, Claus D. Liver transplantation in children: University of Louvain Medical School (Brussels): experience with the first 139 patients. In: Terasaki P, editor. Clinical transplants 1989. Los Angeles, UCLA; 1989:143–52.

29
Biliary atresia – complications and results of non-transplant surgery

E.R. HOWARD

INTRODUCTION AND PATHOLOGY

Destruction of the bile ducts in the fetus and young infant is the end-result of a progressive inflammatory process. The extent of the destruction varies from case to case and in approximately 25% of patients the gallbladder and common bile duct are spared. The proximal bile ducts in the porta hepatis are completely occluded in 85%[1] but microscopical examination of the duct remnants in these cases may show a variety of features which include duct-like structures, inflammatory cell infiltrates and a variable degree of fibrosis. This variety of biliary atresia is now classified as type 3[2]. The duct-like structures may represent residual lumina of true bile ducts, or non-communicating biliary glands, and this is not always clear from conventional histological examination.

Approximately 10% of cases may possess a residual cystic segment of bile duct in the porta hepatis (type 1) which can be utilized for a conventional type of biliary–enteric anastomosis, and these cases were previously known as 'correctable' atresias. Type 3 cases, on the other hand, were called 'non-correctable' atresias, but investigations by Kasai[3] showed from three-dimensional histological studies that during early infancy most of the patients possess intrahepatic bile ducts which communicate with ductular remnants in the residual tissue of the porta hepatis.

An unusual variety of atresia in which there is partial preservation of the lumina of the right and left hepatic ducts is found in 2–3% of patients, but for practical purposes this type is treated surgically as a type 3 lesion.

Gautier and Eliot classified the histological appearances of the tissue found at the porta hepatis into three types[4] (Fig. 1). A complete absence of biliary ductules within the fibrous tissue was designated as type 1 histology, the presence of small ductules with lumina less than $50\,\mu$m as type 2, and the persistence of remnants of true bile ducts with at least some columnar epithelial lining as type 3. This classification should not be confused with the classification of the macroscopic appearances of the biliary remnants

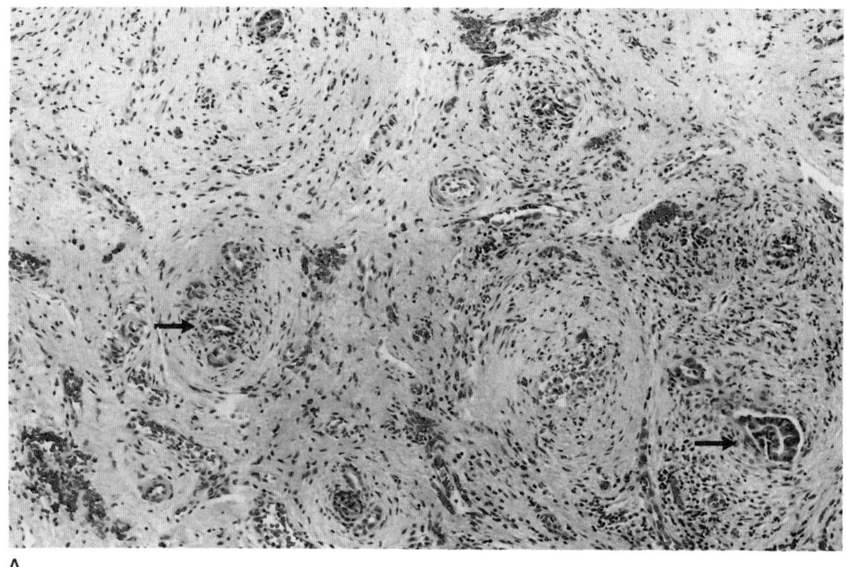

A

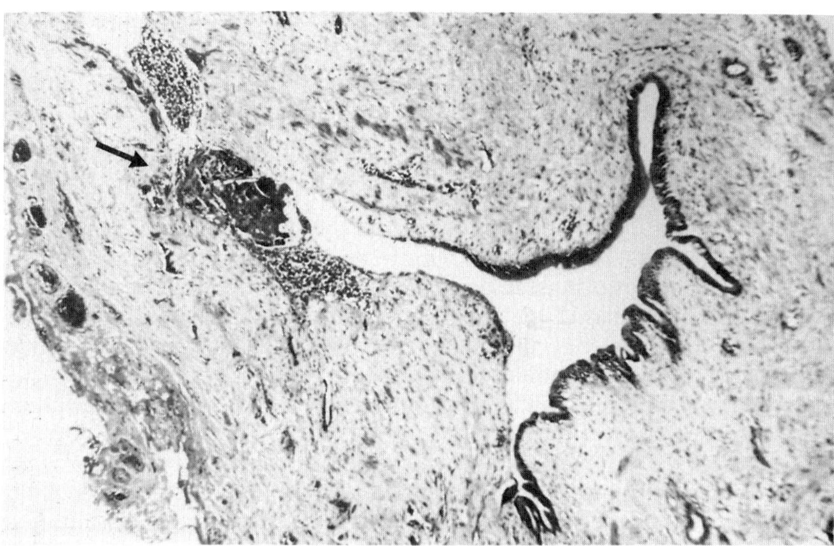

B

Fig. 1 Various appearances of the porta hepatis in biliary atresia. Examples from three patients. **A**: Large bile duct with hyperplastic epithelium. There is partial loss of the epithelium (× 500). **B**: Several small bile ducts are seen in this specimen surrounded by fibrous tissue with a scattering of inflammatory cells (× 500). **C**: A section showing a complete absence of bile ducts in the porta hepatis (× 500)

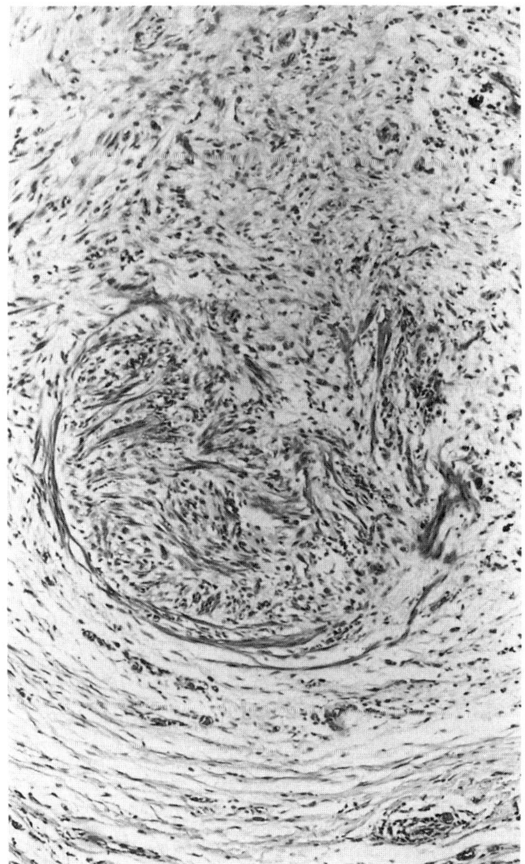

Figure 1C. *Continued*

described previously.

Attempts have been made to relate histological observations to the success of surgical procedures in biliary atresia. There is a greater chance of achieving good bile flow if the size of bile duct remnants exceeds 150 μm[5,6] but good results can also be achieved in children with much smaller ductules[7]. Surgical success or failure also depends on the severity of the intrahepatic disease at the time of operation. The typical changes observed in liver histology include oedema and fibrosis of the portal tracts and proliferation of bile ducts. Progressive hepatocellular damage and multinucleate giant cell formation follow unrelieved cholestasis. It has been suggested that the onset of cirrhosis may be the result of both bile duct obstruction and a cholangiopathic process similar to that seen in the neonatal hepatitis syndrome[8].

Liver histology may improve after successful surgery, particularly for type

Table 1 Examples of some of the associated anomalies described in 87 (11.5%) of 758 patients with biliary atresia (modified from ref. 20)

Anomaly	*No.*
Congenital cardiac	
ventricular septal defect	11
dextrocardia	3
Gastrointestinal	
malrotation	11
situs inversus	5
Vascular	
preduodenal portal vein	5
absent inferior vena cava	3
Splenic	
polysplenia	11
bifid spleen	9
asplenia	1

1 atresia, but the intrahepatic bile ducts never develop a normal morphology[9]. Preoperative liver histology cannot be used as a predictor of surgical success[10] and the resolution of jaundice cannot be related to preoperative measures of hepatic fibrosis, inflammation or giant cell formation[11]. Long-term postoperative studies have shown a disappointing progression of hepatic fibrosis in approximately 70% of patients[5,12], in spite of good bile drainage.

ASSOCIATED ANOMALIES

The aetiology of biliary atresia remains unknown. The incidence throughout the world appears to be between 1 : 12 000 and 1 : 14 000 live births, and there is a small preponderance of female over male infants of 1.4 to 1.0[13]. An association with other congenital anomalies suggests a possible genetic factor in at least a proportion of cases, and it has been described in association with trisomy 17, 18 and 21[14,15]. Twin studies, on the other hand, have not shown any simple genetic relationship. Atresia has been observed only in single siblings of both mono- and dizygotic pairs[16].

Thirteen instances of a familial occurrence of atresia have been reported[17], and this perhaps suggests a combination of genetic susceptibility and environmental insult in the aetiology. A hypothesis of genetic susceptibility is supported by the occurrence of associated anomalies in 10–30% of cases[13,18–20]. These anomalies include polysplenia, situs inversus, and cardiac defects (Table 1). There is a distinct syndromic relationship between splenic defects (either polysplenia or asplenia), situs inversus and anomalies of the portal vein. Splenic malformations were present in 23 (8.6%) of 267 cases under our care[21] and these included polysplenia in 20 (7.1%), a double spleen in one, and asplenia in two. One of our infants also had immotile respiratory cilia, cavernous transformation of the portal vein and malrotation. The association with immotile cilia in the respiratory tract has been recognized previously[22]. A defect in embryonic canalization or an abnormality in the blood supply to the bile ducts have been suggested as aetiological mechanisms for atresia[16].

Surgical results may be affected by these associated anomalies. Severe cardiac problems obviously increase early mortality, whereas anatomical derangements within the abdomen may increase the difficulty and morbidity of surgery in the porta hepatis.

CLINICAL PRESENTATION AND INVESTIGATION

Biliary atresia presents within the first few days of life with jaundice, dark urine and non-pigmented tools. Spontaneous bleeding caused by malabsorption of vitamin K may be the presenting feature in infants with delayed diagnosis. A majority of these children appear to be healthy with satisfactory development, and they do not show any of the chronic stigmata of liver disease in early life. A delay in diagnosis is therefore not uncommon. However, the best surgical results are achieved if operations are carried out before 8 weeks of age, and urgent investigation of any infant with conjugated hyperbilirubinaemia is imperative. A survey of 816 cases treated in more than 100 hospitals in the USA showed a median age at surgery of 10 weeks[13]. Similarly an analysis of 50 cases from our own unit also showed a median age at operation of 10 weeks[23].

Liver function tests are of limited value in the diagnosis of biliary atresia from other causes of infantile cholestasis, as the associated hepatocellular injury is associated with elevated serum transaminase, γ-glutamyl transpeptidase and alkaline phosphatase levels. Ultrasound is of limited value, except for the differential diagnosis of choledochal cyst, because of the absence of intrahepatic duct dilatation. Hepatobiliary excretion scans are used routinely for diagnosis and a complete absence of radioactivity in the gut after 24 h is highly suggestive of atresia of the biliary tract[24]. It must be emphasized that a battery of tests is usually necessary for the firm diagnosis of atresia, and that every test, including percutaneous liver biopsy, has an incidence of false-negative results[25]. Endoscopic retrograde cholangiography is now used in a few centres with a diagnostic success rate of approximately 85%[26,27].

A firm preoperative diagnosis of biliary atresia should be made whenever possible in these children, as the patency of the bile ducts cannot always be proven at laparotomy even with the most careful intraoperative cholangiography. The extrahepatic bile ducts in cases of hepatitis syndrome and biliary hypoplasia are minute, and mistaken diagnosis has led to unnecessary surgery at times[28].

HISTORY OF SURGERY

More than 100 cases of biliary atresia were reported by Holmes in 1916[29], and he observed that approximately 16% might have been suitable for a surgical procedure using a bile duct to bowel anastomosis. This report led to the concept of 'correctable' and 'non-correctable' forms of atresia. Early reports, however, often confused biliary atresia with choledochal cyst, inspissated bile syndrome and neonatal hepatitis syndrome[30] and the overall results of surgical treatment were very poor. There were only 52 reported successes between 1927 and 1970[31], and a variety of unsuccessful surgical techniques were devised during this time. These included resection and anastomosis of the left lobe of the liver[32], the implantation of intrahepatic tubes[33] and the anastomosis of hepatic lymphatics to the bowel[34].

In 1959 Kasai and Suzuki[35] reported the results of detailed histological investigations of the porta hepatis in atresia, and described bile drainage from the liver after resection of all residual bile duct tissue. Anastomosis of a Roux-en-Y loop of jejunum to the cut surface of the porta hepatis, the portoenterostomy operation, is now the standard technique for surgical correction, and effective bile drainage has been described in large numbers of patients during the past 20 years. The oldest survivors are now in their third decade.

SURGICAL PROCEDURES

The bile ducts are explored through a transverse incision in the upper abdomen. The abdominal cavity is examined in detail for the presence of any other anomalies, e.g. polysplenia. A shrunken, fibrotic gallbladder suggests a diagnosis of biliary atresia and precludes the possibility of operative cholangiography. A clear mucoid fluid may be aspirated from the gallbladder, but if aspiration reveals bile then the diagnosis is either of a type 1 atresia or an incorrect diagnosis of another type of cholestatic disease. Operative cholangiography is mandatory after the demonstration of bile in the gallbladder. The demonstration of a communication with the intrahepatic ducts through the cystic duct with no flow into the duodenum confirms the diagnosis of the less usual type 1 atresia. This may be managed with an hepaticojejunostomy which is facilitated by complete mobilization of the liver by dividing the left and right triangular ligaments. This allows the liver to be displaced into the abdominal wound in infants.

A biliary–enteric anastomosis is not possible in a majority of patients with biliary atresia who have no visible bile duct lumen, and in these cases bile drainage can be achieved only with the operation of portoenterostomy[36]. The main points in this technique include full mobilization of the liver to get adequate access to the porta hepatis, complete excision of the gallbladder with all remnants of the extrahepatic bile ducts (Fig. 2), and anastomosis of a loop of jejunum to the portal plate area of the porta hepatis. The critical part of the operation is the removal of bile duct remnants by transecting the tissue in the porta hepatis parallel to the liver capsule. This line of excision extends behind the posterior surface of the bifurcation of the portal vein.

The gallbladder and common bile duct may be spared by the atretic process, and if patency is confirmed with cholangiography they may be used for bile drainage. The gallbladder may be anastomosed to the porta hepatis in place of a Roux loop of bowel and a reduced incidence of postoperative cholangitis has been reported after this procedure (portocholecystostomy)[13].

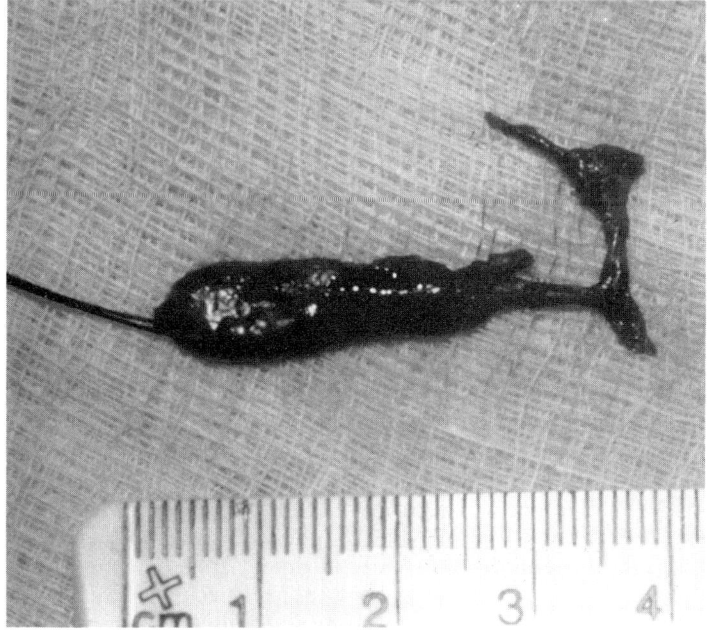

Fig. 2 An atretic gallbladder and residual bile duct tissue excised from a 6-week infant with biliary atresia

Table 2 The effect of biliary diversion (modification of portoenterostomy) on the incidence of cholangitis (modified from ref. 39)

	Diversion	*No diversion*
Number of patients	12.0	19.0
Cholangitis episodes	4.0 (33%)	6.0 (32%)
Two-year survival	7.0 (58%)	14.0 (82%)

However, some of the benefit is offset by an increased risk of technical problems such as gallbladder obstruction and kinking of the common bile duct[37].

Many ingenious cutaneous enterostomies have been devised to divert bile and to reduce intraluminal pressures within the biliary conduits in an attempt to reduce the incidence of ascending cholangitis after portoenterostomy[36]. The beneficial effects of these stomas have not been proven, however[38,39] (Table 2). Furthermore, complications of stomas have included dehydration, hyponatraemia, and bleeding from the stoma edge secondary to portal hypertension. Analysis of 648 cases treated in Japan showed that 43% of the patients suffered attacks of cholangitis in spite of the almost universal use of a stoma[1] and the technique is no longer recommended. The stomas can also seriously complicate hepatic transplantation, which may be required at a later date in some of these patients.

POSTOPERATIVE COMPLICATIONS

The postoperative course of biliary atresia patients may be complicated by attacks of bacterial cholangitis, portal hypertension, a variety of metabolic disorders or by cyst formation within the liver. The liver may also show a relentless progression to severe cirrhosis and liver failure in spite of the successful establishment of bile flow.

Patients who fail to achieve an adequate flow of bile after portoenterostomy undergo a gradual deterioration of liver function, and death commonly occurs between 1 and 2 years of age.

Ascending cholangitis is recognized from the triad of pyrexia, a rise in serum bilirubin and a recurrence of acholic stools. Attacks are more common during the first year after surgery and are rare after 4 years. A late onset of cholangitis should suggest a possible mechanical cause such as stricture or kinking of the biliary conduit. Recurrent infection is very serious as each attack may result in further liver damage. In one series a survival rate of 54% was recorded in patients with recurrent cholangitis compared with a survival rate of 91% in those who remained infection-free[40]. It is generally believed that cholangitis arises from the flora of the bowel but cutaneous diversion of bile (see above) and prophylactic antibiotics have proved disappointing[41]. Diagnosis may be confirmed from blood cultures or, in difficult cases, from the culture of liver biopsy specimens, and treatment is by the administration of broad-spectrum antibiotics.

Oesophageal varices were detected in 67% of patients who underwent oesophagoscopy 2.5 years or more after portoenterostomy[42]. However, only 28% had problems with variceal bleeding and, as in previous reports[43], the problem was worse in those who remained jaundiced after surgery. Measurements of portal pressure at the time of portoenterostomy have shown hypertension secondary to hepatic fibrosis[44], and this has worsened in patients who suffer with recurrent cholangitis. Injection sclerotherapy is generally regarded as the treatment of choice for the bleeding complications of oesophageal varices[42], but portosystemic shunts and oesophageal transection have also been used[45].

Abnormalities in the metabolism of fat, protein, vitamins, iron, calcium, zinc and copper are well known in children with chronic liver disease[46], and infants with biliary atresia are no exception. Careful follow-up and the administration of appropriate supplements is essential in postoperative management.

Cystic changes within the liver may occur at any time in the postoperative course. These have been classified, from an analysis of 24 cases, into either communicating or non-communicating single cysts or multiple cystic dilatations of the intrahepatic bile ducts[47]. Approximately 40% showed cholangitis within 1 year of surgery, and 67% within 3 years. Treatment has included either cystenterostomy or percutaneous drainage[48].

RESULTS OF TREATMENT

Type 1 atresia, treatable by conventional biliary–enteric anastomotic techniques, represents less than 10% of the cases reported in most large series.

Table 3 Improvements in the treatment of biliary atresia are reflected in the increasing numbers of children who lose their jaundice after portoenterostomy; this table shows the improved results obtained in a single centre (modified from ref. 49)

	No. of cases	Jaundice disappeared	Alive – no jaundice	
1953–61	26	3	2	(7.6%)
1962–71	78	19	13	(16.6%)
1972–81	91	60	42	(46.0%)
1982–88	56	40	34	(60.7%)
Total	251	122	91	(36.2%)

Table 4 Liver enzyme values (IU/l) in 24 long-term survivors after portoenterostomy (n = normal values)

Enzyme	Range	Mean
Alkaline phosphatase (n = 60–250)	125–1752	893
Aspartate transaminase (n = 10–45)	45–302	131
Gamma-glutamyl transpeptidase (n = 0–45)	14–1880	481

Although bile flow is achieved rapidly in this group long-term results have been rather disappointing. For example, the correction of 25 type 1 cases between 1953 and 1976 resulted in only 12 long-term jaundice-free survivors[2].

Long-term survival after portoenterostomy for type 2 and 3 atresia is now well documented. Ohi et al.[49], for example, reported a gradual rise in the numbers of long-term jaundice-free survivors from 12% in the period 1953–61 to 85% in 1987–88 (Table 3). Ten year survivors now represent 48% of patients treated between 1973 and 1977.

Age at the time of surgery is probably the most important factor in the improvement of results. In a recent series good bile flow was achieved in 86% of infants treated before 8 weeks of age compared with 36% of older children[24]. A further report showed survival figures of 62.5% for infants treated before 30 days of age, 43.6% for treatment between 31 and 60 days, and only 28.6% for those over 90 days[13]. These results emphasize the value of early surgery.

Liver biopsies from long-term survivors usually show severe disturbances in architecture. Specimens from 20 children who had survived at least 5 years after portoenterostomy showed cirrhosis in all specimens, but the degree of fibrosis and the size of regenerative nodules varied[50]. A surprising observation was the apparent absence of bile ducts within the biopsy specimens. Many long-term survivors continue to show abnormal liver function tests in spite of good bile drainage (Table 4) and in spite of excellent drainage of contrast material during percutaneous cholangiography (Fig. 3).

In summary, long-term survival is possible after non-transplant surgery for biliary atresia. Survival is influenced by the age at which surgery is performed, the histological features of the porta hepatis, the incidence of ascending bacterial cholangitis, the severity of portal hypertension and the

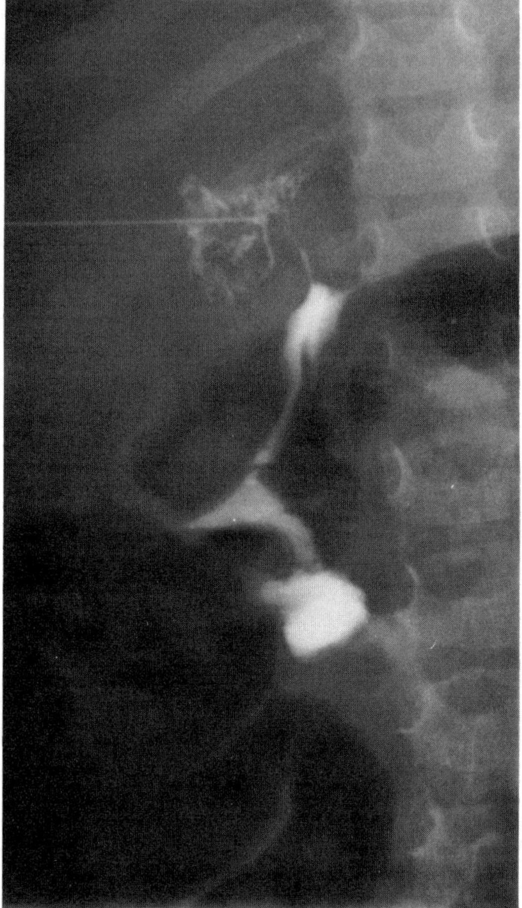

Fig. 3 A percutaneous cholangiogram performed 1 year after portoenterostomy in a child who suffered an attack of cholangitis. Note the excellent flow of contrast from the liver and the peculiar pattern of the bile ducts

progress of intrahepatic disease. The experience of the surgeon also influences the outcome of the portoenterostomy procedure[51]. Liver transplantation should be reserved for children who do not respond to portoenterostomy, or for those who develop intractable complications at a later age.

References

1. Ohi R, Chiba T, Ohkochi N, Yaoita K, Goto M, Ohtsuki S et al. The present status of surgical treatment for biliary atresia: report of the questionnaire for the main institutions in Japan. In: Ohi R, editor. Biliary atresia. Tokyo: Professional Postgraduate Services; 1987:125–30.

2. Hays DM, Kimura K. Biliary atresia: the Japanese experience. Cambridge, Mass: Harvard University Press; 1980.

3. Kasai M, Ohi R, Chiba T. Intrahepatic bile ducts in biliary atresia. In Kasai M, Shiraki K, editors. Cholestasis in infancy. Baltimore, MD: University Park Press, 1980:181–8.

4. Gautier M, Eliot N. Extrahepatic biliary atresia: morphological study of 98 biliary remnants. Arch Pathol Lab Med. 1981:105:397–402.

5. Altman RP, Chandra R, Lilly JR. Ongoing cirrhosis after successful porticoenterostomy in infants with biliary atresia. J Pediatr Surg. 1975;10:685–9.

6. Ohi R, Shikes RH, Stellin GP, Lilly JR. In biliary atresia duct histology correlates with bile flow. J Pediatr Surg. 1984;19:467–70.

7. Lawrence D, Howard ER, Tzanatos C, Mowat AP. Hepatic portoenterostomy for biliary atresia. Arch Dis Child. 1981;56:460–3.

8. Haas JE. Bile duct and liver pathology in biliary atresia. World J Surg. 1978;2:561–9.

9. Ito T, Horisawa M, Ando H. Intrahepatic bile ducts in biliary atresia: a possible factor determining the prognosis. J Pediatr Surg. 1983;18:124–30.

10. Dessanti A, Ohi R, Hanamatsu M, Mochizuchi I, Chiba T, Kasai M. Short term histological liver changes in extrahepatic biliary atresia with good postoperative bile drainage. Arch Dis Child. 1985;60:739–42.

11. Altman RP. The portoenterostomy procedure for biliary atresia. Ann Surg. 1978;188:357–61.

12. Gautier M, Valayer J, Odievre M, Alagille D. Histological liver evaluation 5 years after surgery for extrahepatic biliary atresia: a study of 20 cases. J Pediatr Surg. 1984;19:263–8.

13. Karrer FM, Lilly JR, Stewart BA, Hall RJ. Biliary atresia registry, 1976 to 1989. J Pediatr Surg. 1990;25:1076–81.

14. Danks DM. Prolonged neonatal obstructive jaundice. A survey of modern concepts. Clin Pediatr. 1965;4:499–510.

15. Alpert LI, Strauss L, Hirschhorn K. Neonatal hepatitis and biliary atresia associated with trisomy 17-18 syndrome. N Engl J Med. 1969;280:16–20.

16. Strickland AD, Shannon K, Coln CD. Biliary atresia in two sets of twins. J Pediatr. 1985;107:418 19.

17. Cunningham ML, Sybert VP. Idiopathic extrahepatic biliary atresia: recurrence in sibs in two families. Am J Med Genet. 1988;31:421–6.

18. Chandra RS. Biliary atresia and other structural anomalies in the congenital polysplenia syndrome. J Pediatr. 1974;85:649 55.

19. Lilly JR, Chandra RS. Surgical hazards of co-existing anomalies in biliary atresia. Surg Gynecol Obstet. 1974;139:49–54.

20. Miyamoto M, Kajimoto T. Associated anomalies in biliary atresia patients. In: Kasai M, editor. Biliary atresia and its related disorders. Amsterdam: Excerpta Medica; 1983:13–19.

21. Davenport M, Savage M, Mowat AP, Howard ER. The biliary atresia-splenic malformation syndrome. In: Ohi R, editor. Biliary atresia. Tokyo: ICOM Associates Inc; 1991;11–14.

22. Gershoni-Baruch R, Gottfried E, Pery M. Immotile cilia syndrome including polysplenia, situs inversus and extrahepatic biliary atresia. Am J Med Genet. 1989;33:390–3.

23. Mieli-Vergani G, Howard ER, Portmann B, Mowat AP. Late referral for biliary atresia – missed opportunities for effective surgery. Lancet. 1989;1:421–3.

24. Dick M, Mowart AP. Biliary scintigraphy with DISIDA. A simpler way of showing bile duct patency in suspected biliary atresia. Arch Dis Child. 1986;61:191–2.

25. Manolaki AG, Larcher VF, Mowat AP, Barrett JJ, Portmann B, Howard ER. The prelaparotomy diagnosis of extrahepatic biliary atresia. Arch Dis Child. 1983;58:591–4.

26. Takahashi H, Kuriyama Y, Maiae M, Ohnoma N, Eto T. ERCP in jaundiced infants. In: Ohi R, editor. Biliary atresia. Tokyo: Professional Postgraduate Services; 1987:110–13.

27. Hayman MB, Shapiro HA, Thaler MM. Endoscopic retrograde cholangiography in the diagnosis of biliary malformations in infants. Gastrointest Endosc. 1988;34:449–53.

28. Kahn EI, Daum F. Arterio-hepatic dysplasia: evaluation of the extrahepatic biliary tract, porta hepatis and hepatic parenchyma. In: Daum F, editor. Extrahepatic biliary atresia. New York: Marcel Dekker; 1983.

29. Holmes JB. Congenital obliteration of the bile duct: diagnosis and suggestions for treatment. Am J Dis Child. 1916;11:405–31.

30. Ladd WE. Congenital atresia and stenosis of the bile duct. J Am Med Assoc. 1928;91:1082–4.

31. Bill AH. Biliary atresia. World J Surg. 1978;2:557–9.
32. Longmire WP, Sandford MC. Intrahepatic cholangiojejunostomy for biliary obstruction. Surgery. 1948;24:264–76.
33. Sterling JA, Lowenburg K. Increased longevity in congenital biliary atresia. Ann NY Acad Sci. 1963;111:483–503.
34. Fonkalsrud EW, Kitagawa S, Longmire WP. Hepatic lymphatic drainage to the jejunum for congenital biliary atresia. Am J Surg. 1966;112:188–94.
35. Kasai M, Suzuki S. A new operation for 'non-correctable' biliary atresia: hepatic portoenterostomy. Shujitsu. 1959;13:733–9.
36. Howard ER. Biliary atresia: aetiology, management and complications. In: Howard ER, editor. Surgery of liver disease in children. Oxford: Butterworth–Heinemann; 1991.
37. Freitas, L, Gauthier F, Valayer J. Second operation for repair of biliary atresia. J Pediatr Surg. 1987;22:857–60.
38. Altman RP. Long term results after the Kasai procedure. In: Daum F, editor. Extrahepatic biliary atresia. New York: Marcel Dekker; 1983.
39. Burnweit CA, Coln D. Influence of diversion on the development of cholangitis after hepatoportoenterostomy for biliary atresia. J Pediatr Surg. 1986;21:1143–6.
40. Houwen RHJ, Zwierstra RP, Severijnen RS, Bouquet J, Madern G et al. Prognosis of extrahepatic biliary atresia. Arch Dis Child. 1989;64:214–18.
41. Lilly JR, Karrer FM, Hall RJ, Stellin GP, Vasquez-Estevez JJ, Greenholz SK et al. The surgery of biliary atresia. Ann Surg. 1989;210:289–96.
42. Stringer M, Howard ER, Mowat AP. Endoscopic sclerotherapy in the management of esophageal varices in 61 children with biliary atresia. J Pediatr Surg. 1989;24:438–42.
43. Ohi R, Mochizuki I, Komatsu K, Kasai M. Portal hypertension after successful hepatic portoenterostomy in biliary atresia. J Pediatr Surg. 1986;21:271–4.
44. Kasai M, Okamoto A, Ohi R, Yabe K, Matsumura Y. Changes of portal vein pressure and intrahepatic blood vessels after surgery for biliary atresia. J Pediatr Surg. 1981;16:152–9.
45. Valayer J. Portosystemic shunt surgery. In: Howard ER, editor. Surgery of liver disease in children. Oxford: Butterworth–Heinemann; 1991.
46. Greene HL. Nutritional aspects in the management of biliary atresia. In: Daum F, editor. Extrahepatic biliary atresia. New York: Marcel Dekker: 1983.
47. Tsuchida Y, Komura M, Honna T, Kamii Y. Intra-hepatic cysts and cystic dilatation in biliary atresia after portoenterostomy: implications and management. In: Ohi R, editor. Biliary atresia. Tokyo: ICOM Associates Inc; 1991:147–53.
48. Saito S, Nishina T, Tsuchida Y. Intrahepatic cysts in biliary atresia after successful hepatoportoenterostomy. Arch Dis Child. 1984;59:274–5.
49. Ohi R, Nio M, Chiba T, Endo N, Goto M, Ibrahim M. Long-term follow-up after surgery for patients with biliary atresia. J Pediatr Surg. 1990;25:442–5.
50. Hadchouel M, Gautier M, Valayer J, Odievre M, Alagille D. Histopathology of the liver five years after successful surgery for extrahepatic biliary atresia. In: Daum F, editor. Extrahepatic biliary atresia. New York: Marcel Dekker; 1983.
51. McClement JW, Howard ER, Mowat AP. Results of surgical treatment for extrahepatic biliary atresia in the United Kingdom, 1980–1982. Br Med J. 1985;290:345–7.

30
The effect of phenobarbital in cholestasis

A. STIEHL

INTRODUCTION

Administration of phenobarbital (PB) to experimental animals is followed by an increase in bile flow[1] which is mainly due to an increase in the bile salt-independent fraction of biliary secretion[2]. In addition bile salt excretion may be increased. PB increases uptake storage and excretion of sulpho-bromphthalein and other dyes[3,4], increases the bilirubin-conjugating activity of the liver[5] and the hepatic excretion of bilirubin[6]. In addition PB leads to a proliferation of the hepatic smooth endoplasmatic reticulum[7] with an increase of hepatic cytochrome P-450 activity and an increase of drug hydroxylating proteins[8,9].

The effect of PB on bilirubin metabolism led to its therapeutic use in conjugated hyperbilirubinaemia including neonates[10], Gilbert's syndrome[11], and Crigler–Najjar syndrome[12]. A beneficial effect has been reported in patients with Dubin–Johnson syndrome[13]. The effect of PB on bile flow led to therapeutic trials in various cholestatic liver diseases[14]. A beneficial effect on cholestasis and pruritus has been observed in children with intrahepatic bile duct hypoplasia[15-17], benign intermittent cholestasis[16], and cholestasis of pregnancy[18]. Some patients with primary biliary cirrhosis and primary sclerosing cholangitis responded with improvement of jaundice and pruritus[19]. In extrahepatic cholestasis PB was not effective.

In developing cirrhosis microsomal function is progressively decreased[20], but attempts to treat cirrhosis patients with PB were not successful.

EFFECT OF PB IN BILIARY ATRESIA

Biliary atresia is characterized by a marked reduction of intrahepatic bile ducts and ductules, leading to chronic cholestasis with severe hyperlipidaemia, hyperbileacidaemia, and conjugated hyperbilirubinaemia. Clinical symptoms are pruritus, jaundice and xanthoma formation. Treatment with PB

Table 1 Effect of phenobarbital on cholestasis of childhood

Disease	Jaundice	Pruritus	References
Intrahepatic biliary atresia	↓	↓	14–17
Benign intermittent cholestasis	↓↓	↓	16
Extrahepatic biliary atresia	0	0	16

(10 mg/kg) leads to a marked decrease of serum bile acids and serum bilirubin[14–16]. Faecal ^{131}I-Rose-Bengal excretion is increased[16]. The decline of serum bile acids and serum bilirubin is accompanied by reduction in jaundice and pruritus[14–16]. Following withdrawal of PB, jaundice and pruritus reappear rapidly[16].

EFFECT OF PB IN BENIGN INTERMITTENT CHOLESTASIS

This disease is characterized by recurrent episodes of cholestasis accompanied by pruritus and jaundice. Besides serum bilirubin serum bile acids are also elevated. The only histological abnormality is centrilobular inspissation of bile and mild non-specific inflammatory changes. The episodes may persist for days or months, but eventually cholestasis clears completely. Treatment with PB leads to rapid decrease of serum bile acids and serum bilirubin[16]. Jaundice and pruritus disappear. Faecal ^{131}I-Rose-Bengal excretion increased from 10% to 71%[16], indicating that the biliary and faecal excretion of this cholephilic substance was improved. Following withdrawal of PB, jaundice and pruritus may rapidly recur.

MECHANISM OF ACTION OF PB IN CHOLESTASIS

The mechanism of action whereby PB stimulates the excretion of bilirubin and bile salts is still not completely understood. Obviously PB leads to an increase in bile flow[1,2] and it seems possible that this allows the cholestatic liver to excrete more cholephilic substances.

The effect of PB on bile acid metabolism is of especial interest since the accumulation of these molecules in cholestasis may lead to parenchymal liver damage[21]. Studies in children with bile duct hypoplasia indicate that PB treatment induces a decrease of serum bile acids[16,17] which is accompanied by a decrease in the pools of cholic and chenodeoxycholic acid, with a shifting of the pool from the peripheral to the enterohepatic circulation[22]. Furthermore, PB treatment reduces biological half-life and increases bile acid synthesis[22]. The effect of PB on serum concentration, pool size and biological half-life of cholate was greater than on those of chenodeoxycholate. Thus, PB enhanced the excretion and altered the distribution of the primary bile salts.

In cholestasis the liver hydroxylates common bile acids to form C-1 and C-6 hydroxylated bile acids[23], which are less toxic and more rapidly excreted by the urine than the corresponding original bile acids. PB treatment may induce hydroxylation of bile acids leading to an increased formation of hyocholic acid. Following PB treatment of our children with cholestasis, however, no increase of hydroxylated bile acids was observed[17]. The observed decrease in the plasma concentrations of bile acids was therefore not due to an increased formation of polyhydroxylated bile acids. PB induces bile acid UDP–glucuronyl transferase[24] and increases formation of bile acid glucuronides, leading to an increased urinary and biliary excretion of glucuronidated bile acids[17]. In bile and urine the major bile acid glucuronides were conjugates of di- and trihydroxylated bile acids, whereas only very small amounts of toxic monohydroxy bile acids were excreted. Bile acid glucuronides in bile of children with cholestasis increased only from 4.5% to 8.1% of total bile acids[17] and therefore the increased bile acid glucuronide formation following PB treatment is only of minor importance for the overall biliary and faecal excretion of bile acids. In urine glucuronidated bile acids increased[17] from 5.6 to 7.1 mg/24 h. The increased renal excretion of bile acid glucuronides also may facilitate their excretion. Thus, comparison to the marked effect of PB on bile flow, its influence on formation and excretion of bile acid glucuronides seems less important.

It is of interest that treatment with ursodeoxycholic acid, another substance used in the treatment of cholestatic diseases, also reduces endogenous bile acids in peripheral blood. Furthermore, PB, like ursodeoxycholic acid, leads to an increase in the fractional turnover and synthesis of bile acids. These similarities in the effects of ursodeoxycholic acid and PB may be due to the fact that both substances increase bile flow.

PB treatment of patients with cholestatic disease states does not improve liver enzymes activity in serum, or liver histology. PB seems helpful in reducing pruritus and jaundice in patients with certain forms of cholestasis. However, whether PB treatment prolongs survival and/or reduces morbidity remains unclear.

References

1. Klaassen CD. Biliary flow after microsomal enzyme induction. J Pharmacol Exp Ther. 1969;168:218–23.
2. Berthelot O, Erlinger S, Dhumeaux D et al. Mechanism of phenobarbital-induced hypercholeresis in the rat. Am J Physiol. 1970;219:809–13.
3. Redinger RN, Small DM. Primate physiology. VIII. The effect of phenobarbital upon bile salt synthesis and pool size, biliary lipid secretion, and bile composition. J Clin Invest. 1973;52:161–72.
4. Schellhas H, Hornef W, Remmer H. Beschleunigung der Elimination von Bromsulfthalein durch Phenobarbital. Nauyn Schmiedebergs Arch Pharmakol. 1965;251:111–12.
5. Hart LG, Guarino AM, Adamson RH. Effects of phenobarbital on biliary excretion of organic acids in male and female rats. Am J Physiol. 1969;217:46–52.
6. Catz C, Yaffe SJ. Barbiturate enhancement of bilirubin conjugation and excretion in young and adult animals. Pediatr Res. 1968;2:361–70.
7. Remmer H, Merker HJ. Effect of drugs on the formation of smooth endoplasmatic reticulum and drug metabolizing enzymes. Ann NY Acad Sci. 1965;123:79–97.
8. Conney AH, Davison C, Gastel R et al. Adaptive increases in drug-metabolizing enzymes induced by phenobarbital and other drugs. J Pharmacol Exp Ther. 1960;130.1–8.
9. Marshall WJ, McLean AEM. The effect of oral phenobarbitone on hepatic microsomal

cytochrome P-450 and demethylation activity in rats fed normal and low protein diets. Biochem Pharmacol. 1969;18:153–7.

10. Trolle D. Decrease of total serum bilirubin concentration in newborn infants after phenobarbitone treatment. Lancet. 1968;2:705–8.

11. Kreek MJ, Sleisenger MH. Reduction of serum unconjugated bilirubin with phenobarbitone in adult congenital non-haemolytic unconjugated hyperbilirubinaemia. Lancet. 1968;2:73–8.

12. Arias IM, Gartner LM, Cohen M *et al.* Chronic nonhemolytic unconjugated hyperbilirubinemia with glucuronyl transferase deficiency. Clinical, biochemical, pharmacologic and genetic evidence for heterogeneity. Am J Med. 1969;47:395–409.

13. Shani M, Seligsohn U, Ben-Ezzer J. Effect of phenobarbital on liver functions in patients with Dubin-Johnson syndrome. Gastroenterology. 1974;67:303–8.

14. Thompson RPH, Williams R. Phenobarbitone in intrahepatic biliary atresia. Lancet. 1970;2:466.

15. Sharp HL, Mirkin BL. Effect of phenobarbital on hyperbilirubinemia, bile acid metabolism, and microsomal enzyme activity in chronic intrahepatic cholestasis of childhood. J Pediatr. 1972;81:116–26.

16. Stiehl A, Thaler MM, Admirand WH. The effects of phenobarbital on bile salts and bilirubin in patients with intrahepatic and extrahepatic cholestasis. N Engl J Med. 1972;286:858–61.

17. Stiehl A, Becker M, Czygan P *et al.* Bile acids and their sulphated and glucuronidated derivatives in bile, plasma and urine of children with intrahepatic cholestasis: effects of phenobarbital treatment. Eur J Clin Invest. 1980;10:307–16.

18. Espinozza J, Barnafi L, Schnaidt E. The effect of phenobarbital on intrahepatic cholestasis of pregnancy. Am J Obstet Gynecol. 1974;119:234–8.

19. Bloomer JR, Boyer JL. Phenobarbital effects in cholestatic liver disease. Ann Intern Med. 1975;82:310–17.

20. Gross JB, Reichen J, Zeltner T, Zimmermann A. The evolution of changes in quantitative liver function tests in a rat model of cirrhosis. Hepatology. 1987;7:457–63.

21. Greim H, Trülzsch D, Czygan P *et al.* Mechanism of cholestasis. 6. Bile acids in human livers with or without biliary obstruction. Gastroenterology. 1972;63:846–50.

22. Stiehl A, Thaler MM, Admirand WH. Effects of phenobarbital on bile salt metabolism in cholestasis due to intrahepatic bile duct hypoplasia. Pediatrics. 1973;51:992–7.

23. Bremmelgaard A, Sjövall J. Hydroxylation of cholic, chenodeoxycholic, and deoxycholic acids in patients with intrahepatic cholestasis. J Lipid Res. 1980;21:1072–81.

24. Fröhling W, Ast E, Stiehl A, Czygan P, Kommerell B. Induction and activation of rat liver microsomal bile salt glucuronyl transferase. Biochim Biophys Acta. 1976;444:525–30.

31
Vitamin deficiency and replacement in childhood cholestasis

R. J. SOKOL

INTRODUCTION

Prolonged survival of children with chronic cholestatic liver disease has become possible over the past two decades because of advances in surgical treatment of extrahepatic biliary atresia, improvements in medical treatment and correction of nutritional deficiencies in children with chronic intrahepatic cholestasis, and the advent of orthotopic liver transplantation for those children who progress to end-stage liver disease or suffer from unremitting, severe consequences of cholestasis. For these reasons, attention to all clinically important nutritional deficiencies has become an essential part of the management of children with chronic cholestasis, in order to prevent permanent sequelae and to improve quality of life. The fat-soluble vitamins are particularly prone to deficiency during cholestasis because of the requirement of adequate bile flow for intraluminal solubilization of ingested lipids. Each of the four fat-soluble vitamins is metabolized in a manner differing from the others, requiring a different strategy for evaluating nutritional status for each vitamin as well as for treating deficiencies. This review will focus on the unique physiology and metabolism of each of the fat-soluble vitamins during cholestasis, problems that exist in evaluating nutritional status for each of the vitamins, and recommendations for evaluation and supplementation during cholestasis.

VITAMIN A

Dietary sources of vitamin A include the carotene family, retinyl esters and free retinol. The parent compound of the vitamin A group is called all-*trans*-retinol[1]. Absorption of all these compounds requires adequate bile flow for micellar solubilization of dietary fat; hence malabsorption of vitamin A is common in chronic cholestatic liver disease. In addition, dietary intake of foods containing vitamin A and beta carotene (e.g. dairy products, internal organs, yellow and green leafy vegetables and fruits) may be low in children with liver disease. Pancreatic esterases hydrolyse retinyl esters in the gut lumen prior to absorption. In normal circumstances vitamin A compounds are absorbed in the jejunum. Free retinol absorbed into the enterocyte undergoes esterification with palmitate and other fatty acids, and is then incorporated into newly synthesized chylomicrons, in which vitamin A is transported from the enterocyte into the mesenteric lymphatics. Retinyl esters are neither hydrolysed nor transported to tissues during the metabolism by lipoprotein lipase of circulating chylomicrons. The resulting chylomicron remnants are then taken up by hepatocytes in which retinyl esters are released for hepatocyte metabolism. In the hepatocyte, retinyl esters may be hydrolysed, releasing the free retinol which can be transported into the sinusoids bound in a 1:1 molar ratio with retinol binding protein (RBP). Alternatively, retinyl esters may be stored in the hepatocyte or transported as RBP-bound retinol from the hepatocyte to Itoh cells (perisinusoidal stellate cells; lipocytes), the site for over 80% of hepatic vitamin A storage under normal conditions[2]. A small portion of vitamin A may be oxidized to retinoic acid and conjugated with glucuronides for secretion into the bile. The synthesis and secretion of RBP is dependent on adequacy of zinc, thus in zinc deficiency plasma RBP levels, and hence plasma retinol levels, are depressed[1]. The synthesis of hepatic RBP is also dependent upon adequate protein status and the capacity of the liver to synthesize proteins. Consequently, in protein malnutrition or in hepatic failure the plasma RBP levels may likewise be low[3]. Recent studies indicating that Itoh cells may also synthesize RBP suggest that RBP-retinol may be directly mobilized and secreted from Itoh cells during vitamin A depletion[2]. The circulating retinol bound to RBP in the plasma compartment is taken up by target issues such as the retina by a receptor-mediated process. In the retina, retinol is oxidized to its aldehyde, 11-*cis*-retinaldehyde, an important constituent of the visual photoreceptor pigment, rhodopsin[1]. Retinol is also important for differentiation and the integrity of many epithelial tissues including the bronchial mucosa, the skin and the corneal epithelium. The role of β-carotene in human nutrition is less well characterized; however, blood carotene levels correlate inversely with the risk for development of certain carcinomas in adults, particularly those in the lung[4]. Absorption of β-carotene and the other carotenoids in the diet requires solubilization by intraluminal bile acids in a similar manner to vitamin A.

Several perturbations in hepatic metabolism of vitamin A are present in chronic cholestatic liver disease. The intraluminal solubilization of vitamin A and other carotenoids is compromised by lack of bile flow, resulting in malabsorption and depletion of vitamin A stores[5]. If protein malnutrition, zinc deficiency or depressed hepatic synthetic function is present, hepatic secretion of RBP is diminished, leading to low plasma levels of retinol and impaired delivery to target tissues[1]. Retinol may undergo oxidation when antioxidant protection is low, or possibly in the presence of pro-oxidants such as copper and iron. Finally, it is unclear whether hepatocyte accumulation of bile acids has a direct effect on vitamin A mobilization from the liver.

The clinical evaluation of vitamin A status in children with chronic cholestasis is problematic because of several confounding factors. The standard indices of vitamin A clinical status include serum retinol levels (high-pressure liquid chromatography measurement), serum retinol : RBP molar ratio, dark-field adaptation testing, slit-lamp examination of the cornea and conjunctivae, and liver levels of retinol and retinyl esters. In addition, electron microscopy and special histological staining of the liver may reveal excessive accumulation of vitamin A in Itoh cells in vitamin A overload[2]. A special test to evaluate vitamin A status is the relative dose response (RDR) test[6-8]. For this test a modest dose of vitamin A is given orally or parenterally (450 μg), and serum retinol is measured at 0 and 5 h. The RDR is defined as the difference between the retinol level at 5 h and the retinol level at 0 h divided by the retinol level at 5 h × 100%. An RDR less than 10% indicates vitamin A adequacy and values above 20% indicate A deficiency[6,8]. Thus, an excessive increase in serum retinol occurs after a modest oral dose of vitamin A if deficiency is present, probably due to a large capacity of the RBP in the deficient liver to transport absorbed retinol quickly to target tissues. Finally, conjunctival compression cytology has been used to detect subclinical vitamin A deficiency[9-12]. In this test a small piece of filter paper is applied to the bulbar conjunctiva, patted gently, and peeled off slowly. After staining procedures, morphology of the adherent epithelial cells is evaluated histologically. The abnormalities found in vitamin A deficiency include abnormalities in epithelial cell morphology, decreased number of goblet cells, and mucin spots covering less than 25% of the sample, all consistent with signs of vitamin A deficiency.

If one defines vitamin A deficiency based on low hepatic vitamin A levels (hepatic vitamin A stores less than 20 μg/g wet liver), serum retinol levels are not uniformly indicative of vitamin A status in children with chronic cholestasis, Amadee-Manesme et al.[5] showed that plasma retinol levels below 10 μg/dl are associated with low hepatic concentrations of vitamin A in children with chronic cholestasis. However, plasma levels between 10 and 20 μg/dl, a range that most would consider indicative of vitamin A deficiency, were occasionally associated with normal hepatic concentrations of vitamin A. More importantly, plasma concentrations of retinol greater than 20 μg/dl, a range considered to indicate vitamin A sufficiency, were frequently associated with hepatic vitamin A concentrations well below 20 μg/g wet weight[5]. Thus, children who are vitamin A-deficient based on low hepatic stores frequently have plasma retinol concentrations in the normal range.

The retinol : RBP molar ratio appears promising as a tool to differentiate vitamin A-depleted from vitamin A-sufficient cholestatic children. Mourey et al.[13] recently showed that liver RBP levels were not different between vitamin A-deficient (defined by hepatic vitamin A levels) versus sufficient children with cholestasis or control children. However, plasma RBP levels were lower in the deficient patients. More importantly, the molar ratio of retinol to RBP was 0.62 ± 0.15 in vitamin A-deficient patients but was 1.04 ± 0.06 in vitamin A-repleted patients. This ratio differentiated all but one vitamin A-deficient patient from the vitamin A-sufficient patients. In addition, there was a wide overlap in plasma retinol concentrations among the deficient and sufficient patients, as in previous studies. Therefore, this easily obtained plasma ratio may prove to be a useful non-invasive means of determining vitamin A status during cholestasis. Certainly, further studies need to be conducted to confirm the utility of this ratio, particularly comparing it to liver vitamin A levels in a larger group of children, or comparing it to the RDR in cholestatic children.

The RDR after an oral dose of vitamin A depends upon adequate solubilization and absorption of ingested vitamin A. In cholestasis the intestinal absorption of vitamin A may be severely impaired, so that this test is invalidated. Amadee-Manesme et al.[8] recently showed that intravenous injection of 1000 µg of retinyl palmitate and employment of the RDR formula correctly identified vitamin A status (based on hepatic vitamin A levels) in 12 children with liver disease. This study of a relatively small group of patients demonstrated the possible utility of the intravenous RDR for non-invasive evaluation of vitamin A status in cholestatic children. Clearly, the determination of vitamin A levels in liver biopsy tissue will not prove to be a useful clinical tool. If the RDR can be calculated after an oral dose of vitamin A that is solubilized by a micellar agent, such as water-soluble vitamin E (D-α-tocopheryl polyethylene glycol-1000 succinate; TPGS), then the RDR may prove extremely useful on an outpatient basis. Tests are now being conducted as to the feasibility of this modification of the oral RDR.

It is unknown why plasma retinol levels do not reflect hepatic stores during chronic cholestasis. In cystic fibrosis it has been proposed that impaired RBP secretion by the liver may lead to elevated hepatic concentrations of vitamin A in the face of low circulating vitamin A levels. The opposite appears to be the case during chronic cholestasis wherein normal circulating vitamin A levels are associated with hepatic depletion. It may be that Itoh cells release vitamin A stores as they are transformed to activated cells in response to hepatic injury. Further investigations of the regulation of hepatic and cellular apo- and holo-RBP will possibly yield information to help explain these paradoxes.

The most recent development in evaluating vitamin A status has been the conjunctival impression cytology method[9-12]. This tool has proved useful in field trials because of the stability of conjunctival epithelium on filter paper over time. One study[11] has investigated its use in children with cholestasis, and reported that the impression cytology correctly identified the vitamin A status of the 16 children studied with liver disease. Only eight of these children had chronic cholestasis, four of whom were vitamin A-deficient based on low liver concentration or an intravenous RDR of greater than 20%. If subsequent investigations document a strong correlation between the conjunctival impression cytology and vitamin A status, this simple test could be used to screen and follow patients while on vitamin A therapy. Routine slit-lamp testing by an ophthalmologist would be tedious, and is difficult in young children; however, early ophthalmological findings of xerophthalmia are certainly indicative of preclinical vitamin A deficiency. Dark-field adaptation testing can be very difficult in children, particularly those under the age of 7 or 8 years, and is therefore not particularly helpful for evaluating vitamin A status in young children with chronic cholestasis.

The emphasis on detecting vitamin A deficiency is important for several reasons. Firstly, although blindness and severe ocular findings of vitamin A deficiency are very rare in children with chronic cholestasis, the potential for impairment in vision certainly is present. It is also possible that vitamin A deficiency increases the risk of patients towards infection, and perhaps perturbs biliary epithelization of Roux-Y conduits following hepatic portoenterostomy procedures. Finally, the effect of vitamin A status on predisposition to hepatocellular carcinoma in children with chronic liver disease is unknown. Importantly, overzealous treatment with vitamin A supplements poses a risk for vitamin A hepatotoxicity complicating the underlying cholestatic liver disease. In a recent report, Geubel et al.[14] found that, among 41 patients with vitamin A hepatotoxicity, the smallest continuous daily consumption that led to cirrhosis was 25 000 IU during 6 years of vitamin A supplementation. Thus, doses of vitamin A that are not uncommonly prescribed in children with chronic cholestasis (25 000–50 000 IU per day) have the potential for causing hepatotoxicity if adequately absorbed. Because serum retinol levels may not reflect vitamin A toxicity, the standard means for following vitamin A status in these patients (serum retinol) may not identify those patients who are becoming vitamin A toxic. Rather, monitoring should be performed to detect elevated plasma vitamin A esters indicative of patients at risk for vitamin A toxicity.

Routine supplementation with vitamin A compounds to prevent deficiency has been recommended by several authorities. However, optimal means for monitoring vitamin A repletion, as well as screening for toxicity, have not been agreed upon. The French group recommends intramuscular injections of 100 000 IU (33 000 µg) of retinyl palmitate in an aqueous preparation every 2 months for at least 6 months in patients who have vitamin A deficiency[15]. This form of vitamin A is not uniformly available, the treatment requires intramuscular injections, and the lack of vitamin A toxicity in adequate numbers of patients treated in this way has not been fully documented. Others[16] recommend large oral doses of vitamin A esters (25 000–50 000 IU per day), although there is little documentation of the adequacy or safety of this treatment. The water-soluble vitamin E, TPGS, has been shown to improve intestinal absorption of other lipid-soluble molecules (cyclosporin[17] and vitamin D[18]) during cholestasis. Therefore, oral co-administration of vitamin A supplements and TPGS may be the means of improving solubilization and hence absorption of vitamin A during cholestasis, particularly in patients who are also under therapy for vitamin E deficiency. This would preclude the necessity for intramuscular injections of vitamin A, and would most likely result in the need for smaller oral doses of vitamin A (e.g. 5000–20 000 IU per day). This strategy for oral vitamin A replacement is currently under investigation. Since standard multiple vitamin preparations contain 5000 IU of vitamin A, the recommended administration of two doses of a multiple vitamin per day to children with chronic cholestasis may provide them with adequate (10 000 IU) vitamin A per day if given with TPGS.

VITAMIN D

Vitamin D nutritional status depends on both ingestion of vitamin D2 (ergocalciferol) and biosynthesis of vitamin D3 in the skin upon ultraviolet light exposure[19]. The compound 7-dehydrocholesterol is converted into vitamin D3 (cholecalciferol) through this photochemical reaction. The second source, vitamin D2, is from ingested plants and supplemented milk. The absorption of vitamin D2 is dependent upon adequate bile flow for micellar solubilization, thus vitamin D2 malabsorption during cholestasis has been observed. The two vitamin D compounds are absorbed into the enterocyte in the jejunum and ileum, from which vitamin D is carried by chylomicrons into the bloodstream. Interestingly, the 25-hydroxylated form of vitamin D2 (25-OHD) is absorbed significantly into the portal venous circulation, avoiding to some extent the reliance on micellar solubilization of dietary fat[20]. The vitamin D compounds are protein-bound in the plasma, with vitamin D, 25-OHD, and probably 1,25-dihydroxy vitamin D and 24,25-dihydroxy vitamin D being transported on the same 5–6 kD protein in humans. This vitamin D-binding protein has a higher affinity for 25-OHD than for vitamin D or 1,25-dihydroxy vitamin D. Absorbed vitamin D2 or photosynthesized vitamin D3 undergo 25-hydroxylation in the liver, resulting in the major circulating form of vitamin D, 25-OHD. From the liver, 25-OHD is returned to the circulation where it is transported to the kidney and undergoes 1α-hydroxylation to form 1,25-dihydroxy vitamin D. This is the active form of vitamin D which increases intestinal absorption of calcium and stimulates renal conservation of calcium. Secretion of parathyroid hormone increases 1α-hydroxylase activity and thus stimulates calcium absorption. Finally, a 24-hydroxylation step may result in the synthesis of 24,25-dihydroxy vitamin D, the action of which is not certain; however, it appears to be necessary for adequate bone mineralization[21].

During cholestatic liver disease, absorption of ingested vitamin D2 is most certainly impaired[22]. Consequently, photosynthesized vitamin D3 appears to have greater importance in determining the vitamin D status of the cholestatic child[22]. Initially, it was felt that 25-hydroxylation of vitamin D might be impaired during cholestatic liver disease; however, more recent studies indicate that 25-hydroxylation is intact[23]. Importantly, many children with cholestatic liver disease are not exposed to adequate sunlight because of the chronic debilitation that many suffer, thus diminishing the cutaneous synthesis of vitamin D3. The effect of cholestatic liver disease on the synthesis of the circulating vitamin D binding proteins and its effects on vitamin D status and bone mineralization are unknown.

The clinical evaluation of vitamin D status in children with chronic cholestasis is performed by measuring serum 25-OHD blood levels, taking into account seasonal variations in normal values based on age. The blood level of 1,25-dihydroxy vitamin D is more indicative of calcium status than of vitamin D status, with a high level indicative of calcium deficiency. Vitamin D2 and vitamin D3 blood levels are not useful indices because of the rapid conversion of these compounds to the 25-hydroxylated forms. Thus, it is generally felt that a serum 25-OHD level below 14–15 ng/ml is indicative of vitamin D deficiency. Serum calcium, phosphorus, alkaline phosphatase, and parathyroid hormone levels may identify biochemical deficiency, and bone X-rays and bone densitometry may confirm osteomalacia, osteopenia, rickets or abnormal bone calcification.

Several studies have investigated vitamin D status and absorption in children with chronic cholestatic liver disease. In extrahepatic biliary atresia, 25-hydroxy vitamin D blood levels are significantly lower in children with unsuccessful portoenterostomy procedures compared to those with successful procedures[24]. In children with other forms of chronic cholestasis, 20–50% may have low 25-OHD blood levels. Despite supplementation with large oral doses of vitamin D2, circulating levels of vitamin D2 and 25-OHD-2 have been shown to be significantly lower than levels of vitamin D3 and 25-OHD-3 in children with chronic cholestasis[22]. These data suggest that much of the vitamin D is derived from photochemical reactions in the skin rather than from ingested supplements. However, absorption of 25-OHD is superior to that of vitamin D2 in cholestasis[22,25], even though there is significant malabsorption of 25-OHD compared to control children[22,24,26]. Oral supplementation with 25-OHD in the range of $2-4\,\mu g/kg$ per day has normalized 25-OHD blood levels and presumably vitamin D status in cholestatic children. Despite normal vitamin D status, many children with chronic cholestasis continue to show evidence of metabolic bone disease instead of the classic findings of rickets. Bucuvalas et al.[27] have recently used stable isotope technology to demonstrate that calcium absorption is not significantly impaired in children with chronic cholestasis compared to control children. Calcium balance was also positive in four of the five subjects studied, despite diminished bone density measured by single beam photon absorptiometry of the distal radius. These studies suggest that factors other than calcium malabsorption and decreased serum 25-hydroxy vitamin D levels must contribute to this diminished bone mass. Factors such as limitations in physical activity, fluoride and aluminium status, and other nutrient deficiencies require investigation.

Current recommendations are to evaluate serum 25-OHD blood levels at periodic intervals, particularly if they are found to be low, encourage adequate sunlight exposure of all children with cholestatic liver disease, and encourage normal intake of calcium and phosphorus in the child's diet[28]. If vitamin D deficiency is found, supplementation with 3–10 times the recommended dietary allowance of vitamin D2 or D3 for age can be attempted. Intestinal absorption of these supplements can be improved by the co-administration of oral TPGS-vitamin E as a solubilizing agent[18]. If vitamin D deficiency is recalcitrant to these treatments, oral 25-OHD at a dose of $2-4\,\mu g/kg$ per day should be started, and 25-OHD blood levels remeasured in 1–2 months. Monitoring for vitamin D toxicity should include urine calcium:creatinine ratios, serum calcium and phosphorus, and blood concentrations of 25-OHD. Routine supplementation with large oral doses of vitamin D without proper monitoring and follow-up is discouraged, despite the fact that children with moderate to severe cholestasis will probably absorb little of standard vitamin D preparations. Following these recommendations the incidence of rickets has decreased dramatically in our clinic population of children with biliary atresia and other chronic cholestatic conditions. However, the progressive loss of bone mass and recurrent fractures of long bones have become one of the more frequent complications of chronic cholestasis that have led to liver transplantation. Adequate nutritional or medical treatments to prevent this progression to osteopenia have not been developed, and remain one of the major challenges in the medical management of the child (or adult) with chronic cholestasis.

VITAMIN K

Compounds with vitamin K activity exist as three forms[29]. Phylloquinone (vitamin K1) is synthesized by green plants and is available in most diets. Menaquinones (vitamin K2) are a group of compounds that are synthesized by intestinal bacteria and presumably absorbed through the intestinal mucosa. A third group are the menadiones (K3), synthetic vitamin K compounds which have better water-solubility than the two natural forms. Menadiol sodium diphosphate is manufactured as Synkayvite, which is available in a liquid form for neonates. Phylloquinone is sold as Mephyton or Aquamephyton, as well as several other brand names. The specific action of vitamin K is the post-translational γ-carboxylation of glutamic acid residues on the vitamin K-dependent proteins (gla proteins), creating effective calcium-binding sites on these proteins[29,30]. The vitamin K-dependent proteins include clotting factors II, VII, IX, X, protein C, and protein S. There is also a family of other vitamin K-dependent proteins (gla proteins), which are found in many tissues. The function of these gla proteins is currently unknown.

The absorption of vitamin K is dependent on its incorporation into mixed micelles in the intestinal lumen, thus requiring the presence of both bile acids and pancreatic enzymes[29]. The absorption of vitamin K in normal situations may be up to 50–80%, but it is markedly depressed if bile flow is impaired. Phylloquinone is absorbed from the intestine by an energy-dependent active transport process, whereas menaquinone is absorbed by a passive non-carrier-mediated process. Menaquinone can be absorbed from the distal ileum and colon where bacterial growth is common; however, the concentration of bile acids in the colon may not be sufficient to allow significant absorption of bacterial-derived menaquinones in the intact gut. Menadione is absorbed from both the colon and small intestine by a passive process. The absorbed vitamin K derivatives are incorporated in the enterocyte into chylomicrons, transported to the lymphatics and eventually into the systemic circulation. Phylloquinone appears to be retained in the liver whereas menadione is widely distributed to all tissues and actually may be rapidly excreted, at least in the rat.

Clinical evaluation of vitamin K status is generally achieved by measuring the prothrombin time which is dependent on the vitamin K-dependent clotting factors in the intrinsic coagulation pathway[30]. Prolongation of the prothrombin time indicates deficiency, consumption, or inhibition of the vitamin K-dependent clotting factors as well as several other factors. If the prothrombin time is prolonged in comparison to the partial thromboplastin time, then this indicates most likely a vitamin K deficiency. More recently, newer techniques for the measurement of serum vitamin K concentrations have been developed, although these are generally available only on a research basis. More available are the assays for non-carboxylated vitamin K-dependent proteins, the so-called PIVKA (protein in vitamin K absence) assay[30]. Finally, specific clotting factor levels (factor II, VII, IX and X) can be measured to determine if these vitamin K-dependent proteins are diminished.

The major cause of vitamin K deficiency in children with chronic cholestasis is due to malabsorption of vitamin K. Thus, an intramuscular dose of vitamin K will correct the prolongation of the prothrombin time within 24 h if malabsorption of dietary or supplemental vitamin K is aetiologic. Yanofsky et al.[31] utilized this response to intramuscular vitamin K as well as plasma levels of specific clotting factors to determine the frequency and source of coagulopathy in 43 patients with extrahepatic biliary atresia who had undergone hepatic portoenterostomy. They found that 23.3% of the patients were vitamin K-deficient, 30.2% had coagulopathy due to chronic liver disease, 46.5% had no coagulopathy. Vitamin K deficiency was less common than vitamin E deficiency, although all vitamin K-deficient patients were severely E-deficient.

It is currently recommended that vitamin K supplements of 2.5–5.0 mg be given two to seven times a week to all children with chronic cholestasis who have persistent elevation of serum bilirubin and evidence of poor bile flow[16,28]. Many children will absorb the phylloquinone (Mephyton) form of vitamin K adequately for prevention of coagulopathy. Co-administration of vitamin K with TPGS may theoretically increase solubilization of vitamin K and potentially improve absorption. Use of menadione (Synkayvite) should be discouraged because of the severe toxicity of large doses of menadione, which is particularly toxic to the liver. Menadione creates a redox generation of free radicals which can lead to massive haemolysis as well as hepato-toxicity[32]. Thus, although Synkayvite may be absorbed better than Mephyton, its potential toxicity needs to be considered. If oral vitamin K supplementation is unsuccessful, intramuscular or intravenous injections of vitamin K virtually always correct vitamin K deficiency coagulopathy. Monthly injections of vitamin K may be needed in children with chronic severe cholestasis. Vitamin K should certainly be given to children with coagulopathy prior to any surgical procedures or if massive or life-threatening bleeding episodes occur.

VITAMIN E

One of the interesting stories in the treatment of chronic cholestatic liver disease in childhood in the past decade has been the observation that vitamin E deficiency causes a progressive, neuromuscular degeneration that may result in a crippling combination of ataxia, peripheral neuropathy, muscle weakness, and ophthalmoplegia within the first decade of life[33]. The initial description of this neurological disorder in patients with abetalipoprotein-aemia[34] and associated vitamin E deficiency led to investigations in children with chronic cholestasis in the late 1970s. More recent studies have documented malabsorption of vitamin E as the cause of the deficiency[35], and have shown responsiveness to vitamin E repletion both by the intramuscular route[36,37] and through the administration of TPGS-vitamin E orally[38,39]. Other effects of vitamin E deficiency in cholestatic children are being sought.

The term vitamin E describes a group of eight compounds called the tocopherols and the tocotrienols[40]. These structurally related compounds consist of substituted hydroxylated chromanol ring systems linked to an isoprenoid side-chain. The four major forms of vitamin E (α-, β-, δ- and γ-tocopherol) differ by the number and position of the methyl group substitutions on the chromanol ring. Bioactivity is not uniform among these forms of vitamin E, with activity being highest in α-tocopherol followed by γ- and then β- and δ-tocopherol. γ-Tocopherol has only approximately 20% of the bioactivity of α-tocopherol. Commonly administered vitamin E supplements are tocopherol esterified to acetate, succinate, or nicotinate; however, despite labelling claims, these compounds are not water-soluble. It has recently been recognized that there are eight stereoisomers of vitamin E that can be synthesized for each of the tocopherol compounds based on the rotational direction of the methyl groups at the 2-position on the chromanol ring and the 4' and 8' positions on the isoprenoid side-chain. Only the R–R–R isomers (i.e. D-α-tocopherol) occur abundantly in nature and are called the natural forms of the vitamin. The S rotation in the number 2 position confers much less bioactivity to the molecule than the R rotation. The common dietary sources of vitamin E are the oil-containing grains, plants, and vegetables.

Ingested vitamin E requires intestinal solubilization by bile acids into mixed micelles so that the highly hydrophobic vitamin E can traverse the aqueous environment in the intestinal lumen to reach the surface of the absorptive enterocyte[35], where 20–40% of vitamin E is absorbed[40]. Prior to intestinal absorption, most esters of vitamin E are hydrolysed by esterases either secreted by the pancreas or found in the intestinal mucosa. Vitamin E is absorbed into the intestinal mucosa by a non-saturable, non-carrier-mediated passive diffusion process. Once inside the enterocyte, α- and γ-tocopherol are incorporated with the other products of dietary lipid digestion and apolipoproteins into newly synthesized chylomicrons and very low-density lipoproteins (VLDL) which are transported via mesenteric lymphatics and the thoracic duct into the systemic circulation[40]. During hydrolysis of circulating chylomicrons and VLDL by lipoprotein lipase and hepatic triglyceride lipase, α-tocopherol is transferred to some extent to target tissues[41]. The α- and γ-tocopherol remaining in chylomicron remnants are transported to the liver. In the liver, α-tocopherol is re-secreted as a component of hepatic derived VLDL and perhaps high-density lipoproteins (HDL). γ-Tocopherol is not secreted substantially into hepatic-derived lipoproteins but appears to be metabolized or excreted by the liver. The hepatic tocopherol binding protein (TBP), a 30–32 kD cytosolic protein, may play a role in the hepatic discrimination process by which α-tocopherol is incorporated into lipoproteins, and γ-tocopherol is not. In the fasting state, most circulating α-tocopherol is found in low-density lipoprotein (LDL) and HDL. During receptor-mediated binding and non-specific binding of LDL to various cells, α-tocopherol appears to be transferred to tissues[42].

During cholestatic liver disease, impaired secretion of bile acids by the liver may result in intraluminal bile acid concentrations below the critical micellar concentration, causing severe malabsorption of vitamin E[35]. Because of its extreme hydrophobic nature, almost all forms of vitamin E and vitamin E esters have an absolute requirement for sufficient intraluminal bile acids for absorption. Thus, it has been clearly demonstrated that intraluminal bile acid concentrations can predict the ability of a cholestatic child to absorb vitamin E, and the co-administration of bile acids with vitamin E will enhance the absorption of this vitamin[35]. Prolonged deficiency of vitamin E in cholestatic children leads to a degenerative neuromyopathy involving the spinocerebellar tracts, cranial nerve nuclei 3 and 4, large-calibre myelinated axons in peripheral nerves and the posterior columns of the spinal cord, skeletal muscle and the ocular retina[33]. This degenerative process begins within the first 2 years of life and is usually heralded by hyporeflexia at approximately 18–24 months of life. Within 2–4 years truncal and limb ataxia develop and, if left untreated, severe gait abnormalities, dysmetria, and impairment in balance and coordination will occur[43]. After several more years peripheral neuropathy, muscular weakness, ophthalmoplegia, and retinal dysfunction develop. Thus by 10 years of age the child may have incapacitating neurological symptoms that preclude normal function and that is, unfortunately, irreversible to a significant degree[43]. This irreversibility mandates the aggressive evaluation and correction of vitamin E status early in the course of chronic cholestasis in children.

The clinical evaluation of vitamin E status in children with chronic cholestasis is unique among the various malabsorptive conditions that may lead to vitamin E deficiency because of the hyperlipidaemia that is frequently present. Serum vitamin E levels directly correlate with total serum lipid concentrations and with serum cholesterol levels to a lesser extent[44], most likely because of partitioning of the lipid-soluble vitamin E into the plasma lipoproteins as well as the close relationship between the regulation of plasma vitamin E levels and that of lipoprotein clearance. Thus, hyperlipidaemia in a person with normal vitamin E status will result in elevated plasma vitamin E levels and the opposite is the case for hypolipidaemia. Consequently, in a cholestatic child who is vitamin E-deficient but has severe hyperlipidaemia (e.g. total serum lipids 3000–4000 mg/dl), a normal serum vitamin E level may be attained because of this artifactual elevation caused by the hyperlipidaemia[45]. Therefore, the ratio of serum vitamin E to total serum lipids has been adopted as a more accurate reflection of vitamin E status during hyperlipidaemic states[44,45]. The total serum lipid concentration is considered the sum of the serum cholesterol, triglycerides, and phospholipids. Normal serum vitamin E levels in older children and adults range from 5 to 20 μg/ml, and perhaps a bit lower in infants and young children. Premature infants with very low circulating lipid levels have lower serum vitamin E levels without indicating deficiency. The threshold for biochemical vitamin E deficiency in older children and adults using the vitamin E : total serum lipid ratio is 0.8 mg of total tocopherol per gram of total lipid[44]. In children under age 12 years, 0.6 mg/g may indicate vitamin E adequacy. Thus, in children with cholestatic liver disease, a serum vitamin E level should be accompanied by total serum lipid level for adequate interpretation, lest children with hyperlipidaemia and normal serum vitamin E levels who are actually vitamin E-deficient be thought to be E-sufficient and therefore not receive therapy.

Several functional assays for vitamin E status exist. Red blood cells haemolyse (>10%) when exposed to hydrogen peroxide when they are vitamin E-deficient[46]. Unfortunately, selenium deficiency and other nutritional factors (e.g. polyunsaturated fatty acid status) also affect red blood cell hydrogen peroxide haemolysis, therefore the test is not specific to vitamin E deficiency. Another test has been proposed wherein the amount of malondialdehyde, a lipid peroxidation product that is released by red blood cells exposed to hydrogen peroxide, is measured[47]. Serum lipid peroxide measurements have been made; however, these are difficult to interpret during hyperlipidaemia and may not correct even when vitamin E status is corrected[48]. Expired pentane gas, a sensitive measure of total body lipid peroxidation of linoleic acid, can be used to quantitate antioxidant deficiency[49]. However, selenium deficiency will cause abnormal pentane gas excretion. More importantly the current technology is tedious and expensive. Nevertheless, expired pentane gas may become a useful tool for analysing vitamin E and other antioxidant status if the methodology can be simplified.

Finally, neurological evaluation of the patient, and possibly histological examination of nerve, muscle or other tissues, may be very useful in evaluating vitamin E status. The progressive nature of the clinical signs of vitamin E deficiency have been well described and may help determine if the deficiency has led to organ dysfunction[43]. The chronological development of these symptoms has been outlined, thus the presence or absence of signs of vitamin E deficiency may help confirm borderline biochemical studies, particularly if the child is older than 2 or 3 years. Characteristic, but not necessarily unique, histological and ultrastructural features of peripheral nerve and muscle are present in vitamin E deficiency[33]. Biopsies of these tissues are useful in the research setting, but are not practical for everyday patient care.

For routine evaluation of vitamin E status in cholestatic patients we employ the vitamin E:total lipid ratio, and obtain hydrogen peroxide haemolysis testing or adipose tissue biopsy levels of α-tocopherol if the vitamin E status is in question[50]. Children should be evaluated within the first few months of life if they have persisting cholestasis. Initially, standard oral forms of vitamin E (α-tocopherol, α-tocopheryl acetate, α-tocopheryl succinate) are administered in doses starting at approximately 10–25 IU/kg per day and increased up to 100–200 IU/kg per day (by 25–50 IU/kg per day increments) if there is no response in serum vitamin E:total lipid ratio within 3–4 weeks. The dose of vitamin E is given as a single morning dose at least 2 h after or before any bile acid binding resins, and preferably with breakfast when bile flow is maximal. If vitamin E status fails to normalize by 6–12 months, with the child receiving over 100 IU/kg per day of standard vitamin E forms, we have now begun treating them with a truly water-soluble form of the R–R–R form of vitamin E, D-α-tocopheryl polyethylene glycol-1000 succinate (TPGS) at a dose of 25 IU/kg per day[38]. Out of 60 children with chronic cholestasis failing to respond to large doses of standard forms of vitamin E in a multi-centre trial across the USA, all children responded to 15–30 IU/kg per day of TPGS without detectable side-effects[51].

Alternatively, intramuscular vitamin E can be administered using 0.5–1.0 IU/kg per day given as an intramuscular injection each 3–10 days, depending on the patient's weight[36]. The USA preparation from Hoffman-LaRoche is DL-α-tocopherol at a concentration of 50 mg/ml. The Hoffman-LaRoche Basel preparation is DL-α-tocopheryl acetate at 100 mg/ml. We have found it unnecessary to use these parenteral forms of vitamin E in cholestatic children since the advent of TPGS therapy. Whichever form of therapy is chosen, trough vitamin E levels and total serum lipid levels need to be monitored to avoid achieving excessive serum levels of vitamin E while keeping the vitamin E : total lipid ratio above 0.8 mg/g. Because up to 3–4% of the polyethylene glycol contained in TPGS may be absorbed[38], caution should be paid to the possibility of inducing a hyperosmolar state if the patient has a decreased glomerular filtration rate. Using this treatment protocol, neurological degeneration due to vitamin E deficiency can be completely prevented in children treated from infancy, reversed to normal in children who are treated before age 3–4 years, and improved to some extent in older children[51]. Unfortunately children with significant neurological handicaps show gradual but limited improvement, supporting the notion that vitamin E should be aggressively evaluated early in their course.

Several other reasons for treating vitamin E deficiency in this situation deserve mention. Children with end-stage liver disease, caused by biliary atresia, in several major liver centres have died while awaiting transplantation due to massive hepatic necrosis following an upper gastrointestinal haemorrhage or an episode of septic shock. We postulate that the ischaemia–reperfusion injury to the liver of these children was worsened by the presumed deficiency of vitamin E, a major antioxidant protecting against reperfusion injury[50]. In addition, data from our laboratory indicate that free-radical damage to the liver appears to be involved in the pathogenesis of chronic cholestatic liver injury in the rat, and that vitamin E deficiency combined with a diet containing over 30% calories as fat may exacerbate the cholestatic oxidant hepatic injury[52]. Finally, it is possible that copper, which accumulates during cholestasis, may drive the Haber–Weiss reaction towards producing hydroxyl free radicals from hydrogen peroxide, again requiring vitamin E to scavenge these free radicals and protect the liver from additional injury[53]. Finally, vitamin E deficiency may increase the oxidation of the high levels of circulating lipoproteins in cholestatic patients, potentiating atherosclerotic changes.

The proposed use of TPGS-vitamin E to solubilize and improve intestinal absorption of the other fat-soluble vitamins presents a potentially simple means of correcting fat-soluble vitamin deficiencies in children with chronic cholestasis using currently available oral preparations of the other fat-soluble vitamins. Further studies of the effect of co-administration of TPGS-vitamin E with vitamins A, D, and K, is indicated, to define doses of each of the other vitamins that may be adequate when administered in this manner.

SUMMARY

A substantial effort has been made over the past decade to characterize the metabolism of the fat-soluble vitamins in chronic childhood cholestasis to both improve the clinical care of affected children and to understand the pathophysiology of the vitamin deficiency states. Cholestatic liver disease is a unique cause of fat malabsorption in which standard indices to evaluate vitamin status may be inaccurate. Thus, specific approaches to define vitamin status have been developed and validated by vigorous clinical research. Using the treatment modalities outlined in this review, fat-soluble vitamin deficiency should be a manageable problem and not lead to significant morbidity in children with chronic cholestasis. The more subtle consequences of deficiency of each vitamin remain to be discovered.

Acknowledgements

This work was supported in part by USPHS grants (RR00069 and RR00123) from the General Clinical Research Centers Branch, Division of Research Resources, National Institutes of Health (NIH), NIH First Award (R29 DK38446), NIH Hepatobiliary Research Center (IP30 AM34914), March of Dimes, the Abby Bennett Liver Research Fund, and Eastman Chemical Products, Inc.

References

1. Olson JA. Vitamin A. In: Machlin LJ, ed. Handbook of vitamins–nutritional, biochemical and clinical aspects. New York: Marcel-Dekker; 1984:1–44.
2. Blomhoff R, Wake K. Perisinusoidal stellate cells of the liver: important roles in retinol metabolism and fibrosis. FASEB J. 1991;5:271–7.
3. Underwood BA. Effect of protein quantity and quality on plasma response to an oral dose of vitamin A as an indicator of hepatic vitamin A reserves in rats. J Nutr. 1980;110: 1635–40.
4. Willett WC, Polk BF, Underwood BA *et al.* Relation of serum vitamins A and E and carotenoids to the risk of cancer. N Engl J Med. 1984;310:430–4.
5. Amadee-Manesme O, Furr HO, Alvarez F, Hadchouel M, Alagille D, Olson JA. Biochemical indicators of vitamin A depletion in children with cholestasis. Hepatology. 1985;6:1143–8.
6. Mobarhan S, Russell RM, Underwood BA, Wallingford J, Mathieson RD, Al-Midani H. Evaluation of the relative dose response test for vitamin A nutriture in cirrhotics. Am J Clin Nutr. 1981;34:2264–70.
7. Zachman RD, Chen X. Intramuscular relative dose response (RDR) determination of liver vitamin A stores in rats. J Nutr. 1991;121:187–91.
8. Amadee-Manesme O, Mourey MS, Hanck A, Therasse J. Vitamin A relative dose response test: validation by intravenous injection in children with liver disease. Am J Clin Nutr. 1987;46:286–9.
9. Natadiastra G, Wittpenn JR, Muhilal, West KP, Mele L, Sommer A. Impression cytology: a practical index of vitamin A status. Am J Clin Nutr. 1988;48:695–701.
10. Scheffer C, Tseng G. Staging of conjunctival squamous metaplasia by impression cytology. J Ophthalmol. 1985;92:728–33.
11. Amadee-Manesme O, Luzeau R, Wittpenn JR, Hanck A, Sommer A. Impression cytology detects subclinical vitamin A deficiency. Am J Clin Nutr. 1988;47:875–88.
12. Gadomski AM, Kjolhede CL, Wittpenn J, Bulux J, Rosas AR, Forman MR. Conjunctival impression cytology (CIC) to detect subclinical vitamin A deficiency: comparison of CIC with biochemical assessments. Am J Clin Nutr. 1989;49:495–500.
13. Mourey MS, Siegenthaler G, Amadee-Manesme O. Regulation of metabolism of retinol-binding protein by vitamin A status in children with biliary atresia. Am J Clin Nutr.

1990;51:638–43.
14. Geubel AP, DeGalocsy C, Alves N, Rahier J, Dive C. Liver damage caused by therapeutic vitamin A administration: estimate of dose-related toxicity in 41 cases. Gastroenterology. 1991;100:1701–9.
15. Alagille D. Management of chronic cholestasis in childhood. Sem Liver Dis. 1985;5: 254–62.
16. Balistreri WF. Neonatal cholestasis. J Pediatr. 1985;106:171–84.
17. Sokol RJ, Johnson KE, Karrer FM, Narkewicz MR, Smith D, Kam I. Improvement of cyclosporin absorption in children after liver transplantation by means of water-soluble vitamin E. Lancet. 1991;338:212 15.
18. Argao EA, Heubi JE, Hollis BW. D-alpha-tocopheryl-polyethylene glycol-1000 succinate (TPGS) enhances absorption of vitamin D in infants and children with chronic cholestasis. Hepatology. 1990;12:886 (abstr.).
19. Norman AW, Miller BE. Vitamin D. In: Machlin LJ, ed. Handbook of vitamins–nutritional, biochemical and clinical aspects. New York: Marcel-Dekker; 1984:45–98.
20. Sitrin MD, Pollack KL, Bolt MJG, Rosenberg IH. Comparison of vitamin D and 25-hydroxyvitamin D absorption in the rat. Am J Physiol. 1982;242:G236–32.
21. Ornoy A, Goodwin D, Noff D, Edelstein S. 24,25-dihydroxyvitamin D is a metabolite of vitamin D essential for bone formation. Nature. 1978;276:517–19.
22. Heubi JE, Hollis BW, Specker B, Tsang RC. Bone disease in chronic childhood cholestasis. I. Vitamin D absorption and metabolism. Hepatology. 1989;9:258–64.
23. Skinner RK, Long RG, Sherlock S, Wills MR. 25-hydroxylation of vitamin D in primary biliary cirrhosis. Lancet. 1977;1:720–1.
24. Heubi JE, Hollis BW, Tsang RC. Bone disease in chronic childhood cholestasis. II. Better absorption of 25-OH vitamin D than vitamin D in extrahepatic biliary atresia. Pediatr Res. 1990;27:26–31.
25. Sitrin MD, Bengoa JM. Intestinal absorption of cholecalciferol and 25-hydroxycholecalciferol in chronic cholestatic liver disease. Am J Clin Nutr. 1987;46:1011–15.
26. Sokol RJ, Farrell MK, Heubi JE, Tsang RC, Balistreri WF. Comparison of vitamin E and 25-hydroxy vitamin D absorption during childhood cholestasis. J Pediatr. 1985;103: 712–17.
27. Bucuvalas JC, Heubi JE, Specker BL, Gregg DJ, Yergey AL, Vieira NE. Calcium absorption in bone disease associated with chronic cholestasis during childhood. Hepatology. 1990;12:1200–5.
28. Sokol RJ. Medical management of the infant or child with chronic liver disease. Sem Liver Dis. 1987;7:155–67.
29. Suttie JW. Vitamin K. In: Machlin LJ, ed. Handbook of vitamins–nutritional, biochemical and clinical aspects. New York: Marcel-Dekker; 1984:147–98.
30. Lane PA, Hathaway WE. Vitamin K in infancy. J. Pediatr. 1985;106:3:351–9.
31. Yanofsky RA, Jackson VG, Lilly JR, Stellin G, Klingensmith III WC, Hathaway WE. The multiple coagulopathies of biliary atresia. Am J Hematol. 1984;16:171–80.
32. Mirabelli F, Salis A, Perotti M, Taddei F, Bellomo G, Orrenius S. Alterations of surface morphology caused by the metabolism of menadione in mammalian cells are associated with the oxidation of critical sulfhydryl groups in cytoskeletal proteins. Biochem Pharmacol. 1988;37:18:3423–7.
33. Sokol RJ. Vitamin E deficiency and neurologic disease. Ann Rev Nutr. 1988;8:351–73.
34. Muller DPR, Lloyd JK, Bird AC. Long-term management of abetalipoproteinemia. Possible role for vitamin E. Arch Dis Child. 1977;52:209–14.
35. Sokol RJ, Heubi JE, Iannaccone S, Bove ST, Balistreri WF. Vitamin E deficiency with normal serum vitamin E concentrations in children with chronic cholestasis. N Engl J Med. 1984;310:1209–12.
36. Sokol RJ, Guggenheim MA, Iannaccone ST, Barkhaus PE, Miller C et al. Improved neurologic function following long-term correction of vitamin E deficiency in children with chronic cholestasis. N Engl J Med. 1985;313:1580 6.
37. Alvarez F, Landrieu P, Feo C et al. Vitamin E deficiency is responsible for neurologic abnormalities in cholestatic children. J Pediatr. 1985;107:422–5.
38. Sokol RJ, Heubi JE, Butler-Simon N et al. Treatment of vitamin E deficiency during chronic childhood cholestasis with oral d-alpha tocopheryl polyethylene glycol-1000 succinate.

Gastroenterology. 1987;93:975–85.
39. Sokol RJ, Butler-Simon N, Bettis D *et al.* Tocopheryl polyethylene glycol 1000 succinate therapy for vitamin E deficiency during chronic childhood cholestasis: neurologic outcome. J Pediatr. 1987;111:830–6.
40. Machlin LJ. Vitamin E. In: Machlin LJ, ed. Handbook of vitamins–nutritional, biochemical and clinical aspects. New York: Marcel-Dekker; 1984:99–146.
41. Traber MG, Olivercrona T, Kayden HJ. Bovine milk lipoprotein lipase transfers tocopherol to human fibroblasts during triglyceride hydrolysis *in vitro*. J Clin Invest. 1985;75:1729–34.
42. Traber MG, Kayden HJ. Vitamin E is delivered to cells via the high affinity receptor for low density lipoprotein. Am J Clin Nutr. 1984;40:747–51.
43. Sokol RJ, Farrell MK, Heubi JE, Tsang RC, Balistreri WF. Comparison of vitamin E and 25-hydroxy vitamin D absorption during childhood cholestasis. J Pediatr. 1983;103:712–17.
44. Horwitt MK, Harvey CC, Dahm Jr CH, Searcy MT. Relationship between tocopherol and serum lipid levels for determination of nutritional adequacy. Ann NY Acad Sci. 1972;203:223–36.
45. Sokol RJ, Heubi JE, Iannaccone S, Bove KE, Balistreri WF. Mechanism causing vitamin E deficiency in children with chronic cholestasis. Gastroenterology. 1983;85:1172–82.
46. Gordon HH, Nitowsky HM, Cornblath M. Studies of tocopherol deficiency in infants and children: I. Hemolysis of erythrocytes in hydrogen peroxide. Am J Dis Child. 1955;90:669–81.
47. Cynamon HA, Isenberg JN, Nguyen CH. Erythrocyte malondialdehyde release in vitro: a functional measure of vitamin E status. Clin Chim Acta. 1985;151:169–76.
48. Lemmonnier F, Cresteil D, Feneant M *et al.* Plasma lipid peroxides in cholestatic children. Acta Paediatr Scand. 1987;76:928–34.
49. Tappel AL, Dillard CJ. *In vivo* lipid peroxidation: measurement via exhaled pentane and protection by vitamin E. Fed Proc. 1981;40:174–8.
50. Sokol RJ. Vitamin E and neurologic deficits. Adv Pediatr. 1990;37:119–48.
51. Solol RJ, Butler-Simon N, Conner C, Heubi JE, Sinatra F, Heyman M, Ferrault J, Riely C, Suchy F, Levy J, Rothbaum R. Multicenter trial of d-alpha-tocopherol polyethylene glycol-1000 succinate (TPGS) therapy for vitamin E deficiency in chronic childhood cholestasis. Gastroenterology. 1991;100:A799 (abstr.).
52. Sokol RJ, Devereaux MW, Khandwala RA. Effect of dietary lipid and vitamin E on hepatic mitochondrial lipid peroxidation in the bile duct-ligated rat. J Lipid Res. 1991;32:1349–57.
53. Sokol RJ, Devereaux MW, Mireau G, Hambidge KM, Shikes RH. Oxidant injury to hepatic mitochondrial lipids in rats with dietary copper overload: modification by vitamin E deficiency. Gastroenterology. 1990;99:1061–71.

32
Colchicine treatment of paediatric chronic cholestatic liver disease

J. C. COLLINS, R. MORECKI, J. McPHILLIPS and L. M. GARTNER

INTRODUCTION

Colchicine is an antifibrogenic drug with possible efficacy in adults with cirrhosis[1,2]. Beginning in 1979 we offered colchicine in a double-blind, placebo-controlled, randomized trial to patients with chronic cholestatic liver disease beginning in infancy. Goals of this pilot trial were: (a) to determine if long-term colchicine was safe and tolerable; (b) to compare clinical course and outcome in patients who received drug or placebo.

METHODS

Patients eligible for the colchicine protocol were those with predicted chronic and progressive liver disease on the basis of diagnosis, clinical course and liver histology (Table 1). The study was approved by the Committee on Clinical Investigation of the Albert Einstein College of Medicine. All appropriate standard medical and surgical treatments were instituted and patients stabilized, to the extent possible, prior to obtaining informed consent for entry into the colchicine protocol.

Colchicine was given once daily by mouth (0.025 mg/kg) a regimen based on familial Mediterranean fever prophylaxis[3]. Older patients received 0.6 mg per day in tablet form. Placebo solution (quinine) and placebo tablets appeared and tasted like the drug.

Patients were examined monthly for three visits, then quarterly, with CBC, chemistry profile and urinalysis recorded. After 12 months and again after 5 years, repeat abdominal ultrasonogram, DISIDA scan, evaluation for varices (barium swallow or endoscopy as necessary) and, where possible, percutaneous liver biopsy were obtained.

Endpoints were hepatic transplantation or death. The study was also terminated if ursodeoxycholic acid (Actigall) was added to a patient's regimen. No patients have been lost to follow-up, and some continue receiving colchicine in an un-blinded fashion.

Table 1 Patient characteristics

Treatment	Diagnosis	Age	Sex	Pre-existing complications	Duration of treatment	Outcome
Group I						
Colchicine	1. α_1-Antitrypsin	3 months	M	—	12 months	Well
	2. Hepatic fibrosis	8 months	F	Portal hypertension	5 months	OLT
	3. Neonatal hepatitis	3 months	M	Hepatic failure	5 months	Died
	4. Neonatal hepatitis	1 month	M	Hepatic failure	3 months	Well
	Mean	4 months		Mean	6 months	
Placebo	1. Biliary atresia	2 months	F	Non-draining stoma	8 months	Died
	2. Choledochal cyst	7 months	M	—	4 months	Died
	3. Alagille syndrome	8 months	F	—	20 months	Died
	4. Choledochal cyst	3 months	F	—	8 months	Well
	Mean	5 months		Mean	10 months	
Group II						
Colchicine	1. Polycystic/fibrosis	8 years	M	Portal hypertension, severe	5 years	Unchanged
	2. Biliary atresia	7 years	F	Splenorenal shunt, splenectomy	10 years	Inactive for OLT, primary amenorrhoea
	3. Bile duct stenosis	18 years	M	Multiple surgery, splenectomy	8 years	Active for OLT
	4. α_1-Antitrypsin	23 years	F	Portacaval shunt	14 months	Died, primary amenorrhoea
	Mean	14 years		Mean	6.5 years	
Placebo	1. Biliary atresia	3 years	M	Sarcoid, portal hypertension, mild	10 years	OLT
	2. Neonatal hepatitis	7 years	F	—	9 years	OLT
	3. Biliary atresia	6 years	F	Portal hypertension, mild	8 years	Portal hypertension (severe); first degree amenorrhoea
	4. Intrahepatic hypoplasia	18 years	M	—	7 years	Portal hypertension (mild)
	5. Biliary atresia	3 years	F	—	3 years	OLT
	Mean	7 years		Mean	7.5 years	

OLT = orthotopic liver transplant

RESULTS

Nineteen patients enrolled in the colchicine trial; however, two patients were excluded from analysis for non-compliance or diarrhoea. The 17 patients who completed the protocol are described in Table 1. Although all had onset of liver disease in the neonatal period, they are retrospectively grouped into those entering protocol between 1 and 8 months of age (group I, eight patients) and those treated between ages 3 and 23 years (group II, nine patients).

Group I patients began colchicine or placebo at mean age 4 or 5 months (ranges 1–8 and 2–8 months, respectively), treatment continuing for a mean of 6 months (range 3–12 months) in the colchicine group and 10 months (range 4–20 months) in the placebo group. Group I patients randomized to placebo differed from the colchicine group in that three had surgically treatable disease (biliary atresia and choledochal cyst) causing neonatal cholestasis.

Two group I patients (one colchicine, one placebo) are well at least 6 years after stopping the drug. One, with severe neonatal hepatitis, has stabilized during colchicine treatment (3 months) and remains on therapy, now with added ursodeoxycholic acid. Three patients taking placebo died, while one receiving colchicine died and another underwent successful hepatic transplant.

Children in group II began colchicine or placebo at ages considerably removed from the initial insult to the liver (Table 1). Patients in the colchicine group averaged 14 years of age (range 7–23 years) while placebo patients averaged 7 years (range 3–18 years). Both groups contained patients treated for the full 10 years, with mean duration of treatment 6.5 and 7.5 years, and minimum treatment 14 months and 3 years, respectively. The two long-term placebo recipients (9 10 years) were transplanted shortly thereafter. One other placebo patient has been transplanted, while two have stable cirrhosis and portal hypertension. For both these patients portal hypertension developed or worsened during the period of observation. The outcome of colchicine-treated patients includes one death (hepatic failure and sepsis after 14 months on colchicine), one patient activated for transplant, one patient evaluated, but on the inactive list, for transplant, and patient IIC1, who has not deteriorated in the 5 years after terminating colchicine therapy.

DISCUSSION

Paediatric patients who participated in this pilot trial of colchicine, while diagnostically diverse, all had neonatal onset of chronic liver disease, which was characterized by (a) clinical severity, (b) anticipated or actual chronicity, and (c) hepatic fibrosis or cirrhosis. Only two are asymptomatic, one with AST twice normal, in 5–10-year follow-up, while nine of 19 (47%) have died or undergone successful orthotopic liver transplantation. Long-term colchicine treatment appeared safe. However, in this heterogeneous population colchicine did not appear to significantly prevent hepatic failure, prevent or resolve portal hypertension, or alter outcome. Based on this pilot study we recommend further study of colchicine to include a larger sample of patients strictly categorized by diagnosis and histology (inter-institutional collaborative trial), use of the drug in the early acute phase of neonatal cholestasis, and development of other potentially more powerful antifibrogenic drugs.

Acknowledgements

This work was supported by a grant from the Gail I. Zuckerman Foundation for Research in Chronic Liver Diseases of Children. We thank M. Abish, PharmD, and F. Ricz, PharmD, Weiler Hospital of the Albert Einstein College of Medicine, for their valuable assistance with the project.

References

1. Kershenobich D, Uribe M, Suarez GI *et al.* Treatment of cirrhosis with colchicine: a double-blind randomized trial. Gastroenterology. 1979;77:532–6.
2. Kershenobich D, Vargas F, Garcia-Tsao G *et al.* Colchicine in the treatment of cirrhosis of the liver. N Engl J Med. 1988;318:1709–13.
3. Sohar E, Gafni J, Pras M, Heller H. Familial Mediterranean fever: survey of 470 cases and review of the literature. Am J Med. 1967;43:227–52.

33
The impact of cholestatic liver disease on oral vitamin E loading tests in cystic fibrosis

B. M. WINKLHOFER-ROOB, D. H. SHMERLING, M. G. SCHIMEK and P. E. TUCHSCHMID

INTRODUCTION

Patients with chronic cholestatic liver disorders exhibit particularly severe vitamin E deficiency, leading to a progressive neuromuscular disease[1] that is probably caused by an inadequate delivery of tocopherol to the affected tissues[2]. Patients with cystic fibrosis (CF) are also frequently vitamin E-deficient[3], which is attributed to exocrine pancreatic insufficiency. There is a certain proportion of CF patients with a pathogenetically not yet fully eludicated cholestatic liver disease (CLD)[4,5], which may further contribute to the development of vitamin E deficiency in these patients.

Vitamin E most efficiently blocks free radical-mediated lipid peroxidation, thus playing a major role within the antioxidant protective system in biomembranes and lipoproteins[6,7]. In CF patients, free radical generation is likely to be enhanced due to chronic inflammatory processes in the lungs as well as in other tissues. Under these conditions it appears to be particularly deleterious that dietary vitamin E is less well absorbed in these patients. Consequently, therapeutic regimes focus on an efficient vitamin E supply. In this context it has attracted attention that vitamin E deficiency in patients with chronic cholestasis is difficult to correct orally[1].

All-rac-α-tocopheryl acetate is the usual commercially available and most frequently applied vitamin E preparation in central Europe, although it has been shown that the natural RRR-α-tocopherol form generally exhibits a higher bioavailability[2,8].

To our knowledge there are no data in the literature discriminating CF patients with and without CLD with regard to a response to single-dose vitamin E loading. We have previously studied the uptake of a high oral loading dose of all-rac-α-tocopheryl acetate in plasma and erythrocytes of CF patients over an observation period of 24h[9]. We focus here on the differences between CF patients with and without CLD, to answer the question if CF patients with CLD less efficiently respond to all-rac-α-tocopheryl acetate loading in a test situation with controlled exocrine pancreatic insufficiency compared with CF patients without CLD.

PATIENTS AND METHODS

Ten CF patients, aged 1.5–19.7 years (median 5.7 years), showing erythrocyte α-tocopherol values below the lower limit of normal (4.5 μmol/l) were enrolled in the study, as reported in ref. 9. Five had CLD, based on sonographic criteria and pathological biochemical findings (elevated γ-glutamyltransferase, alkaline phosphatase and/or total serum bile acids). The patient data upon inclusion in the study are listed in Table 1.

Vitamin E loading tests were performed as previously described in detail[9]. Briefly, after an overnight fast, plasma and erythrocyte α-tocopherol, as well as plasma lipids, were determined before, 1, 3, 6, 9, 12 and 24 h after an oral loading dose of 100 mg/kg body weight of all-rac-α-tocopheryl acetate (Ephynal[®], F. Hoffmann-La Roche & Co., Switzerland), given in milk together with pancreatic enzymes in amounts corresponding to individual requirements, established before study entry for correcting exocrine pancreatic insufficiency. The applied analytical and statistical methods have been recently reported[9].

RESULTS

Applying randomization tests, patients with CLD did not show significantly lower preloading plasma and erythrocyte α-tocopherol concentrations than patients without (NCLD) ($\alpha = 0.01$, one-sided). Peak plasma α-tocopherol concentrations and plasma α-tocopherol:cholesterol ratios were most frequently found at 6 h after the loading dose in patients with CLD and at 9 h in those without, whereas erythrocyte α-tocopherol most frequently peaked at 9 h in both groups.

In Fig. 1 the medians and regression curve estimates based on these medians for the erythrocyte α-tocopherol concentrations of group A, B and A combined with B (Σ) are displayed. Differences were observed both for the maximal values reached and the time elapsed between the application of the loading dose and saturation.

Randomization tests ($\alpha = 0.01$, one-sided) revealed significantly lower erythrocyte α-tocopherol for the 9 h and 24 h observations for patients with CLD compared with those without. Significantly lower plasma α-tocopherol concentrations were found with the same test ($\alpha = 0.01$, one-sided) for the CLD group at 9, 12 and 24 h.

DISCUSSION

The data presented demonstrate that CF patients with associated liver disease cannot be as efficiently supplied with oral all-rac-α-tocopheryl

Table 1 Patient data upon inclusion in the study

Patient no.	Age (years)	Sex	EC α-T (μmol/l)	P α-T (μmol/l)	P α-T : Chol (mmol/mol)	Chol (mmol/l)	GGT (μkat/l)	ALP (μkat/l)	BA (μmol/l)	Sonography
Patients with CLD										
1	20.7	F	1.5	7.43	1.81	4.1	3.12	22.21[a]	22.0	NS, PH, SM
2	16.3	F	4.1	17.65	5.19	3.4	0.35	12.46[a]	2.7	HM, GS, SM
3	13.8	M	< 1.0	8.59	2.53	3.4	0.27	16.52	7.3	HM, GS
4	13.1	F	3.5	11.84	2.42	4.9	2.09	31.26[a]	39.7	HM, NS, PH, SM
5	7.6	F	1.9	5.11	1.70	3.0	2.09 ·	20.37[a]	7.5	HM, NS, PH, SM
Patients without CLD										
6	5.8	F	2.1	9.75	2.79	3.5	0.48	12.22	7.0	normal
7	2.1	M	2.3	5.80	1.71	3.4	0.15	12.24	4.7	normal
8	2.2	M	< 1.5	8.13	2.03	4.0	< 0.02	13.88	5.5	normal
9	5.2	F	3.1	17.18	4.77	3.6	0.05	5.31	7.5	normal
10	1.5	M	1.7	5.57	2.53	2.2	0.12	12.96	5.6	normal
Normal			> 4.5[b]	> 20.00[c]	> 2.71 children, > 3.41 adults[d]	age dependent[b]	< 0.60[b]	age dependent[b]	< 10.0[b]	

[a]Elevated. [b]Normal values established by our laboratory. [c]for normal values see reference 9. [d]for normal values see reference 8. Abbreviations: EC = erythrocyte, P = plasma, α-T = α-tocopherol, Chol = cholesterol, GGT = γ-glutamyltransferase, ALP = alkaline phosphatase, BA = serum bile acids, NS = nodular structure, GS = granular structure, PH = portal hypertension, SM = splenomegaly, HM = hepatomegaly.

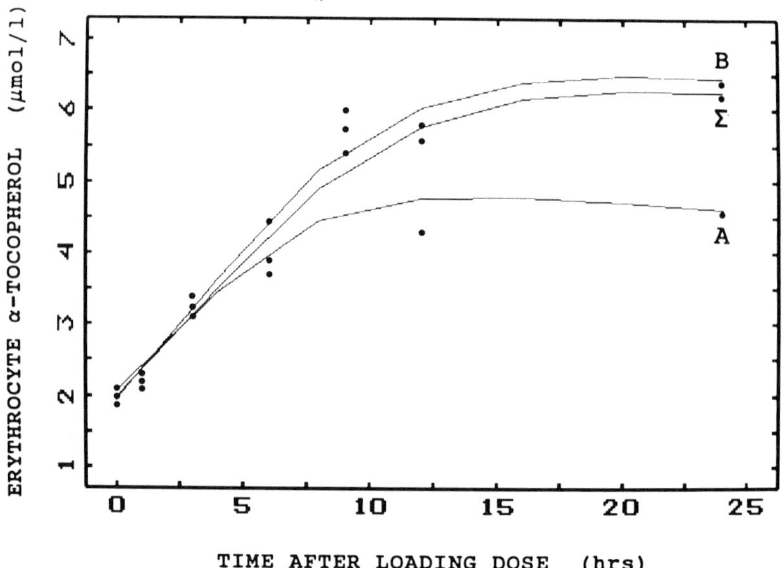

Figure 1 Erythrocyte α-tocopherol concentrations after administration: observations and curve estimates for the total sample (Σ) and the groups with CLD (**A**) and without CLD (**B**). (Obtained from ref. 9 with permission)

acetate as those without, even in a test situation with simultaneous administration of pancreatic enzymes in amounts sufficient to correct exocrine pancreatic insufficiency. This finding is consistent with impaired oral vitamin E absorption reported for patients with several chronic cholestatic disorders[10-12]. However, it should be pointed out that CLD in CF patients represents a distinct type of liver disease[4,5] with a substantial proportion of patients presenting with less severe cholestasis[13,14], as suggested by only slightly elevated liver enzymes. Table 1 demonstrates that this phenomenon was also evident in the present study.

Sokol et al.[10] performed oral vitamin E tolerance tests in three patient groups (vitamin E-deficient cholestatic subjects [group A], vitamin E-sufficient cholestatic controls [group B], and vitamin E-sufficient non-cholestatic controls [group C]), and demonstrated the best results for group B, followed by group C. Group A showed practically no response to oral 100 mg/kg body weight of emulsified all-rac-α-tocopheryl acetate. However, in group A all six patients exhibited steatorrhoea, in group C two of five patients, yet none of group B. Consequently, it is difficult to conclude from these results whether fat malabsorption, caused by bile acid deficiency due to cholestasis, might have been the most important or unique determinant of vitamin E malabsorption. Yet individual patients with CLD from the same study showed smaller areas under the curve (AUC) (CLD 11.25 vs. NCLD 693.96 μg/ml per hour, CLD 51.60 vs. NCLD 428.13 μg/ml per hour), compared with those without CLD with similar coefficients of fat excretion (CLD 22.4 vs. NCLD 20.6%, CLD 28.8 vs. NCLD 26.8%), strongly suggesting that CLD itself influences the test results. This is consistent with our findings of a less efficient vitamin E loading of CF patients with CLD.

In another study on adults with primary biliary cirrhosis (PBC) the AUC was inversely correlated with PBC stage and with markers of cholestasis[11]. Another group found significantly lower AUC, peak values, and maximal rise in vitamin E levels for patients with PBC compared with controls, yet no correlation between standard biochemical liver tests, fasting serum cholylglycine and vitamin E levels[12].

Oral vitamin E absorption tests in CF patients have been reported by Skopnik et al.[15,16]. They applied 100 mg/kg α-tocopheryl acetate orally, yet it is not specified whether an all-rac or RRR-form had been used. Patients were assigned according to their weight percentiles to group I ($<$ 10 p), group II (10–50 p) or group III ($>$ 50 p)[15]. The AUC was found to be highest for group III and lowest for group I. Patients with liver disease were included in all three groups: 5/10 (group I), 2/5 (group II) and 1/4 (group III) had elevated fasting cholylglycine concentrations and two patients of group II had markedly elevated liver enzymes. Because the influence of CLD was not further analysed, one might argue from these data that CLD could have contributed to the differences between the three groups. The same authors demonstrated improved responses to oral vitamin E loading after taurine supplementation in CF patients, three with and eight without CLD[16], yet they did not analyse the CLD patients separately in this investigation either.

In our study, however, the differences between CLD and NCLD patients were restricted to the 9 h to 24 h observations. This may indicate a different handling of vitamin E after the initial intestinal absorption phase, cither with respect to the delivery of vitamin E from the liver into nascent very low-density lipoproteins (VLDL)[17] or to the exchange between the lipoprotein classes and the tissues.

Data concerning the biokinetics and bioavailability of all-rac-α-tocopheryl acetate, the preparation used in our loading tests, are now available from stable isotope studies in addition to data from high-dose vitamin E loading tests. Horwitt et al.[18] studied plasma α-tocopherol concentrations in normal humans after large oral doses of both RRR-α-tocopherol and RRR-α-tocopheryl acetate and found only insignificantly higher concentrations for RRR-α-tocopherol in the presence of large interindividual variations. Burton et al.[19] observed no differences between d3-RRR-α-tocopherol compared with d6-RRR-α-tocopheryl acetate in a competitive uptake study, using deuterated α-tocopherol in adult humans, i.e. both were equally well absorbed and transported into the plasma. Nevertheless, CF patients may less efficiently hydrolyse the ester bond of the acetate form in the intestinal lumen because of a lack of esterases due to exocrine pancreatic insufficiency.

An investigational RRR-α-tocopheryl polyethylene glycol 1000 succinate preparation proved to provide a better response to oral vitamin E supplementation than all-rac-α-tocopherol or all-rac-α-tocopheryl acetate in patients with severe chronic cholestasis[20]. The addition of polyethylene glycol appears to enable patients with compromised bile secretion to absorb the RRR-α-tocopherol form more efficiently and to allow a prolonged α-tocopherol loading effect. Because an unesterified RRR-α-tocopherol preparation was not included in this study, it remains to be determined whether the RRR-form in the polyethylene glycol preparation could have been contributing to the remarkably better response.

Competitive uptake studies of a single dose of a 1:1 mixture of d3-SRR-α-tocopheryl acetate and d6-RRR-α-tocopheryl acetate in humans showed at 9 h the latter preferentially incorporated in the VLDL, LDL, and HDL fractions[17]. During the post-absorption phase the ratio of deuterated/total tocopherol concentration in VLDL dropped twice as fast for d3-SRR-α-tocopherol as for d6-RRR-α-tocopherol. The authors conclude that the two forms of tocopherol are not different during intestinal absorption, but during hepatic secretion of α-tocopherol in VLDL. This is known to represent the mechanism of delivery of α-tocopherol into lipoproteins[21], thereby providing for the maintenance of plasma α-tocopherol concentrations. In addition, patients with familial isolated vitamin E deficiency showed no differences in the plasma concentrations of d6-RRR-α-tocopheryl acetate during the first 12 h after a test dose compared with controls, yet significantly lower concentrations in VLDL of the patients at 24 h[22]. The decline of d6-RRR-α-tocopherol in the plasma of patients was significantly faster compared with that of controls. Traber and co-workers suggest that the secretion of α-tocopherol in VLDL is impaired because of a lack of, or a defect in, the liver tocopherol transfer protein.

It may be speculated that there could be an analogy for CF patients with CLD, who may exhibit a compromised delivery of all-rac-α-tocopherol to VLDL, attributable to mechanisms related to their liver disease. If so, this could explain the differences between CF patients with and without CLD found in this study. Studies with deuterated tocopherol preparations are required to further elucidate this peculiarity.

In conclusion, the data presented show that under controlled exocrine pancreatic insufficiency plasma and erythrocytes of CF patients with CLD cannot be loaded as efficiently with α-tocopheryl acetate as those of patients without CLD. Differences become obvious at 9 h and the following observations, possibly indicating a less efficient delivery of all-rac-α-tocopherol from the liver in VLDL of CF patients with CLD or, otherwise, a different equilibration pattern between plasma and the tissues, which might be attributable, for example, to increased consumption of vitamin E in patients with CLD.

Acknowledgements

We acknowledge the skilful cooperation of Mr H. Frischknecht in performing erythrocyte α-tocopherol determinations, and thank the Laboratories of F. Hoffmann-La Roche AG, Basle, for the plasma α-tocopherol determinations. This study was supported by the Fonds zur Foerderung der wissenschaftlichen Forschung, Vienna, Austria (Erwin-Schroedinger Research Grant J0378 and J0511 of BMWR), the Roche Research Foundation, Basle, Switzerland and the KaliChemie AG, Berne, Switzerland.

References

1. Guggenheim MA, Ringel SP, Silverman A, Grabert BE. Progressive neuromuscular disease in children with chronic cholestasis and vitamin E deficiency: diagnosis and treatment with alpha tocopherol. J Pediatr. 1982;100:51–8.
2. Burton GW, Traber MG. Vitamin E: antioxidant activity, biokinetics, and bioavailability. Annu Rev Nutr. 1990;10:357–82.
3. Sokol RJ, Reardon MC, Accurso FJ, Stall C, Narkewicz M, Abman SH, Hammond KB. Fat-soluble vitamin status during the first year of life in infants with cystic fibrosis identified by screening of newborns. Am J Clin Nutr. 1989;50:1064–71.
4. Di Sant'Agnese PA, Blanc WA. A distinctive type of biliary cirrhosis of the liver associated with cystic fibrosis of the pancreas: recognition through signs of portal hypertension. Pediatrics. 1956;18:387–409.
5. Hultcrantz R, Mengarelli S, Strandvik B. Morphological findings in the liver of children with cystic fibrosis: a light and electron microscopical study. Hepatology. 1986;6:881–9.
6. Esterbauer H, Dieber-Rotheneder M, Striegl G, Waeg G. Role of vitamin E in preventing the oxidation of low-density lipoprotein. Am J Clin Nutr. 1991;53:314S–21S.
7. Burton GW, Ingold KU. Vitamin E as an in vitro and in vivo antioxidant. Ann NY Acad Sci. 1989;570:7–22.
8. Horwitt MK. Relative biological values of d-α-tocopheryl acetate and all-rac-α-tocopheryl acetate in man. Am J Clin Nutr. 1980;33:1856–60.
9. Winklhofer-Roob BM, Shmerling DH, Schimek MG, Tuchschmid PE. Short-term changes in erythrocyte α-tocopherol content of vitamin E-deficient patients with cystic fibrosis. Am J Clin Nutr. 1992;55:100–3.
10. Sokol RJ, Heubi JE, Iannaccone S, Bove KE, Balistreri WF. Mechanism causing vitamin E deficiency during chronic childhood cholestasis. Gastroenterology. 1983;85:1172–82.
11. Sokol RJ, Kim YS, Hoofnagle JH, Heubi JE, Jones EA, Balistreri WF. Intestinal malabsorption of vitamin E in primary biliary cirrhosis. Gastroenterology. 1989;96:479–86.
12. Munoz SJ, Heubi JE, Balistreri WF, Maddrey WC. Vitamin E deficiency in primary biliary cirrhosis: Gastrointestinal malabsorption, frequency and relationship to other lipid-soluble vitamins. Hepatology. 1989;9:525–31.
13. Feigelson J, Pecau Y, Cathelineau L, Navarro J. Additional data on hepatic function tests in cystic fibrosis. Acta Paediatr Scand. 1975;64:337–44.
14. Schwarz HP, Kraemer R, Thurnheer U, Rossi E. Liver involvement in cystic fibrosis. Helv Paediatr Acta. 1978;33:351–64.
15. Skopnik H, Karl M, Kusenbach G, Bergt U, Geron M, Heimann G. Einfluss des Ernährungsstatus auf die Absorptionskinetik von Vitamin E bei Mukoviszidose (CF). Klin Paediatr. 1990;202:43–9.
16. Skopnik H, Kusenbach G, Bergt U, Friedrichs F, Stuhlsatz H, Döhmen H, Heimann G. Taurin-Supplementierung bei cystischer Fibrose (CF): Einfluss auf die Absorptionskinetik von Vitamin E. Klin Paediatr. 1991;203:28–32.
17. Traber MG, Burton GW, Ingold KU, Kayden HJ. RRR- and SRR-α-tocopherols are secreted without discrimination in human chylomicrons, but RRR-α-tocopherol is preferentially secreted in very low density lipoproteins. J Lipid Res. 1990;31:675–85.
18. Horwitt MK, Elliott WH, Kanjananggulpan P, Fitch CD. Serum concentrations of α-tocopherol after ingestion of various vitamin E preparations. Am J Clin Nutr. 1984;40:240–5.
19. Burton GW, Ingold KU, Foster DO et al. Comparison of free α-tocopherol and α-tocopheryl acetate as sources of vitamin E in rats and humans. Lipids. 1988;23:834–40.
20. Sokol RJ, Heubi JE, Butler-Simon N, McClung HJ, Lilly JR, Silverman A. Treatment of vitamin E deficiency during chronic childhood cholestasis with oral d-α-tocopheryl polyethylene glycol-1000 succinate. Gastroenterology. 1987;93:975–85.
21. Cohn W, Loechleitner F, Weber F. α-Tocopherol is secreted from rat liver in very low density lipoproteins. J Lipid Res. 1988;29:1359–66.
22. Traber MG, Sokol RJ, Burton GW et al. Impaired ability of patients with familial isolated vitamin E deficiency to incorporate α-tocopherol into lipoproteins secreted by the liver. J Clin Invest. 1990;85:397–407.

Section 6
Treatment of Cholestatic Disorders:

2: Ursodeoxycholate

34
Mechanisms of hepatoprotection by ursodeoxycholic acid

R. POUPON, Y. CALMUS and R. E. POUPON

INTRODUCTION

Although an increasing body of data suggests that ursodeoxycholic acid (UDCA) has therapeutically beneficial effects in a number of chronic cholestatic disorders, data from controlled trials are so far available only for patients with primary biliary cirrhosis (PBC). In PBC, continuous administration of UDCA improves clinical, biochemical and immune parameters and most of the histological features of the disease, and significantly reduces the incidence of clinical events considered to be indicators of entry to the terminal phase[1-3].

RATIONALE FOR THE USE OF UDCA IN CHOLESTATIC DISORDERS

The drugs which have so far been evaluated in controlled trials for the medical therapy of PBC or sclerosing cholangitis have been used for their immunosuppressive or anti-inflammatory properties to decrease portal inflammation and thus to limit bile duct destruction.

In contrast, when we proposed UDCA as a novel therapeutic approach to these chronic cholestatic disorders[1] the rationale was based on the following arguments. In chronic biliary obstruction bile acids (BA) accumulate in the liver[4,5]; in our experience chenodeoxycholic acid (CDCA) and cholic acid (CA) concentrations average 500–600 nmol/g of liver in end-stage PBC or sclerosing cholangitis.

Endogenous human BA are hepatotoxic. Since the pioneering work of Holsti[6], we have learned that primary and secondary human BA are potentially cytotoxic and cholestatic. These deleterious properties are apparently influenced by three major determinants: (a) the chemical structure and the degree of hydrophobicity of the BA, as quantified by reversed-phase HPLC; (b) the nature of the cells or tissue exposed to the BA and (c) the

"

concentration–time product in or around the cells or tissue. In contrast, UDCA is a hydrophilic, non-hepatotoxic bile acid both *in vitro* and in humans. However, in some species, UDCA administered chronically can induce ductular proliferation and hepatic fibrosis. In this setting lithocholate, the major bacterial metabolite of UDCA and CDCA, accumulates in the enterohepatic circulation[7]. Because hepatotoxicity is correlated with the degree of accumulation of lithocholate in the enterohepatic circulation, and because lithocholate is hepatotoxic, it is accepted as the agent responsible for the hepatotoxicity of UDCA. Humans detoxify and rapidly excrete lithocholate[8], which does not therefore accumulate in bile; hepatotoxicity has never been reported.

In some experimental models, UDCA can prevent both cholestasis and cell damage induced by biliary obstruction or BA administration. This was first clearly demonstrated by Kitani *et al.*[9], who found that in rats with chronic bile fistulae, simultaneous intravenous administration of UDCA to animals receiving high doses of taurocholate preserved bile flow and hepatocellular viability. Similar findings have been confirmed recently with co-infusion of tauro-UDCA and CDCA[10,11] and tauro-CDCA and lithocholate[12].

In the light of these data, we postulated that changes in the concentrations and composition of the BA perfusing the liver might be beneficial in patients with chronic cholestatic disorders. To test the hypothesis, we designed an open pilot study in an exemplary, slowly progressive cholestatic disorder, PBC. Major improvements occurred during the continuous administration of UDCA, 13–15 mg/kg per day, given twice daily for 2 years[1]. These findings were confirmed and extended by a subsequent controlled double-blind trial[2,3].

MECHANISMS OF ACTION OF UDCA

Three basic mechanisms might account for the beneficial effects of UDCA: (a) an effect on the enterohepatic circulation of endogenous BA; (b) a cytoprotective effect towards hepatocytes and, more precisely, an inhibition of BA-induced hepatocyte injury; (c) an effect on the immune system.

EFFECT OF UDCA ON THE ENTEROHEPATIC CIRCULATION OF ENDOGENOUS BA

Continuous administration of UDCA (13–15 mg/kg per day, twice daily) induces marked changes in plasma BA composition and distribution in PBC[13-15]. Whatever the histological stage of the disease, UDCA – mostly glyco-UDCA – becomes the major circulating BA. The levels and proportions of CA and CDCA, the two major BA in the serum and liver tissue of these patients, decreased markedly. Atypical BA, such as 3β-monohydroxyl $\Delta 5$-cholenoic acid, also decreased significantly. In contrast, the total proportion of secondary BA did not change significantly. During UDCA therapy liver cells are thus exposed on the one hand to UDCA and, on the other hand, to reduced concentrations of primary BA.

Two mechanisms might explain the reduced levels of CA and CDCA, i.e. an effect on active intestinal reabsorption and/or an effect on the intrinsic hepatic clearance of these two BA.

Active ileal absorption is the major mechanism of BA pool conservation. *In vitro* and *in vivo* experimental studies have revealed mutual inhibition of this active intestinal transport between pairs of BA[16]. To test the hypothesis that UDCA might promote intestinal excretion of primary BA by inhibiting the active ileal transport of endogenous BA conjugates, we used the SeHCAT test (tauro23[^{75}Se] Selena-25 homotaurocholic acid), a structural analogue of taurocholate which is not deconjugated by bacteria and which is highly sensitive and specific in the investigation of active ileal absorption of BA). During UDCA administration the percentage of retention of [^{75}Se]HCAT fell significantly from $45.9 \pm 6.8\%$ to $20.5 \pm 5.7\%$ ($p < 0.01$), while no change occurred during placebo administration[17]. Similar results have been obtained by Stiehl *et al.*[18] in patients with ileostomies, who served as a model to investigate the effects of UDCA and CDCA on the ileal excretion of primary BA.

A second mechanism by which UDCA influences the enterohepatic circulation of BA is through an increase in the intrinsic ability of hepatocytes to excrete BA. Kitani and Kanai[19] have shown that UDCA clearly affects excretion of other BA by hepatocytes in a situation mimicking cholestasis – i.e. an increased load of BA in liver cells. When taurocholate was infused simultaneously with UDCA to rats, not only was the cholestasis caused by excess taurocholate prevented, but canalicular excretion of both taurocholate and total BA was higher. The exact mechanism of this effect is not known. It has been generally assumed that it was related to a cytoprotective effect of UDCA on hepatocytes. One alternative is that UDCA, a BA with very high intrinsic hepatic clearance[20], might increase the vectorial transport of BA by facilitating intracellular or canalicular flux, thereby decreasing their concentration, and thus the toxicity of these BA.

CYTOPROTECTIVE EFFECT OF UDCA

UDCA lacks the membrane and metabolic toxicity seen with other BA and might also counteract the deleterious properties of hydrophobic BA. CDCA caused enzyme release and urea synthesis inhibition above $500\,\mu mol/l$, whereas UDCA has no significant toxicity in terms of enzyme release up to $1500\,\mu mol/l$[21]. Leuschner *et al.* evaluated the effect of bile salts on red blood cell membranes *in vitro*[22]. Electron spin resonance values of the erythrocyte membranes were unchanged by exposure to $20\,mmol/l$ of UDCA or its taurine conjugate. In contrast, CDCA and, to a lesser extent, its conjugates significantly increased electron spin resonance (an effect abolished in the presence of $2\,mmol/l$ of UDCA). Using primary cultures of human hepatocytes, Galle and co-workers have also shown that UDCA slightly reduces the hepatotoxic effect of glyco-CDCA, suggesting that UDCA can have a hepatoprotective effect by itself[23].

We have also used human hepatocytes in primary culture to investigate the cytoprotective properties of UDCA. In this model CDCA, but not UDCA or tauro-UDCA, induced in a dose-dependent manner the release of LDH, and reduced protein synthesis. However, the cytotoxic effect of CDCA was not reversed when incubated with equimolar concentration of UDCA or tauro-UDCA. A possible explanation for such discrepancies includes, at least in part, marked differences in experimental design, particularly with regard to the test concentrations and the contact time between the cells or membranes and BA. So the relevance of *in vitro* conditions to the *in vivo* situation may be questionable and, in our opinion, it is not clearly established that UDCA *per se* is cytoprotective.

EFFECT OF UDCA ON THE IMMUNE SYSTEM

Unexpectedly our controlled trial showed that some of the immune markers of PBC improved during UDCA treatment. This finding suggests that BA and/or UDCA interfere with immune regulation in this disease. HLA molecules, particularly class I, are the main targets of the cytotoxic reaction. In the liver, HLA expression is normally limited and hepatocytes do not express HLA molecules. In contrast, abnormal expression of class I molecules on hepatocytes is a salient feature of PBC. A first study was undertaken to evaluate the effects of UDCA therapy on this expression[24]. Twelve untreated patients with PBC were compared to eight patients treated for at least a year with 13–15 mg/kg per day of UDCA, and eight control patients without hepatobiliary disease. MHC expression was studied using an immunofluorescence technique. No class I molecules were expressed on hepatocytes from control subjects, contrasting with strong expression on hepatocytes from untreated PBC patients. UDCA treatment induced a dramatic reduction in HLA class I expression. Similarly, no class II molecules were expressed in bile ducts of controls, but there was a strong class II expression in bile ducts of PBC patients, with no significant difference in expression between treated and untreated patients. These results suggest that cholestasis itself can induce aberrant expression of MHC class I molecules on hepatocytes. The beneficial effect of UDCA on this expression could result from an improvement in cholestasis or a direct effect of UDCA on hepatocytes.

To further investigate the role of BA in HLA overexpression on hepatocytes, we used human hepatocytes in primary culture. Normal human hepatocytes were isolated from five patients undergoing surgical liver resection, by two-step collagenase perfusion. Hepatocytes were placed in medium containing the following: (a) CDCA (a model of endogenous bile acids), 100–150 μmol/l; (b) UDCA 100–500 μmol/l; (c) tauroursodeoxycholic acid (tauro-UDCA) 100–500 μmol/l; (d) CDCA 100 μmol/l and UDCA 100 μmol/l; (e) CDCA 100 μmol/l and tauro-UDCA 100 μmol/l. After 4 days of culture in the presence of the bile acids the monolayer of flattened hepatocytes was incubated in EDTA to detach the cells. Cytofluorimetric analysis was performed using monoclonal anti-class I or anti-class II antibodies. MHC class I expression was found on 25% of control hepatocytes. CDCA induced overexpression of class I MHC molecules, which was dose-dependent for concentrations ranging from 100 to 500 μmol/l. In contrast, UDCA and tauro-UDCA had no significant effect. CDCA, UDCA and tauro-UDCA had no effect on hepatocyte MHC class II expression, which did not exceed 10% of cells. Furthermore, the addition of UDCA (100 μmol/l) or tauro-UDCA (100 μmol/l) to CDCA (100 μmol/l) suppresses overexpression of HLA class I on human hepatocytes[25].

These results suggest that the reduction in hepatocyte MHC class I antigen expression induced by UDCA could block periportal and lobular cell necrosis by suppressing the cytotoxic T cell target and thus slow the progression of PBC.

CONCLUSIONS

UDCA inhibits, at least in part, the biological and toxic effects of the endogenous BA, firstly by reducing their concentrations in and around the liver cells and secondly because UDCA itself is devoid of any toxicity and behaves virtually as a neutral BA. This probably accounts for the therapeutic effects of UDCA in chronic cholestatic disease.

References

1. Poupon R, Chrétien Y, Poupon RE, Ballet F, Calmus Y, Darnis F. Is ursodeoxycholic acid an effective treatment for primary biliary cirrhosis? Lancet. 1987;1:834–6.
2. Poupon RE, Eschwege E, Poupon R and the UDCA-PBC Study Group. Ursodeoxycholic acid for the treatment of primary biliary cirrhosis. Interim analysis. J Hepatol. 1990;11;16–21.
3. Poupon RE, Balkau B, Eschwege E, Poupon R. A multicenter controlled trial of ursodiol for the treatment of primary biliary cirrhosis. N Engl J Med. 1991;324:1548–54.
4. Akashi Y, Miyazaki H, Yanagisawa J, Nakayama F. Bile acid metabolism in cirrhotic liver tissue-altered synthesis and impaired hepatic secretion. Clin Chim Acta. 1987;168:199–206.
5. Greim H, Czygan P, Schaffner F, Popper H. Determination of bile acids in needle biopsies of human liver. Biochem Med. 1973;8:280–6.
6. Holsti P. Experimental cirrhosis of the liver in rabbits induced by gastric instillation of dessicated whole bile. Acta Pathol Microbiol Scand. 1956;112:1–67.
7. Cohen BI, Hofmann AF, Mosbach EH, Stenger RJ, Rothschild MA, Hagey LR, Bum Yoon Y. Differing effects of nor-ursodeoxycholic or ursodeoxycholic acid on hepatic histology and bile acid metabolism in the rabbit. Gastroenterology. 1986;91:189–97.
8. Cowen AC, Korman MG, Hofmann AF, Cass OW, Coffin SB. Metabolism of lithocholate in healthy man. Gastroenterology. 1975;69:62–76.
9. Kitani K, Kanai S. Tauroursodeoxycholate prevents taurocholate induced cholestasis. Life Sci. 1982;30:515–23.
10. Schmucker DL, Ohta M, Kanai S, Sato Y, Kitani K. Hepatic injury induced by bile salts: correlation between biochemical and morphological events. Hepatology. 1990;12:1216–21.
11. Heuman DM, Mills AS, McCall J, Hylemon PB, Pandak WM, Vlahcevic ZR. Conjugates of ursodeoxycholate protect against cholestasis and hepatocellular necrosis caused by more hydrophobic bile salts. Gastroenterology. 1991;100:203–11.
12. Schölmerich J, Baumgartner U, Miyai K, Gerok W. Tauroursodeoxycholate prevents taurolithocholate-induced cholestasis and toxicity in rat liver. J Hepatol. 1990;10:280–3.
13. Chrétien Y, Poupon R, Gherardt MF, Chazouillères O, Labbé D, Myara A, Trivin F. Bile

acid glycine and taurine conjugates in serum of patients with primary biliary cirrhosis: effect of ursodeoxycholic treatment. Gut. 1989;30:1110–15.

14. Poupon RE, Chrétien Y, Paumgartner G, Poupon R and the UDCA-PBC Study Group. Serum bile acid levels and distribution in primary biliary cirrhosis (PBC): effect of ursodeoxycholic acid (UDCA) therapy. Gastroenterology. 1991;100:786 (abstr.).

15. Stiehl A, Rudolph G, Raedsch R, Moller B, Hopf U, Lotterer E, Bircher J, Fölsch U, Klaus J, Endele R, Senn M. Ursodeoxycholic acid-induced changes of plasma and urinary bile acids in patients with primary biliary cirrhosis. Hepatology. 1990;12:492–7.

16. Wilson FA. Intestinal transport of bile acids. Am J Physiol. 1981;241:G83–92.

17. Marteau P, Chazouillères O, Myara A, Jian R, Rambaud JC, Poupon R. Effect of chronic administration of ursodeoxycholic acid on the ileal absorption of endogenous bile acids in man. Hepatology. 1990;12:1206–8.

18. Stiehl A, Raedsch R, Rudolph G. Acute effects of ursodeoxycholic and chenodeoxycholic acid on the small intestinal absorption of bile acids. Gastroenterology. 1990;98:424–8.

19. Kitani K, Kanai S. Interactions between different bile salts in the biliary excretion of the rat. Chem Pathol. Pharmacol. 1983;39:139–52.

20. Poupon R, Chrétien Y, Parquet M, Rey C, Ballet F, Infante R. Hepatic transport of bile acids in the isolated perfused rat liver: structure–kinetics relationship. Biochem Pharmacol. 1988;37:207–12.

21. Schölmerich J, Becher MS, Schmidt K *et al.* Influence of hydroxylation and conjugation of bile salts of their membrane-damaging properties: studies on isolated hepatocytes and lipid membrane vesicles. Hepatology. 1984;4:661–6.

22. Leuschner U, Fischer H, Kurtz W, Güldütuna S, Hübner K, Hellstern A, Gatzen M, Leuschner M. Ursodeoxycholic acid in primary biliary cirrhosis: results of a controlled double-blind trial. Gastroenterology. 1989;97:1268–74.

23. Galle PR, Theilmann L, Raedsch R, Otto G, Stiehl A. Ursodeoxycholate reduces hepatotoxicity of bile salts in primary human hepatocytes. Hepatology. 1990;12:486–91.

24. Calmus Y, Gane P, Rouger P, Poupon R. Hepatic expression of class I and class II major histocompatibility complex molecules in primary biliary cirrhosis: effect of ursodeoxycholic acid. Hepatology. 1990;11:12–15.

25. Hillaire S, Calmus Y, Boucher E, Gane P, Ballet F, Franco D, Houssin D, Poupon R. Bile acids modulate hepatocyte HLA class I expression in human hepatocytes by a transcriptional mechanism. Hepatology. 1991;14:99 (abstr.).

35
Metabolism of ursodeoxycholic acid

G. PAUMGARTNER, U. BEUERS, M. NEUBRAND, U. SPENGLER and S. FISCHER

INTRODUCTION

For many years ursodeoxycholic acid (UDCA) has been established as an efficacious and safe agent for dissolution of cholesterol gallstones. It is now increasingly used in the treatment of certain cholestatic liver diseases[1]. Recent studies suggest that UDCA counteracts the hepatotoxic effects of more hydrophobic bile acids such as taurochenodeoxycholic acid (TCDCA) and taurodeoxycholic acid (TDCA) by a direct effect on the liver[2,3]. One of its main advantages is that it is safe, well tolerated and virtually free from side-effects.

UDCA differs in its pharmacokinetics and metabolism from most other drugs. It is an enterohepatic drug that occurs naturally in small quantities in human bile. It is formed by epimerization of the primary bile acid chenodeoxycholic acid (CDCA) through the action of intestinal bacteria. A large amount of data is available on the kinetics and the metabolism of UDCA in patients with normal liver function. Less is known about the metabolism of UDCA in patients with liver disease.

ABSORPTION OF UDCA

UDCA is absorbed from the intestine mainly by non-ionic passive diffusion[4]. The unconjugated, protonated acid is poorly soluble in water. Before absorption from the intestine can occur it must be brought into molecular or micellar solution. Its solubility is very poor below pH 8 and improves markedly when the pH is raised above 8. Above pH 8 the concentration of the ionized species increases so that the critical micellar concentration is reached. Once micelles are formed, the entire crystalline dispersion can change to a micellar solution provided that sufficient excess of base is available. This process can be accelerated by micelles of endogenous bile acids in bile. Lack of endogenous bile acid micelles may lead to differences in UDCA absorption between patients with liver disease and healthy subjects.

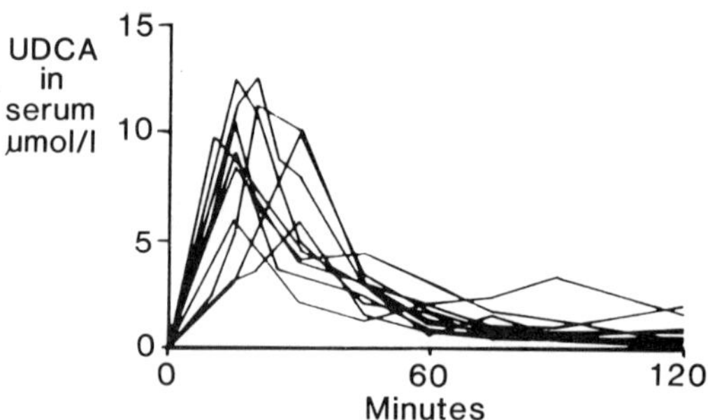

Fig. 1 Concentration of unconjugated UDCA in serum following oral administration of 1.5 mg/kg of UDCA in 10 healthy subjects; 1.5 mg UDCA was dissolved in 1 ml of a solution containing 15 mg of bicarbonate per ml. The volume was adjusted to 200 ml with tap water[5]

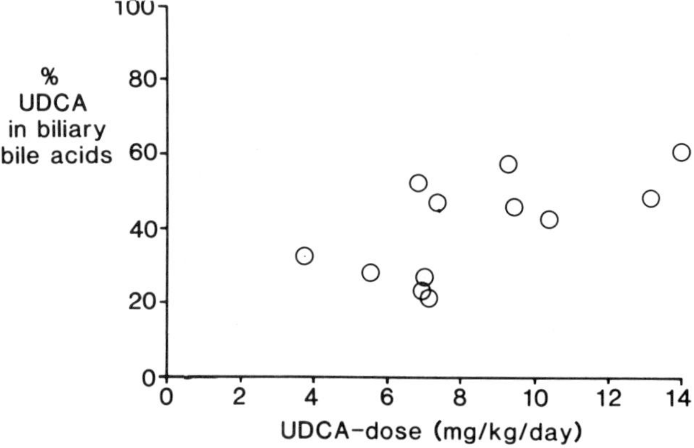

Fig. 2 Enrichment of biliary bile acids with UDCA in relation to the dose of UDCA in patients with gallstone[7]

When a single dose of UDCA dissolved in bicarbonate solution is ingested by healthy subjects, unconjugated UDCA peaks in serum between 15 and 30 min after intake[5] (Fig. 1). During chronic administration, UDCA becomes the major bile acid in serum and bile[4,6].

ENRICHMENT WITH UDCA

The enrichment of biliary bile acids with UDCA, up to a certain dose, is dose-dependent. However, the relationship between percentage enrichment and dose is not linear but decreases with increasing dose. In patients with gallstones maximal enrichment of 40–60% was reached with daily doses between 10 and 14 mg kg^{-1} (Fig. 2)[7].

Maximal enrichment of biliary bile acids with administered bile acid is lower during UDCA (40–60%) than during CDCA therapy (80–90%)[7]. This difference cannot sufficiently be explained by differences in absorption of

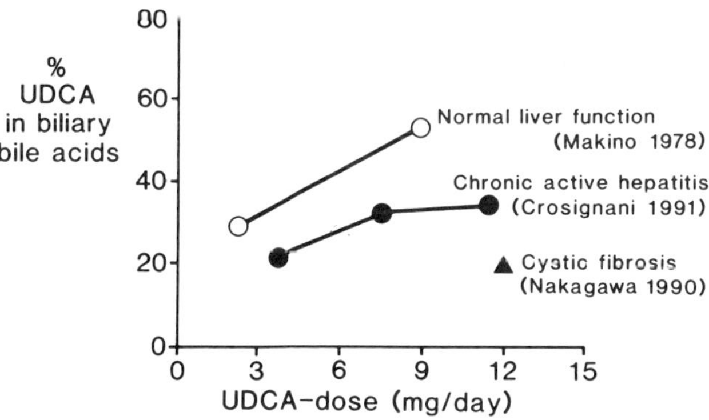

Fig. 3 Enrichment of biliary acids with UDCA during UDCA administration in gallstone patients[6], patients with chronic active hepatitis[11] and patients with cystic fibrosis and hepatic dysfunction[12]

these two bile acids. Enrichment of the bile acid pool with UDCA is limited by lack of inhibition of endogenous bile acid synthesis by UDCA. In contrast, CDCA inhibits endogenous bile acid synthesis[8]. Furthermore, intestinal conservation of UDCA conjugates is less efficient than that of CDCA conjugates[4]. Finally, epimerization of UDCA to CDCA[9,10] limits the enrichment of UDCA in the total bile acid pool.

Even less enrichment of biliary bile acids with UDCA has been observed during UDCA therapy in patients with liver disease. Crosignani *et al.*[11] reported only 34% enrichment in patients with chronic active hepatitis on a daily dose of nearly $12\,mg\,kg^{-1}$, and Nakagawa *et al.*[12] found only 19% enrichment with UDCA in patients with cystic fibrosis and hepatic dysfunction receiving similar doses of UDCA (Fig. 3). In patients with chronic liver disease, absorption of UDCA may be impaired because of a decrease of endogenous bile acid micelles in duodenal bile. In patients with cystic fibrosis, impairment of pancreatic bicarbonate secretion may result in a low intestinal pH, which decreases absorption of UDCA. This may partly be overcome by administration of higher doses (20 mg/kg per day)[13].

BILIARY BILE ACIDS UNDER UDCA ADMINISTRATION

To compare the bile acid composition in gallbladder bile and serum during UDCA administration, we have performed bile acid determinations in gallbladder bile and serum of patients with cholesterol gallstones who underwent gallbladder puncture prior to gallstone dissolution with methyl-*tert*-butyl ether. Thirteen patients were randomized to either UDCA treatment (10–12 mg/kg per day; $n = 7$) or no treatment (controls; $n = 6$). At 2–3 weeks after the start of the treatment, simultaneous samples of gallbladder bile and blood were obtained in the fasting state. Group separation into free, amidated, sulphated and glucuronidated bile acid species was performed according to Setchell and Matsui[14]. Bile acids were measured by gas–liquid chromatography as described elsewhere[15,16]. Atypical bile acids were

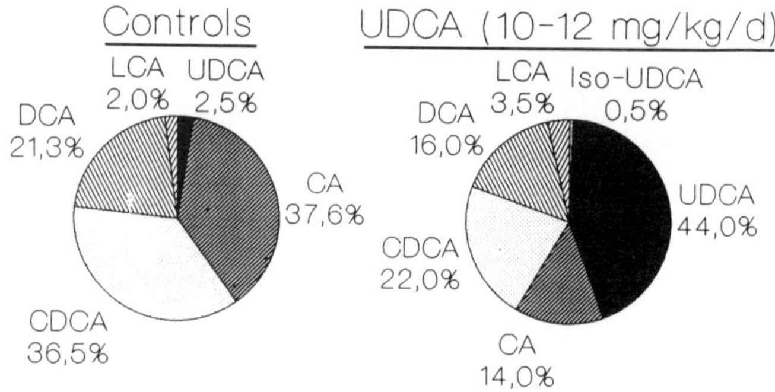

Fig. 4 Bile acids in gallbladder bile of patients with cholesterol gallstones under no medication (controls, $n = 6$) and under administration of 10–12 mg/kg per day UDCA ($n = 7$)

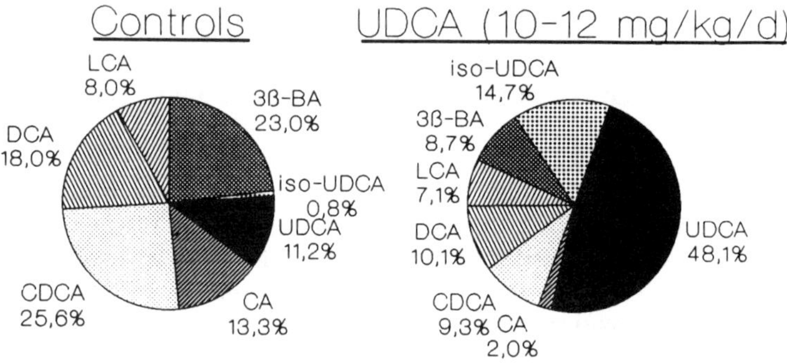

Fig. 5 Bile acids in serum of patients with cholesterol gallstones under no medication (controls, $n = 6$) and under administration of 10–12 mg/kg per day UDCA ($n = 7$); 3β-BA = iso-LCA + iso-CDCA + iso-DCA + 3β-hydroxy-Δ5-cholenoic acid

analysed by gas–liquid chromatography mass spectrometry[16].

In control patients UDCA amounted to 2.5% of total bile acids in bile. Under UDCA administration it increased to 44% and became the major bile acid in bile. This increase of UDCA occurred mainly at the expense of cholic acid (CA) which decreased from 38% to 14%. Interestingly, deoxycholic acid (DCA) decreased only from 21% to 16%. At the same time the concentration of lithocholic acid (LA) rose from 2.0% to 3.5% (Fig. 4). The disproportionate decrease of CA and DCA may be explained by competition of UDCA with CA for ileal absorption, increased loss of CA into the colon and increased formation of DCA from CA by the colonic microflora.

SERUM BILE ACIDS UNDER UDCA ADMINISTRATION

During oral administration, UDCA became the major bile acid also in serum, amounting to 48% of total serum bile acids (Fig. 5). It is noteworthy that the 7β-epimer of UDCA, iso-UDCA[17–19], was the second-largest fraction of serum bile acids, constituting 15% of all serum bile acids, although it was present in bile only in trace amounts (0.5%) (Fig. 4). Beuers *et al.*[16] could prove the precursor–product relationship between UDCA and iso-UDCA by administration of $[^{13}C]$-UDCA to a healthy subject. Furthermore, the putative intermediate, 3-oxo-7β-hydroxy-5β-cholanoic acid could be identified in the serum of patients with cholestatic liver disease by gas–liquid chromatography/mass spectrometry[16]. The most likely site for the epimerization of UDCA to iso-UDCA appears to be the intestine. Thus, we could decrease the concentration of iso-UDCA in serum of healthy subjects during UDCA administration by antibiotic treatment with 100 mg doxycycline daily for 2 weeks[16].

The pathway of the conversion of UDCA to iso-UDCA seems to be analogous to that of the epimerization of UDCA to CDCA (Fig. 6). First, the 3-oxo derivative is formed by intestinal bacteria. This intermediate is then reduced to the 3α or 3β-hydroxy bile acid. Hypothetically, the liver could also be involved in the reduction of the 3-oxo compound since it contains a microsomal 3β-hydroxy-steroid dehydrogenase and the formation of 3β-hydroxy-5β-cholanoic acid from 3-oxo-5β-cholanoic acid has been demonstrated in microsomal preparations of human liver supplemented with NADH[20].

During UDCA administration patients with primary biliary cirrhosis or primary sclerosing cholangitis have less iso-UDCA in their serum than healthy subjects[16]. This may be due: (1) to differences in their intestinal microflora, (2) to decreased biliary secretion of UDCA in patients with cholestasis providing less substrate for the intestinal microflora or (3) to reduced hepatic transformation of the intermediate 3-oxo bile acid to iso-UDCA.

In contrast to UDCA, hepatic conjugation with taurine or glycine is not a major metabolic route for iso-UDCA (Fig. 7). In our gallstone patients treated with UDCA we found that the largest portion of iso-UDCA in serum, namely 47%, was found in the unconjugated fraction. The second-largest fraction of iso-UDCA in serum was the sulphate fraction with 36%, followed by glucuronides amounting to 13%. Glycine and taurine conjugates of iso-UDCA together represented only 3% of total iso-UDCA in serum. Possibly the stereochemical structure of iso-UDCA, like that of other iso-bile acids, is unfavourable for interaction with hepatic conjugating enzymes[21]. Consequently, sulphation[18] or glucuronidation occur, with a relatively large portion of sulphates and glucuronides of iso-UDCA being excreted into the urine[22,23].

Another metabolic pathway for iso-UDCA is conjugation with *N*-acetyl-glucosamine, which appears to be rather selective for 7β-hydroxy-bile acids[24]. Finally, iso-UDCA may be re-epimerized in the liver to UDCA. Thus, interconversion between the 3α- and 3β-isomers may exist, as has been established for the 7α- and 7β-epimers of 3,7-dihydroxy-5β-cholanoic acid. Dehydroxylation of the 3,7-dihydroxy-bile acids in the intestine yields LCA and small amounts of iso-LCA. This may contribute to the increase in LCA

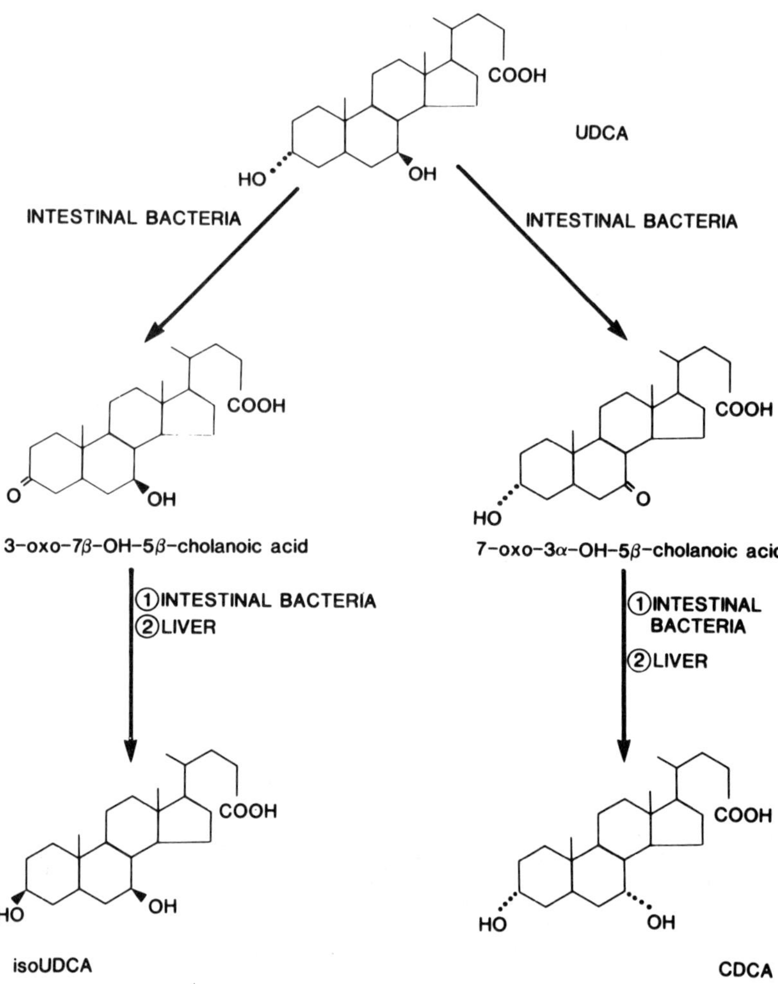

Fig. 6 Epimerization of UDCA in humans

observed during UDCA administration. In addition, small amounts of UDCA may be hydroxylated at C1, C6, C12 and C21[19,23].

CONCLUSIONS

During oral administration, UDCA is enriched in the bile acids of bile and serum. A portion of UDCA undergoes epimerization to CDCA and iso-UDCA, dehydroxylation to LCA and hydroxylation at C1, C6, C12 or C21. The extent to which these metabolic conversions occur depends on the intestinal microflora, hepatic function and enterohepatic circulation of bile acids. The type and extent of conjugation and the rate of biliary secretion of these metabolites differ.

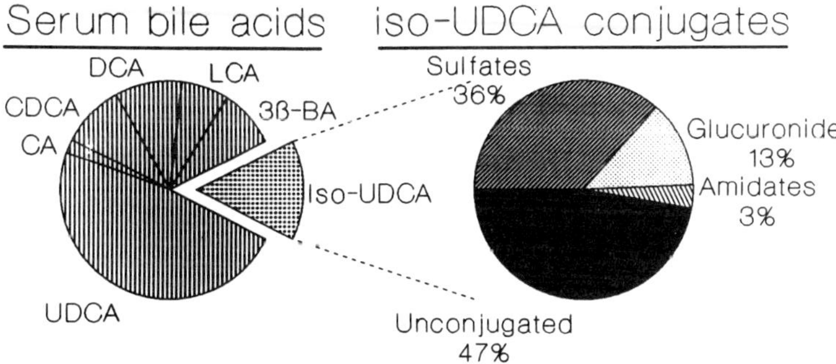

Fig. 7 Conjugates of iso-UDCA in serum of patients with cholesterol gallstones ($n = 7$) under treatment with UDCA (10–12 mg/kg per day)

One may hypothesize that the various metabolites of UDCA differ in their hydrophobicity and hepatotoxicity, and may therefore influence the effects of UDCA in patients with liver disease.

References

1. Poupon RE, Balkau B, Eschwège E, Poupon R and the UDCA-PBC Study Group. A multicenter, controlled trial of ursodiol for the treatment of primary biliary cirrhosis. N Engl J Med 1991;324:1548–54.
2. Schmucker DL, Ohta M, Kanai S, Sato Y, Kitani, K. Hepatic injury induced by bile salts: correlation between biochemical and morphological events. Hepatology. 1990;12:1216–21.
3. Heuman DM, Mills AS, McCall J, Hylemon PB, Pandak WM, Vlahcevic ZR. Conjugates of ursodeoxycholate protect against cholestasis and hepatocellular necrosis caused by more hydrophobic bile salts. *In vitro* studies in the rat. Gastroenterology. 1991;100:203–11.
4. Hofmann AF. Pharmacology of chenodeoxycholic and ursodeoxycholic acid in man. In: Paumgartner. G, Stiehl A, Gerok W, eds, Bile acids and cholesterol in health and disease. Lancaster: MTP Press; 1983:301–36.
5. Miescher G, Paumgartner G, Preisig R. Portal-systemic spill-over of bile acids: a study of mechanisms using ursodeoxycholic acid. Eur J Clin Invest. 1983;13:439–45.
6. Makino I, Nakagawa S. Changes in biliary lipid and biliary bile acid composition in patients after administration of ursodeoxycholic acid. J Lipid Res. 1978;19:723–8.
7. Thistle JL, LaRusso NF, Hofmann AF, Turcotte J, Carlson GL, Ott BJ. Differing effects of ursodeoxycholic or chenodeoxycholic acid on biliary cholesterol saturation and bile acid metabolism in man: a dose response study. Dig Dis Sci. 1982;12:161.
8. Nilsell K, Angelin B, Leijd B, Einarsson K. Comparative effects of ursodeoxycholic acid and chenodeoxycholic acid on bile acid kinetics and biliary lipid secretion in humans. Gastroenterology. 1983;89:1248–56.
9. Fedorowski T, Salen G, Colallilo A, Tint GS, Mosbach EH, Hall JC. Metabolism of ursodeoxycholic acid in man. Gastroenterology. 1977;73:1131–7.
10. Hirano S, Masuda N, Oda H. *In vitro* transformation of chenodeoxycholic acid and ursodeoxycholic acid by human intestinal flora, with particular reference to the mutual conversion between the two bile acids. J Lipid Res. 1981;22:735–43.
11. Crosignani A, Battezzati PM, Setchell KDR, Camisasca M, Bertolini E, Roda A, Zuin M, Podda M. Effects of ursodeoxycholic acid on serum liver enzymes and bile acid metabolism in chronic active hepatitis: a dose–response study. Hepatology. 1991;13:339–44.
12. Nakagawa M, Colombo C, Setchell KDR. Comprehensive study of the biliary bile acid composition of patients with cystic fibrosis and associated liver disease before and after UDCA administration. Hepatology. 1990;12:322–34.

13. Reichen J, Paumgartner G, Cotting J, Lentze MJ. Effect of long-term ursodeoxycholate on liver function, nutritional state, and serum bile acids in cystic fibrosis with long-standing cholestasis. In: Paumgartner G, Stiehl A, Gerok W, eds, Bile acids as therapeutic agents. From basic science to clinical practice. Dordrecht: Kluwer; 1991:335–43.
14. Setchell KDR, Matsui A. Serum bile acid analysis: the application of liquid-gel chromatographic techniques and capillary column gas chromatography and mass spectrometry. Clin Chim Acta. 1983;127:1–17.
15. Stellard F, Sackmann M, Sauerbruch T, Paumgartner G. Simultaneous determination of cholic acid and chenodeoxycholic acid pool sizes and fractional turnover rates in human serum using ^{13}C-labeled bile acids. J Lipid Res. 1984;25:1313–19.
16. Beuers U, Fischer S, Spengler U, Paumgartner G. Formation of iso-ursodeoxycholic acid during administration of ursodeoxycholic acid in man. J Hepatol. 1991;13:97–103.
17. Setchell KDR, Lawson AM, Blackstock EJ, Murphy GM. Diurnal changes in serum unconjugated bile acids in normal man. Gut. 1982;23:637–42.
18. Maeda M, Ohama H, Takeda H, Yabe M, Nambu M, Namihisa T. Identification of $3\beta,7\beta$-dihydroxy-5β-cholan-24-oic acid in serum from patients treated with ursodeoxycholic acid. J Lipid Res. 1984;25:14–26.
19. Batta AK, Arora R, Salen G, Tint GS, Eskreis D, Katz S. Characterization of serum and urinary bile acids in patients with primary biliary cirrhosis by gas-liquid chromatography-mass spectrometry: effect of ursodeoxycholic acid treatment. J Lipid Res. 1989;30:1953–62.
20. Björkhem I, Einarsson K, Hellers G. Metabolism of mono- and dihydroxylated bile acids in preparations of human liver. Eur J Clin Invest. 1973;3:459–65.
21. Shefer S, Salen G, Hauser S et al. Metabolism of iso-bile acids in the rat. J Biol Chem. 1982;257:1401–6.
22. Salvioli G, Lugli R, Pradelli JM, Frignani A, Boccalletti V. Urinary excretion of bile acids during acute administration in man. Eur J Clin Invest. 1988;18:22–8.
23. Stiehl A, Rudolph G, Raedsch R, Moller B, Hopf U, Lotterer E, Bircher J, Fölsch U, Klaus J, Endele R, Senn M. Ursodeoxycholic acid-induced changes of plasma and urinary bile acids in patients with primary biliary cirrhosis. Hepatology. 1990;12:492–7.
24. Marschall H-U, Wietholtz H, Matern H, Matern S, Sjövall J. Conjugation with N-acetylglucosamine – a reaction selective for 7β-hydroxy bile acids? Hepatology. 1990;12:891 (abstr.).

36
Ursodeoxycholic acid therapy in paediatric patients with chronic cholestasis

W. F. BALISTRERI, H. H. A-KADER, F. C. RYCKMAN, J. E. HEUBI,
K. D. R. SETCHELL and the UDCA Study Group

INTRODUCTION

There is currently no effective or specific therapy available for paediatric patients with severe chronic cholestatic hepatobiliary diseases, such as intrahepatic cholestasis (IHC) with or without bile duct paucity[1]. Affected children are plagued by increasing disability, failure to grow, pruritus, sleeplessness and hypercholesterolaemia. Certain forms of IHC are associated with a low mortality rate, while others may progress to end-stage liver disease[1,2]. Therapeutic attempts to date have been aimed at management of complications of chronic cholestasis or cirrhosis, with hope for long-term survival provided by access to liver transplantation.

It has been postulated that intrahepatic accumulation of toxic endogenous bile acids may initiate or perpetuate the liver disease of children with chronic cholestasis; therefore, replacement of the bile acid pool with a *non-toxic*, choleretic bile acid such as ursodeoxycholic acid (UDCA; 3α-7β-dihydroxy-5β-cholanoic acid) may be beneficial[1–3]. There are significant parallels between these diseases and related diseases in adults, such as primary biliary cirrhosis and primary sclerosing cholangitis, in which UDCA has been shown to be beneficial in improving clinical and biochemical symptoms[4–10]. Our hypothesis, therefore, was that UDCA would prove to be effective in inducing choleresis and in ameliorating clinical symptoms in children with chronic IHC.

STUDY DESIGN

Patients

Sixty patients (age range 7 months–27 years) with chronic intrahepatic cholestasis (IHC) were entered into a multi-centre, open-label, pilot trial of

UDCA therapy; the study was carried out in collaboration with members of the UDCA Study Group (see Acknowledgements). Preliminary results of this trial have been reported[3]. The inclusion criteria included chronic IHC, as manifested by growth failure, biochemical derangements including elevated serum bilirubin, aminotransferase activity, serum bile acids, or hypercholesterolaemia and clinical symptoms of pruritus. Thirty-three patients met the criteria for syndromatic IHC (the Alagille syndrome), defined by the variable presence of IHC with bile duct paucity, posterior embryotoxon, vertebral arch defects, unique facies, and cardiac abnormalities (peripheral pulmonic stenosis)[11]. Twenty-seven patients were classified as having 'idiopathic' forms of IHC; this group included many patients with progressive familial IHC (Byler's disease)[12]. All patients had persistent generalized *pruritus* of varying degrees (active scratching with or without evident skin abrasions, or cutaneous mutilation, haemorrhage, and scarring evident), which had been refractory to multiple medications and, in some cases, to partial external biliary drainage[13]. In most cases the pruritus had been of such severity as to interfere with daily activities and with sleep.

Experimental design

All patients received UDCA in an initial dose of 15 mg/kg per day as Ursofalk[R], either as tablets or in solution (3% bicarbonate). All other antipruritic medications, including bile acid binding resins, choleretics and sedatives, were discontinued. Serial monitoring for clinical response was carried out; if there was no improvement in pruritus after 2–3 weeks the dose was serially increased to 30 mg/kg per day and then to 45 mg/kg per day. In addition, fasting blood samples were obtained at baseline and at each of the follow-up evaluations for measurement of standard liver indices, serum cholesterol levels and bile acid concentrations; urine samples were obtained to determine UDCA content and compliance. Compliance was monitored by measurement of UDCA enrichment of serum or bile and by a novel, non-invasive, simple method based on the detection of UDCA sulphate in urine using the techniques of fast atom bombardment ionization–mass spectrometry (FAB-MS)[14]. The data were expressed as the mean ($\pm$ standard error of the mean) and mean values were compared using Student's t-test and the Mann–Whitney U-test. The study was approved by the Children's Hospital Medical Center Institutional Review Board and informed consent was obtained.

RESULTS

All patients tolerated UDCA therapy without noticeable side-effects. The only complaint voiced was related to the bitter taste of the *liquid* preparation; if the taste precluded compliance UDCA was offered in the form of crushed tablets. In the majority of patients with chronic intrahepatic cholestasis who received UDCA for at least 1 month there was clinical and biochemical improvement[3,15–19].

Two of the 33 patients with the Alagille syndrome were non-compliant and were eliminated from further data analysis[3,19]. Of the 31 remaining patients, 15 (48%) had a beneficial clinical response after 1 month of UDCA therapy as documented by a decrease in the degree of pruritus. For the 16 non-responsive patients the UDCA dose was increased and pruritus was ameliorated in an additional 11; therefore overall there were five (16%) *non-responsive* patients. In two of these five non-responsive patients partial external biliary diversion was carried out[13]; diversion combined with UDCA therapy was effective in totally relieving the pruritus. Of the 27 patients with idiopathic intrahepatic cholestasis 23 (85%) noted an improvement in the degree of pruritus[3] at the initial dose of 15 mg/kg. For the four non-responsive patients the dose was increased and one additional patient had an amelioration in the severity of the pruritus. In one of the three refractory patients UDCA, combined with partial external biliary diversion, was effective in reducing pruritus. In the patients with Alagille syndrome the serum alanine aminotransferase declined from a mean baseline level of 222.1 ± 25.6 to $159.4 \pm 17.4 \, \text{IU/l}$, the aspartate aminotransferase decreased from 221.9 ± 26.2 to $180.7 \pm 16.5 \, \text{IU/l}$; the total bilirubin decreased from a mean baseline of 7.0 ± 0.9 to $5.3 \pm 0.8 \, \text{mg/dl}$, and the conjugated bilirubin decreased from 4.8 ± 0.7 to $4.3 \pm 0.7 \, \text{mg/dl}$ (all $p < 0.05$). UDCA was effective in decreasing the serum cholesterol level in patients with Alagille syndrome from a mean value of entry of $627.0 \pm 96.8 \, \text{mg/dl}$ to $467.4 \pm 64.1 \, \text{mg/dl}$ after 3–4 weeks of therapy ($p < 0.02$) and to 396.4 ± 53.5 at 3 months ($p < 0.05$).

Bile was obtained from four patients with IHC after 30 days of therapy; UDCA enrichment ($7.5 \pm 5\%$ tauro-UDCA and $20.5 \pm 17.0\%$ glyco-UDCA) was documented[3], and UDCA-sulphate was found in the urine of all patients treated with UDCA[14].

DISCUSSION

Our preliminary data indicate that UDCA therapy may bring about an improvement in refractory pruritus in patients with chronic IHC. The drug was well tolerated by our patients and readily accepted by parents in view of the relief of symptoms and the ability of the child to have restful evenings. The hepatocytoprotective and choleretic effects were demonstrated by a decrease in aminotransferase and serum bilirubin levels in the patients with the Alagille syndrome. The decline in markedly elevated serum cholesterol was also striking. At the present time we feel that UDCA should be the treatment of choice for cholestatic pruritus.

Rationale for UDCA in liver disease

UDCA (3α-7β-dihydroxy 5β cholanoic acid) will ameliorate liver cell injury and cholestasis induced by bile acids in animal models[20–22], therefore it has been postulated that UDCA may be of benefit in the treatment of patients with chronic cholestasis. The *rationale* for the use of UDCA is that this naturally occurring bile acid has the ability to induce qualitative changes in the bile acid pool[23-27]. Intracellular accumulation of endogenous bile acids, which might initiate or perpetuate injury, is thereby reduced. *In vitro* and *in vivo* studies suggest that the degree of cytotoxicity of a bile acid is directly correlated with hydrophobicity[28-31]. If the biliary bile acid pool is relatively *hydrophobic*, enrichment with UDCA, a *hydrophilic* bile acid, may protect against liver injury. The hepatoprotective effect of UDCA has been well documented[21,30,32-34]. The mechanism of enrichment of the bile acid pool with UDCA is related to the ability of UDCA to compete with endogenous bile acids for active transport at the terminal ileum[35]. UDCA enrichment of the circulating bile acid pool results in a reciprocal *decrease* in the proportion of potentially toxic, endogenous dihydroxy bile acids, thereby reducing the risk of bile acid–induced damage to liver cell membranes[21,22,36-38]. UDCA also induces a *hypercholeresis* with the incremental increase in bile flow closely coupled to biliary HCO_3 concentration and output[39-45].

Use of UDCA hepatobiliary disease

The initial suggestion that UDCA may be beneficial in patients with liver disease was based on a serendipitous observation by Leuscher *et al.*[46]; they noted biochemical improvement in gallstone patients with coexistent liver disease treated with UDCA. Preliminary uncontrolled observations by David *et al.*[47] and by Fisher and Paradine[48], of the effect of UDCA (10–15 mg/kg per day for 6 months) in a total of 16 patients with primary biliary cirrhosis (PBC) suggested an improvement in aminotransferase and alkaline phosphatase levels.

Poupon *et al.* also described the salutary effects of UDCA, in doses of 13–15 mg/kg body weight per day given for a 2-year period, in a pilot open trial of 15 patients with PBC[5]. There was clinical (pruritus ameliorated) and biochemical improvement, with exacerbation when UDCA was discontinued, followed by an improvement with reinstitution of UDCA. Leuschner *et al.* reported the results of a 9-month double-blind, randomized trial of UDCA (10 mg/kg per day) vs. placebo in 20 PBC patients[6]. In the patients treated with UDCA there was biochemical improvement, documented by decreased aminotransferase, alkaline phosphatase, and GGTP activity; however, there was no change in bilirubin or albumin levels or in the prothrombin time. Liver histology was reported to improve in six, while deterioration was noted in four patients in the placebo group. There was a return to pretreatment biochemical values when UDCA was discontinued. Podda *et al.* observed a linear relationship between the dose of UDCA and the degree in decline of aminotransferase values in patients with PBC[49-51]. However, it was cautioned by Hadziyannis *et al.* in a preliminary communication that the early improvement in clinical and biochemical features noted in patients with PBC treated with UDCA may not be maintained at 2 years[52].

The results of a multi-centre, double-blind trial of UDCA (13–15 mg/kg per day) vs. placebo in patients with PBC were recently reported by Poupon *et al.*[7,53]. In the UDCA recipients there were fewer treatment *failures* (defined as a doubling of bilirubin levels or the occurrence of a severe complication), while pruritus improved, and the serum bilirubin, alkaline phosphatase, aminotransferase, GGTP, cholesterol, and IgM levels, and the AMA titre all decreased[7]. There was histological improvement; however, there was no effect of UDCA therapy on fibrosis. Thus while UDCA appeared to be beneficial and safe, especially in those without advanced disease, the long-term effects remain undefined.

Several other studies have documented a similar beneficial effect of UDCA in a variety of chronic hepatobiliary diseases, including primary sclerosing cholangitis (PSC)[9,54,55] and chronic active hepatitis[56-59]. Preliminary observations by Stiehl *et al.*[60] and O'Brien *et al.*[61] suggested that in patients with PSC there is improvement in clinical symptoms and a reduction in enzyme levels during UDCA therapy; they also documented worsening after withdrawal. Chazouilleres[9], in an uncontrolled trial of 15 patients with PSC who received varying doses of UDCA, showed an improvement in pruritus and a decrease in biochemical parameters. Once again there was an exacerbation when UDCA was discontinued. Hayashi *et al.*[62] noted similar results in a single patient; there were no cholangiographic or histological changes.

UDCA has been shown to decrease aminotransferase and alkaline phosphatase activity in patients with chronic active hepatitis[56,57,59,63] and in a wide variety of other hepatobiliary diseases such as post-liver transplant[64], cholestasis of pregnancy[65], and in chronic graft versus host disease (GVHD) following bone marrow transplantation[66]. It is of interest, however, that UDCA has not been effective in patients with benign recurrent intrahepatic cholestasis[67,68].

Effect of UDCA on clinical and biochemical features of intrahepatic cholestasis

There are significant parallels between IHC and PBC/PSC. The *pathogenesis* is unknown and the *initiating process* is unidentified; however, the progressive nature of the injury suggests ongoing injury of the hepatocytes, perhaps mediated or exacerbated by the retention of *hepatotoxic* bile acids. The mechanism which initiates and perpetuates destruction of the interlobular bile ducts, leading to clinical and biochemical alterations and, in many cases cirrhosis, has been ascribed to various viral aetiologies, immune mechanisms, and disorders of hepatic excretory function. In particular disturbances in bile acid metabolism or hepatic excretory function may be operant in these syndromes. *Non-specific* alterations in serum and urinary bile acid patterns have been identified[69-74] and *prototypic defects* in bile acid synthetic or degradative pathways lead to either the absence or choleretic primary bile acids, or the accumulation of potentially cholestatic bile acids[2,75]. The accumulation in the liver of toxic endogenous bile acids may alter hepatic structure and function[76]. There may be an additional deleterious effect of retained abnormal bile acids on *intestinal* function, inciting a decrease in intestinal absorption of sodium, glucose, and glycine[77,78].

In view of the lack of specific, practical and definitive therapy for patients with IHC, empirical therapy for the consequences of cholestasis is mandated; this is especially true for the most disabling and troublesome feature noted in patients with chronic cholestasis – refractory pruritus[79-81]. The pathogenesis of cholestatic pruritus is not known, and the nature of the pruritogen which accumulates in plasma during cholestasis and interacts with dermal nerve endings is undefined. Pruritus associated with cholestasis has been attributed to an increased availability of opiate agonist ligands at opiate receptors in the brain[82]. In attempts to reduce pruritus, multiple modalities have been utilized. The most common approach is the use of cholestyramine resin; however, this agent is difficult to administer to children because of its texture and taste, as well as the potential for side-effects such as constipation and hypercholeraemic acidosis. In the majority of our patients cholestyramine had been ineffective or only partially effective. Other palliative measures include medications such as antipruritics, antihistamines or sedatives, local measures such as moisturizers, topical steroids, and topical anaesthetics[79,80], phototherapy combined with cholestyramine[81] and plasma perfusion[83]. Partial external diversion of bile has also been utilized for the treatment of intractable pruritus[13]. Our preliminary observation suggests that UDCA should be given an *adequate* trial prior to the use of surgical measures or medications which present significant side-effects.

Effect of UDCA on serum cholesterol levels

The effect of UDCA in lowering serum cholesterol levels in our patients was dramatic; however, the mechanisms and implications remain undefined. Hypercholesterolaemia is frequently associated with cholestasis; the major cholesterol containing plasma lipoprotein is lipoprotein-X (LPX)[84,85]. UDCA has several documented effects on cholesterol and lipoprotein metabolism, directly stimulating receptor-dependent low-density lipoprotein uptake in the liver and decreasing HMG-CoA reductase activity[86-89]. There may also be decreased cholesterol absorption from the intestine because of diminished micelle formation and an additional effect of UDCA on cholesterol excretion[23,87,90]. Regardless of the mechanism of cholesterol reduction by UDCA, there may be direct clinical implications; namely, a reduction of plasma viscosity[91,92] and perhaps a reduction in the atherosclerotic propensity[91-93].

SUMMARY

These preliminary results suggest that a short-term administration of UDCA to children with chronic intrahepatic cholestasis may result in improvement of clinical symptoms as well as biochemical indices. The most remarkable improvement seen in these children was in the quality of life; this was dramatically reflected in the marked improvement or disappearance of pruritus in almost all of these patients. The drug was well tolerated by our patients; there were no side-effects noted. A randomized placebo-controlled trial and a dose–response study are under way to further assess the therapeutic value of UDCA in children with chronic cholestatic liver disease.

Acknowledgements

The work was funded by FD-R-000357-03, and UDCA was supplied by the Falk Foundation, Freiburg, Germany. The authors wish to thank the members of the *UDCA Study Group* for enrollment of their patients in our study: John Barnard, MD, William Belknap, MD, Ellen Blank, MD, Andres Blei, MD, John Bucuvalas, MD, Daniel Caplan, MD, Joseph Clark, MD, Mitchell Cohen, MD, Stanley Cohen, MD, A. R. Colon, MD, James Daniel, MD, John Dalzell, MD, Frederic Daum, MD, Lynn Duffy, MD, Michael Farrell, MD, Donald George, MD, Harry Greene, MD, David Gremse, MD, Janet Harnsberger, MD, Mel Hyman, MD, Richard Katz, MD, Stuart Kaufman, MD, John Kerner, MD, Benny Kerzner, MD, Barbara Kirschner, MD, Steven Lichtman, MD, James Markowitz, MD, Juhling McClung, MD, Robert Murray, MD, Prathiba Nanjundiah, MD, Michael Narkewicz, MD, Gerald Odell, MD, Jean Perrault, MD, David Piccoli, MD, Simon Rabinowitz, MD, Anthony Repucci, MD, Mark Rhodes, MD, Philip Rosenthal, MD, Robert Rothbaum, MD, Colin Rudolph, MD, Bradley Schaeffer, MD, Kathy Schwarz, MD, Michael Shelton, MD, Frank Sinatra, MD, Ronald Sokol, MD, Judy Splawski, MD, Robert Squires, MD, Rita Steffen, MD, Robert Stone, MD, Frederick Suchy, MD, Daniel Thomas, MD, John Thompson, MD, Ramon Torres-Pinedo, MD, William Treem, MD, Neil Tucker, MD, Martin Ulshen, MD, Jon Vanderhoof, MD, John Watkins, MD, Peter Whitington, MD, Russell Zweiner, MD. We also wish to thank Colin D. Rudolph, MD, PhD for his assistance in statistical analysis, and Ms Patti Gubser for her assistance in manuscript preparation.

References

1. Balistreri WF. Neonatal cholestasis. J Pediatr. 1985;106:171–84.
2. Balistreri WF. (Foreword) Neonatal cholestasis; lessons from the past, issues for the future. In: Balistreri WF, editor. Seminars in liver disease: neonatal cholestasis, vol. 7, no. 2, May. New York: Thieme Medical Publishers; 1987.
3. Balistreri WF, A-Kader HH, Ryckman FC, Whitington PF, Heubi JE, Setchell, KDR. Biochemical and clinical response to ursodeoxycholic acid administration in pediatric patients with chronic cholestasis. In: Paumgartner G, Stiehl A, Gerok W, editors. Bile acids as therapeutic agents. Lancaster: Kluwer; 1991:323–33.
4. Hofmann AF, Popper H. Ursodeoxycholic acid for primary biliary cirrhosis. Lancet. 1987;2:398–9.
5. Poupon R, Poupon RE, Calmos Y *et al.* Is ursodeoxycholic acid an effective treatment for primary biliary cirrhosis? Lancet. 1987;2:834–6.
6. Leuschner U, Fischer H, Kurtz W, Guldutuna S, Hubner K, Hellstern A, Gatzen M, Leuschner M. Ursodeoxycholic acid in primary biliary cirrhosis: results of a controlled double-blind trial. Gastroenterology. 1989;97:1268–74.

7. Poupon RE, Balkau B, Eschwege E, Poupon R, and the UDCA-PBC Study Group. Multicenter, controlled trial of ursodiol for the treatment of primary biliary cirrhosis. N Engl J Med. 1991;324:1548–54.
8. Oka H, Toda G, Ikeda Y, Hashimoto N, Hasumura Y, Kamimura T, Ohta Y, Tsuji T, Hattori N, Namihisa T, Nishioka M, Ito K, Sasaki H, Kakumu S, Kuroki T, Fujisawa K, Nakanuma Y. A multi-center double-blind controlled trial of ursodeoxycholic acid for primary biliary cirrhosis. Gastroenterol Jpn. 1990;25:774–80.
9. Chazouilleres O, Poupon R, Capron JP, Metman EH, Dhumeaux D, Amouretti M, Couzigou P, Labayle D, Trinchet JC. Ursodeoxycholic acid for primary sclerosing cholangitis. J Hepatol. 1990;11:120–3.
10. Matsuzaki Y, Tanaka N, Osuga T, Aikawa T, Shoda J, Doi M, Nakano M. Improvement of biliary enzyme levels and itching as a result of long-term administration of ursodeoxycholic acid in primary biliary cirrhosis. Am Gastroenterol. 1990;85;15–23.
11. Alagille D, Odievre M, Gartier M *et al.* Hepatic ductular hypoplasia associated with characterization facies, vertebral malformations, retarded physical, mental, and sexual development and cardiac murmur. J Pediatr. 1984;86:63–72.
12. Reily CA. Familial intrahepatic cholestatic syndromes. Sem Liver Dis. 1987;7:119–33.
13. Whitington PF, Whitington GL. Partial external diversion of bile for the treatment of intractable pruritus associated with intrahepatic cholestasis. Gastroenterology. 1988;95:130–6.
14. Setchell KDR, Watson D, Balistreri WF, Yamashita H. A simple rapid and non-invasive test of compliance to oral ursodeoxycholic acid (UDCA) therapy – detection of UDCA sulfate, a specific urinary metabolite. Hepatology 1991; 14:216A.
15. Balistreri WF, Heubi JE, Whitington P, Perrault J, Bancroft J, Setchell KDR. Ursodeoxycholic acid therapy in pediatric hepatobiliary disease. Hepatology. 1989;10:602, (abstr.).
16. Balistreri WF, A-Kader HH, Heubi JE, Setchell KDR, Whitington P. Ursodeoxycholic acid decreases serum cholesterol levels, ameliorates symptoms, and improves biochemical parameters in pediatric patients with chronic intrahepatic cholestasis. Gastroenterology. 1990;96:A566.
17. Balistreri WF, A-Kader HH, Heubi JE, Setchell KDR. Effect of ursodeoxycholic acid on pruritus with cholestasis associated syndromic paucity of intrahepatic bile ducts (Alagille syndrome). Hepatology. 1990;12:994, (abstr.).
18. A-Kader HH, Heubi JE, Setchell KDR, Ryckman FC, Balistreri WF. The effect of ursodeoxycholic acid therapy in patients with extrahepatic biliary atresia. Gastroenterology. 1990;98:A564.
19. Balistreri WF, A-Kader HH, Setchell KDR. Ursodeoxycholic acid (UDCA) therapy in patients with the Alagille syndrome (syndromic paucity of intrahepatic bile ducts): results of a multicenter pilot trial. Pediatr Res. 1991;29:A99.
20. Hertz R, Paumgartner G, Preisig R. Inhibition of bile formation by high dose of taurocholate in the perfused rat liver. Scand J Gastroenterol. 1976;11:741–6.
21. Kitani K. Hepatoprotective effect of ursodeoxycholate in experimental animals. In: Paumgartner G, Stiehl A, Gerok W, eds. Strategies for the treatment of hepatobiliary disease. Lancaster: Kluwer; 19:43–56.
22. Ota S, Tsukahara H, Terano A, Hata Y, Hiraishi H, Mutoh H, Sugimoto T. Protective effect of tauroursodeoxycholate against chenodeoxycholate-induced damage to cultured rabbit gastric cells. Dig Dis Sci. 1991;36:409–26.
23. Tint GS, Salen G, Shefer S. Effect of ursodeoxycholic acid and chenodeoxycholic acid on cholesterol and bile acid metabolism. Gastroenterology. 1986;91:1007–18.
24. Batta AK, Arora R, Salen G, Tint GS, Eskreis D, Katz S. Characterization of serum and urinary bile acids in patients with primary biliary cirrhosis by gas–liquid chromatography–mass spectrometry: effect of ursodeoxycholic acid treatment. Lipid Res. 1989;30:1953–62.
25. Roda E, Mazzella G, Bazzoli F, Villanova N, Minutello A, Simoni P, Ronchi M, Poggi C, Festi D, Aldini R, Roda A. Effect of ursodeoxycholic acid administration on biliary lipid secretion in primary biliary cirrhosis. Dig Dis Sci. 1989;34:52S–8S.
26. Stiehl A, Rudolph G, Raedsch R, Moller B, Hopf U, Lotterer E, Bircher J, Fosch U, Klaus J, Endele R, Senn M. Ursodeoxycholic acid-induced changes of plasma and urinary bile acids in patients with primary biliary cirrhosis. Hepatology. 1990;12:492–7.
27. Crosignani A, Podda M, Battezzati PM, Bertolini PM, Bertolini E, Zuin M, Watson D,

Setchell KDR. Changes in bile acid composition in patients with primary biliary cirrhosis induced by ursodeoxycholic acid administration. Hepatology. 1991;14:1–8.

28. Attili AF, Angelico M, Cantafora A, Alvaro D, Capocaccia L. Bile acid-induced liver toxocity: relation to the hydrophobic–hydrophilic balance of bile acids. Med Hypoth. 1986;19:57–68.

29. Schlomerich J, Baumgartner U, Miyai K, Gerok W. Tauroursodeoxycholate prevents taurolithocholate-induced cholestasis and toxicity in rat liver. J Hepatol. 1990;10:280–3.

30. Schlomerich J, Kitamura S, Baumgartner U, Miyai K, Gerok W. Taurocholate, taurocholate and tauroursodeoxycholate, but not tauroursocholate and taurodehydrocholate counteract effects of taurolithocholate in rat liver. Res Exp Med. 1990;190:121–9.

31. Mizoguchi Y, Kodama C, Sakagami Y, Seki S, Kobayashi K, Yamamoto S, Morisawa S. Effects of bile acids on liver cell injury by cultured supernatant of activated liver adherents cells. Gastroenterol Jpn. 1989;24:25–30.

32. Miyai K, Toyota N, Jones HM, Gochman N. Protective effect of ursodeoxycholic acid against cholestasis and hepatotoxic effects of lithocholic acid. Hepatology. 1982;2:705, (abstr.).

33. Kitani K, Kanai S. Tauroursodeoxycholate prevents taurocholate induced cholestasis. Life Sci. 1982;30:515–23.

34. Galle PR, Theilmann L, Radesch R, Otto G, Stiehl A. Ursodeoxycholate reduces hepatotoxicity of bile salts in primary human hepatocytes. Hepatology. 1990;12:486–91.

35. Stiehl A, Radesch R, Rudolph G. Acute effects of ursodeoxycholic and chenodeoxycholic acid on the small intestinal absorption of bile acids. Gastroenterology. 1990;98:424–8.

36. Miyazaki K, Nakayama F, Koga F, Koga A. Effect of chenodeoxycholic and ursodeoxycholic acids on isolated adult human hepatocytes. Dig Dis Sci. 1984;19:1123–30.

37. Batta AK, Salen G, Arora R, Shefer S, Tint GS, Abroon J, Eskreis D, Katz S. Effect of ursodeoxycholic acid on bile acid metabolism in primary biliary cirrhosis. Hepatology. 1989;10:414–19.

38. Fisher RL, Hofmann AF, Rossi S et al. Pathogenesis of morphological damage and major serum aminotransferase elevations in NCGS patients: enhanced liver cell sensitivity not defective lithocholate metabolism. Hepatology. 1986;6:1169, (abstr.).

39. Scharschmidt BF, Lake JR. Hepatocellular bile acid transport and ursodeoxycholic acid hypercholeresis. Dig Dis Sci. 1989;34:5S–15S.

40. Renner EL, Lake JR, Cragoe, Jr EJ, Van Dyke RW, Scharschmidt BF. Ursodeoxycholic acid choleresis: relationship to biliary HCO_3 and effects of Na^+-H_+ exchange inhibitors. Am J Physiol. 1988;254:G232–41, Part 1.

41. Dumont M, Erlinger S, Uchman S. Hypercholeresis induced by ursodeoxycholic acid and 7-ketolithocholic acid in the rat: possible role of bicarbonate transport. Gastroenterology. 1980;798:82–9.

42. Anwer MS, Hondalus MK, Atkinson JM. Ursodeoxycholate-induced changes in hepatic Na^+-H^+ exchange and biliary HCO_3 excretion. Am J Physiol. 1989;257:G371–9.

43. Moseley RH, Ballatori N, Smith DJ, Boyer JL. Ursodeoxycholate stimulates Na^+-H^+ exchange in rat liver basolateral plasma membrane vesicles. J Clin Invest. 1987;80:684–90.

44. Erlinger S. Hypercholeretic bile acids: a clue to the mechanism? Hepatology. 1990; 11:888–90.

45. Takikawa H, Sano N, Narita T, Yamanaka M. The ursodeoxycholate dose-dependent formation of ursodeoxycholate-glucuronide in the rat and the choleretic potencies. Hepatology. 1990;11:743–9.

46. Leuschner U, Leuschner M, Hubner K. Gallstone dissolution in patients with chronic active hepatitis. Gastroenterology. 1981;80:A1208.

47. David R, Kurtz W, Strohm WD, Leuschner U. Die wirkung von Ursodeoxycholasure bei Chronischen Lebererkrankunge. Eine Pilot Studie. Z Gastroenterol. 1985;23:420.

48. Fisher WW, Paradine ME. Influence of ursodeoxycholic acid on biochemical parameters in cholestatic liver disease. Gastroenterology. 1986;90:A1725.

49. Podda M, Battezzati PM, Crosignani A et al. Ursodeoxycholic acid (UDCA) for symptomatic primary biliary cirrhosis (PBC): a double-blind multi-center trial. Hepatology. 1989;10:639, (abstr.).

50. Podda M, Battezzati PM, Bertolini E, Zuin M, Crosignani A, Petrolini MI, Rizzoli R, Roda A. Effects of ursodeoxycholic acid (UDCA) on liver function tests and bile acid

metabolism in anicteric primary biliary cirrhosis (PBC): a dose–response study. Hepatology. 1988;8:1266, (abstr.).

51. Podda M, Ghezzi C, Battezzati PM, Bertolini E, Crosignani A, Petroni ML, Zuin M. Effect of different doses of ursodeoxycholic acid in chronic liver disease. Dig Dis Sci. 1989;34: 59S–65S.

52. Hadziyannis SJ, Hadziyannis ES, Makris A. A randomized controlled trial of ursodeoxycholic acid in primary biliary cirrhosis. Hepatology. 1989;10:580.

53. Poupon RE, Eschwege E, Poupon R and the UDCA-PBC Study Group. Ursodeoxycholic acid for the treatment of primary biliary cirrhosis – interim analysis of a double-blind multicenter randomized trial. J Hepatol. 1990;11:16–21.

54. James OFW. Ursodeoxycholic acid treatment for chronic cholestatic liver disease. J Hepatol. 1990;11:5–8.

55. Salvioli G, Carati L, Lugli R. Steatorrhoea in cirrhosis – effect of ursodeoxycholic acid administration. J Int Med Res. 1990;18:289–97.

56. Bateson MC. Ursodeoxycholic acid therapy in chronic active hepatitis. Postgrad Med J. 1990;66:781–83.

57. Rolandi E, Franceschini R, Cataldi A, Cicchetti V, Carati L, Barreca T. Effects of ursodeoxycholic acid (UDCA) on serum liver damage indices in patients with chronic active hepatitis. Eur J Clin Pharmacol. 1991;40:473–6.

58. Podda M, Ghezzi C, Battezzati PM, Crosignani A, Zuin M, Roda A. Effects of ursodeoxycholic acid and taurine on serum liver enzymes and bile acids in chronic hepatitis. Gastroenterology. 1990;98:1044–50.

59. Crosignani A, Battezzati PM, Setchell KDR, Camisasca M, Bertolini E, Roda A, Zuin M, Podda M. Effects of ursodeoxycholic acid on serum liver enzymes and bile acid metabolism in chronic active hepatitis: a dose–response study. Hepatology. 1991;13:339–44.

60. Stiehl A, Raedsch R, Rudolph G, Theilmann L. Treatment of primary sclerosing cholangitis with UDCA: first results of a controlled study. Hepatology. 1989;10:A602 (abstr.).

61. O'Brien C, Senior JR, Batta AK, Arora R, Tint GS, Salen G. Ursodeoxycholic acid treatment produces marked clinical and biochemical amelioration of primary sclerosing cholangitis. Gastroenterology. 1989;96:A640.

62. Hiyashi H, Higuchi T, Ichimiya H, Hishida N, Sakamoto N. Asymptomatic primary sclerosing cholangitis treated with ursodeoxycholic acid. Gastroenterology. 1990;99:533–5.

63. Bellentani S, Tabarroni G, Barchi T, Ferretti I, Fratti N, Villa E, Manenti F. Effects of ursodeoxycholic acid treatment on alanine aminotransferase and γ-glutamyltranspeptidase serum levels in patients with hypertransaminasemia. Results from a double-blind controlled trial. J Hepatol. 1989;8:7–12.

64. Friman S, Persson H, Svanvik J, Schersten T, Karlberg I. Does adjuvant ursodeoxycholic acid prevent early rejection in liver transplant recipients? Gastroenterology. 1990;98:A587.

65. Palma J, Reyes H, Ribalta J, Iglesias J, Gonzalez M, Hernandez I, Alvarez C, Molina C, Danitz AM. Effects of ursodeoxycholic acid in patients with intrahepatic cholestasis of pregnancy. In: Paumgartner G, Stiehl A, Gerok W, editors. Bile acids as therapeutic agents; from basic science to clinical practice. Lancaster: Kluwer; 1991:319–33.

66. Fried RH, Wilson RA, Fisher LD, Sullivan KM, Murakami CS, Hinda M, McDonald GB. Ursodeoxycholic acid therapy of chronic graft-versus-host disease of the liver following allogeneic bone marrow transplantation. Hepatology. 1990;12:633, (abstr.).

67. Bijleveld CMA, Vonk RJ, Kuipers F, Havinga R, Boverhof R, Koopman BJ, Wolthers GB, Fernandes J. Benign recurrent intrahepatic cholestasis: altered bile acid metabolism. Gastroenterology. 1989;97:427–32.

68. Crosignani A, Podda M, Bertolini E, Battezzati PM, Zuin M, Setchell KDR. Failure of ursodeoxycholic acid to prevent a cholestatic episode in a patient with benign recurrent intrahepatic cholestasis: a study of bile metabolism. Hepatology. 1991;13:1076–83.

69. Balistreri WF, Heubi JE, Suchy FJ. The immaturity of the enterohepatic circulation in early life: factors predisposing to 'physiologic' maldigestion and cholestasis. J Pediatr Gastroenterol Nutr. 1983;2:346–54.

70. Balistreri WF. Fetal and neonatal bile acid synthesis and metabolism – clinical implications. J Inher Metab Dis. 1991;14:459–77.

71. Sondheimer JM, Bryan H, Andrews W, Forstner GG. Cholestatic tendencies in premature infants on and off parenteral nutrition. Pediatrics. 1978;62:984–9.

72. Tazawa Y, Yamada M, Nakagawa M, Konno Y, Tada K. Unconjugated, glycine-conjugated, taurine-conjugated bile acid nonsulfates and sulfates in urine of young infants with cholestasis. Acta Pediatr Scand. 1984;73:392–7.
73. Kuipers F, Bijleveld CM, Kneepkens CM, van Zanten A, Fernandes J, Vonk RJ. Sulphated lithocholic acid conjugates in serum from children with hepatic and intestinal diseases. Scand J Gastroenterol. 1985;20:1255–61.
74. Balistreri WF, Suchy FJ, Farrell MK, Heubi JE. Pathologic versus physiologic cholestasis elevated serum concentration of a secondary bile acid in the presence of hepatobiliary disease. J Pediatr. 1981;98:399–402.
75. Setchell KDR, Street JM. Inborn errors of bile acid synthesis. Sem Liver Dis. 1987;7: 85–99.
76. Akashi Y, Miyazaki H, Yanagisawa J et al. Bile acid metabolism in cirrhotic liver tissue-altered synthesis and impaired hepatic secretion. Acta. 1987;168:199–206.
77. Freel RW, Hatch M, Earnest DL, Goldner AM. Dihydroxy bile salt-induced alterations in NaCl transport across the rabbit colon. Am J Physiol. 1983;245:G808–15.
78. Berant M, Diamon E, Alon U, Mordochovitz D. Effect of infusion of bile salts into the mesenteric artery in site on jejunal mucosal transport function in dogs. J Pediatr Gastroenterol Nutr. 1988;4:588–93.
79. Zysset T, Reichen J. Anticholestatic agents: experimental and clinical aspects. In: Liver drugs, Boca Raton, FL: CRC Press; 1989:113–32.
80. Garden JM, Ostrow D, Roenigk Jr HH. Pruritus in hepatic cholestasis. Arch Dermatol. 1985;121:1415–20.
81. Cerio R, Murphy GM, Sladen GE, MacDonald DM. A combination of phototherapy and cholestyramine for the relief of pruritus in primary biliary cirrhosis. Br J Dermatol. 1987;116:265–7.
82. Jones EA, Bergasa NV. Hypothesis; the pruritus of cholestasis: from bile acids to opiate agonists. Hepatology. 1990;11:884–7.
83. Lauterberg BH, Pineda AA, Burgstaler EA et al. Treatment of pruritus of cholestasis by plasma perfusion through USP-charcoal-coated glass beads. Lancet. 1980;2:53–5.
84. Seidel D. Lipoproteins in liver disease. J Clin Chem Clin Biochem. 1987;25:541–51.
85. Seidel D, Alaupovic P, Furman RH. A lipoprotein characterizing obstructive jaundice. I. Method for quantitative separation and identification of lipoproteins in jaundiced subjects. J Clin Invest. 1969;48:1211–23.
86. Fromm H. Bile acid lipoprotein interactions: effects of ursodeoxycholic acid (ursodiol). Dig Dis Sci. 1989;34:21S–3S.
87. Armstrong MJ, Carey MC. The hydrophobic–hydrophilic balance of bile salts. Inverse correlation between reverse-phase high performance liquid chromatographic mobilities and micellar cholesterol solubilizing capacities. J Lipid Res. 1982;23:70–80.
88. Carulli N, Loria T, Bertoletti M et al. Effects of acute changes of bile acid pool composition on biliary lipid secretion. J Clin Invest. 1984;74:614–24.
89. Lanzini A, Northfield TC. Effects of ursodeoxycholic acid on biliary lipid coupling and on cholesterol absorption during fasting and eating in subjects with cholesterol gallstones. Gastroenterology. 1985;95:408–16.
90. Shefer L, Nguyen L, Salen G, Batta AK, Brooker D, Zaki FG, Rani I, Tint GS. Feedback regulation of bile-acid synthesis in the rat. J Clin Invest. 1990;85:1191–8.
91. Rosenson RS, Baker AL, Chow MJ, Hay RV. Hyperviscosity syndrome in a hypercholesterolemic patient with primary biliary cirrhosis. Gastroenterology. 1990;98:1351–7.
92. Rosenson RS, Black DD. Influence of lipoprotein-X on plasma viscosity in cholestatic disorders of childhood. Clin Res. 1990;38:817A.
93. Beuers U, Ritter MM, Richter WO, Paumgartner G. Lipoprotein (a) serum levels in chronic cholestatic liver disease during treatment with ursodeoxycholic acid. Arch Intern Med. 1990;150:1542.

37
Ursodeoxycholate in the treatment of cholestasis in cystic fibrosis – a 2-year experience and review of the literature

J. COTTING, J. F. DUFOUR, M. J. LENTZE, G. PAUMGARTNER and J. REICHEN

INTRODUCTION

Mean survival of patients with cystic fibrosis has dramatically increased during the past 50 years. Thus, in the 1940s over 80% of children with cystic fibrosis did not reach age 5[1]; in the 1960s survival had increased to 14 years and it averaged 23 years in the 1980s[2]. This dramatic progress was mainly due to pancreatic enzyme substitution and vigorous physiotherapy and antibiotic treatment of lung disease. The most recent therapeutic advance, lung or heart–lung transplantation[3], has yet to show whether it will further improve survival.

As more and more patients with cystic fibrosis reached adulthood it has become apparent that hepatobiliary disease may become more prevalent and even limit survival. Thus, the incidence of clinically apparent cirrhosis ranges from 0.5% to 6% in children but from 5% to 20% in adolescents and young adults[4].

Following the report on beneficial effects of the tertiary bile acid, ursodeoxycholate, in primary biliary cirrhosis[5], it appeared logical to evaluate this bile acid on its effect on the cholestasis associated with cystic fibrosis. Indeed, two open trials reporting on 6 months follow-up demonstrated beneficial effects[6,7] in open studies and a placebo-controlled study was presented at a Falk Bile Acid meeting[8].

PATIENTS AND METHODS

The inclusion criteria have been published previously[6]. Briefly, they included the diagnosis of cystic fibrosis by typical pulmonary and digestive symptoms and elevated sweat chloride, by the presence of progressive cholestasis manifested by elevated liver enzymes for more than 1 year and by the absence of surgically treatable causes of cholestasis.

Nine patients fulfilled the above criteria and were followed up for more than 2 years. Their ages ranged from 10 to 24 years with a mean of 19 years. Five patients demonstrated failure to thrive, five had experienced variceal bleeding and three had had a splenorenal shunt. One patient died during the study from intractable pulmonary haemorrhage after 19 months of therapy.

Before enrollment, patients underwent a physical examination. Standard liver tests were performed after 12 h of fasting by routine autoanalyser methods. A blood sample was obtained and the serum frozen for later bile acid determination. Liver function was assessed by determination of the galactose elimination capacity as a measure of functional liver cell mass, by the aminopyrine breath test for microsomal capacity and by the sulphobromophthalein (BSP) clearance as previously described and referenced[6]. Stools were collected for 3 days to quantify steatorrhoea and a 24 h urine collection was performed to quantify creatinine excretion as an index of muscular mass. Serum bile acids were measured by gas–liquid chromatography after solvolysis and hydrolysis[9].

Ursodeoxycholic acid (UDCA) was given at a total dose 20 mg/kg per day (range 18–24 mg/kg) in four divided doses. The measurements described above were repeated every 6 months. Vitamins and pancreas enzyme substitution were deliberately left unchanged during the study period. The study had been approved by the Ethics Committee of the University of Bern. Informed consent was obtained after explanation of the study to the patients and their parents.

All results will be reported as mean $\pm$ 1 SEM. Treatment effects were analysed by analysis of variance and by the Student's t-test with the Bonferroni correction[10].

RESULTS

The effects of ursodeoxycholate on liver inflammation as estimated by transaminase activities and on cholestasis as measured by 5′-nucleotidase activity are shown in Fig. 1. In all patients a sustained decrease in both ASAT and ALAT was observed; ALAT had decreased by 59%, 60% and 58% after 6 months, 1 and 2 years. This effect was highly significant ($p < 0.001$) and sustained. Similarly 5′-nucleotidase activity decreased in all patients, namely by 72%, 77% and 78% after 6, 12 and 24 months, respectively ($p < 0.001$). Both alkaline phosphatase and γ-GT showed a similar and significant evolution (data not shown).

Functional evolution of liver function as assessed by dynamic tests is shown in Fig. 2. The galactose elimination capacity, a measure of functional liver cell mass, decreased from 7.2 mg/kg per min to 6.6 over 2 years. However, this decrease was not significant when tested by variance analysis ($p = 0.14$). In contrast, the aminopyrine breath test, a measure of microsomal

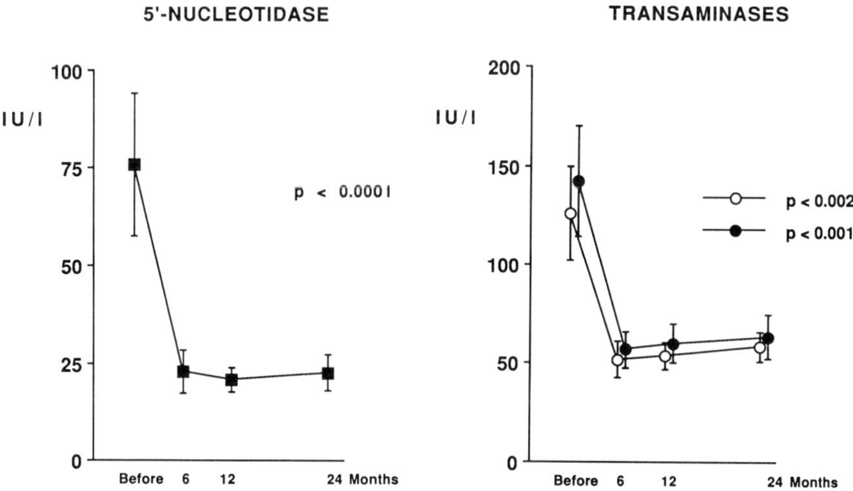

Fig. 1 Effect of UDCA treatment on markers of cytolysis (right panel: ASAT (○) and ALAT (●)) and cholestasis (left panel: 5′-nucleotidase (■)) in young adults with cystic fibrosis and chronic cholestasis. Both cytolysis and cholestasis were significantly improved by UDCA treatment (20 mg/kg per day). The effect persisted after 2 years. Mean ± 1 SEM are indicated. Normal ranges are: ASAT: 0–27 IU/l; ALAT 0–27 IU/l and 5′-nucleotidase 0–18 IU/l

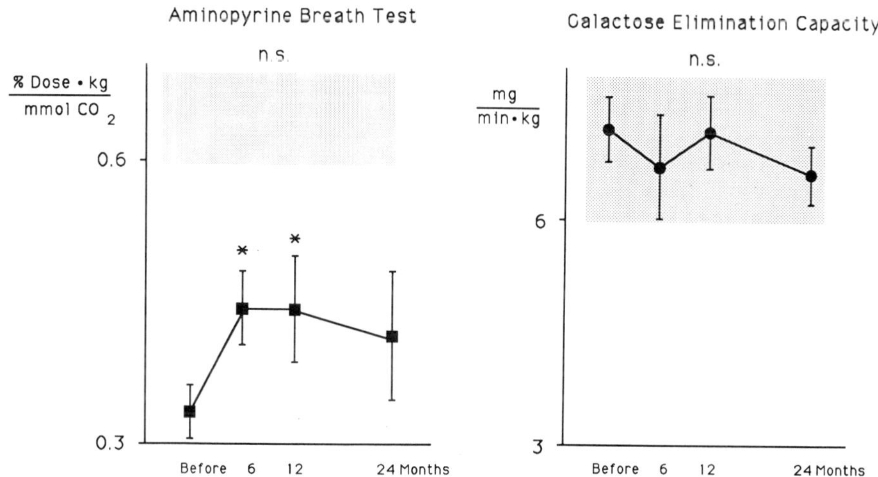

Fig. 2 Functional liver cell mass as estimated by the galactose elimination capacity (right panel) remained stable during the 2 years administration of UDCA. The microsomal reserve, estimated by the aminopyrine breath test (left panel) was improved at 6 and 12 months, then a decrease at 24 months was observed. Normal range is indicated by the shaded area

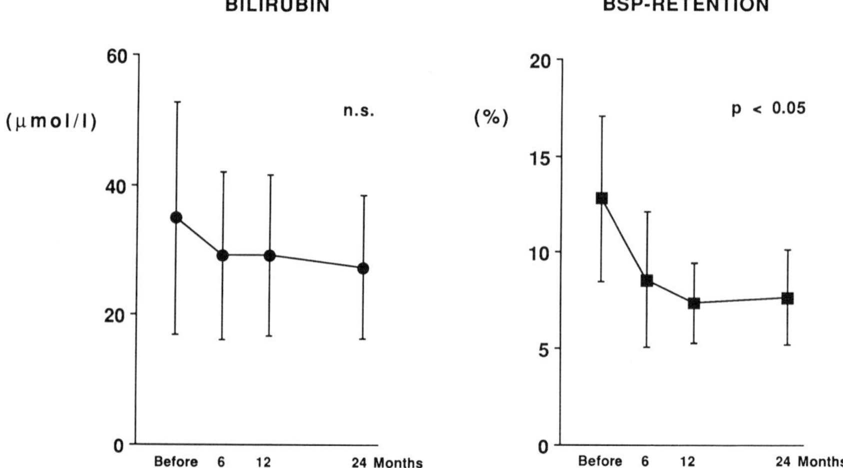

Fig. 3 UDCA had no consistent effect on serum bilirubin (left panel). In contrast a significant improvement was observed for 45-min retention of sulphobromophthalein (BSP) (right panel)

capacity, was lower than normal value before therapy, then showed a slight but significant improvement at 6 months ($p < 0.05$) and at 1 year ($p < 0.05$). Values at 2 years were not significantly different from those before therapy.

The effects of ursodeoxycholate on excretory liver function are shown in Fig. 3. Serum bilirubin levels showed no statistical change for the whole group, but decreased in the four patients with abnormal values before therapy. All patients exhibited abnormal values of BSP retention at 45 min before therapy. During the 2 years of observation the analysis of variance showed a slight but significant effect of treatment ($p < 0.05$). After 6 months of UDCA therapy an improvement in BSP retention was seen in all patients ($p < 0.05$), but one of the eight patients presented with a worsening of his BSP retention at 2 years compared to the value before therapy.

The effect of UDCA on nutrition is shown in Fig. 4. Body weight increased by an average of 2.7 and 4.1 kg at 1 year ($p < 0.05$) and at 2 years ($p < 0.05$), respectively. Even when the three pre-pubertal patients are excluded the increase in body weight remained significant with an increase of 2 and 2.5 kg at 1 and at 2 years, respectively. By expressing this effect of UDCA therapy in term of body mass index the improvement was also significant ($p < 0.01$).

Plasma albumin improved during treatment ($p < 0.002$) from 31 ± 1.2 g/l before therapy to 32.8 ± 1.3 and 34.4 ± 1.3 at 6 and 12 months, respectively; at 2 years there was a decrease compared with values after 1 year (32 ± 3.1 g/l), but the difference with pre-treatment values remained significant ($p < 0.05$). Daily creatinine excretion corrected for body height as an index of the muscular mass could be measured in seven patients; it increased from 31 ± 5 to 47 ± 9 μmol/cm per day after 1 year ($p < 0.05$). By contrast, steatorrhoea did not show any improvement during UDCA therapy.

Results of the plasma concentrations of the different bile acids, including ursodeoxycholate, are presented in Table 1. Total plasma bile salt concen-

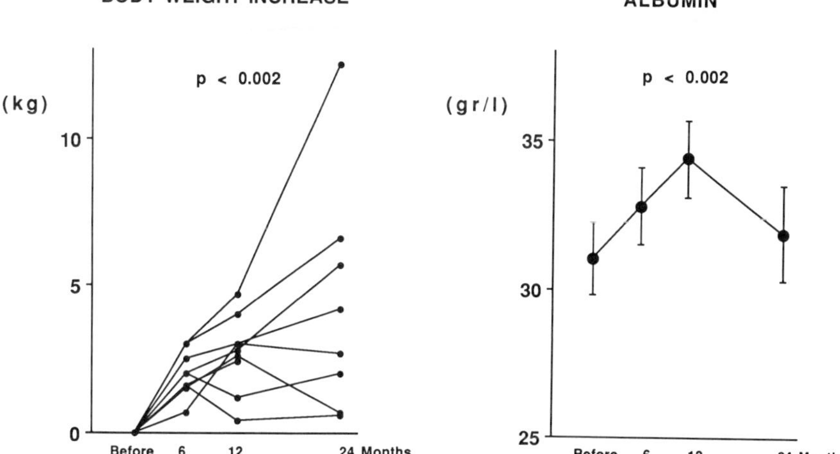

Fig. 4 UDCA improved nutritional state: both body weight (left panel) and plasma albumin (right panel) showed a significant increase during therapy. Even when pre-pubertal patients were excluded from analysis, the improvement in body weight remained significant

Table 1 Serum concentrations of individual serum bile acids (μmol/l) before, after 6 and 24 months of treatment with ursodeoxycholate

	Before	*After 6 months*	*After 24 months*
Chenodeoxycholate	14.9 ± 6.2	16.0 ± 4.7	14.6 ± 3.6
Cholate	13.7 ± 5.5	11.1 ± 3.6	8.2 ± 2.0
Deoxycholate	1.2 ± 4.0	1.5 ± 0.5	3.6 ± 1.0
Ursodeoxycholate	0.9 ± 0.2	31.0 ± 20.8*	27.8 ± 6.7*
Lithocholate	0.3 ± 0.1	0.9 ± 0.5*	0.7 ± 0.4
3β-5Δ-Cholenoate	0.6 ± 0.1	1.1 ± 0.4*	0.7 ± 0.2
Iso-chenodeoxycholate	0.5 ± 0.1	0.5 ± 0.1	0.5 ± 0.1
Iso-deoxycholate	0.1 ± 0.1	0.1 ± 0.1	0.3 ± 0.1
Iso-lithocholate	0.1 ± 0.1	0.2 ± 0.1	0.3 ± 0.1*
Iso-ursodeoxycholate	0.1 ± 0.1	1.1 ± 0.4*	1.1 ± 0.3*

Mean ± SEM are presented; differences with pre-treatment values are indicated; *$p < 0.05$

tration increased from 26 ± 5 to 64 ± 21 ($p < 0.01$) and $54 \pm 12\,\mu$mol/l ($p < 0.01$) after 6 months and 2 years, respectively. The relative concentrations of the major bile salts are presented in Fig. 5. In contrast to other cholestatic conditions the absolute concentration of the primary bile salts did not decrease during therapy. The relative condition of UDCA to serum bile acids increased from 2.9% to 48.8% and 48.2% at 6 months and 2 years, respectively. This increase in ursodeoxycholate led to the decrease in the relative contributions of primary bile acid shown in Fig. 5. One patient (P.M.) had a plasma level of ursodeoxycholate of only 0.7 μmol/l at 2 years, confirming the clinical suspicion that he was not compliant. At this time a marked worsening of transaminases, of 5'-nucleotidase activity and of the BSP clearance was noted.

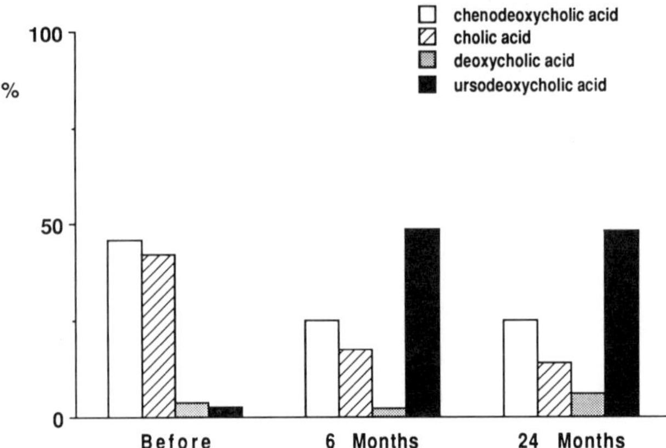

Fig. 5 Changes in the relative composition of serum bile acids before and during UDCA treatment in cystic fibrosis are presented. During treatment relative plasma enrichment of UDCA averaged 50% and this was sustained at 2 years

DISCUSSION

Liver disease in cystic fibrosis is thought to be primarily caused by accumulation in the intrahepatic ducts of inspissated bile; when left untreated this will irrevocably progress to biliary cirrhosis[11–13]. As a secondary effect of cholestasis, accumulation of potentially toxic endogenous bile salts such as lithocholic and chenodeoxycholic acid have been implicated in the pathogenesis of biliary cirrhosis[14]. Both of these pathophysiological scenarios provide a rationale for treatment of this form of liver disease with UDCA. Thus, the bicarbonate bile-rich secretion elicited by ursodeoxycholate[15] could prevent accumulation of inspissated bile. Another important mechanism of action of ursodeoxycholate is the prevention of liver damage induced by the build-up of endogenous toxic bile acids. This could be due to displacement of primary and secondary bile acid[15] and/or to inhibition of ileal absorption of these potentially toxic compounds[16,17].

The present study confirms the improvement of conventional liver tests previously described after shorter observation periods[6–8], and demonstrates that this effect persists after 2 years of therapy in an otherwise progressive disease. By comparing the available data of these three studies performed in patients with cystic fibrosis and chronic cholestasis (see Table 2), different age groups of patients were followed using different doses: Colombo et al.[7] studied younger and less ill patients with slightly lower doses and pre-treated their patients with taurine (30 mg/kg per day). They then continued taurine in co-administration with UDCA. The group of Bittner[8] studied a similar group to ours, but used lower doses. This study was placebo-controlled and showed a significant difference for the transaminases, alkaline phosphatase, γ-GT and GLDH compared to the placebo-treated patients[8].

Comparing the different studies in Table 2 it appears that higher doses of ursodeoxycholate are needed in the treatment of cystic fibrosis. We used the highest dose (of 20 mg/kg per day) and found a decrease of ALT of 60%,

Table 2 Comparison of the effects of ursodeoxycholate treatment in cystic fibrosis patients with cholestasis; all parameters were evaluated after 6 months of treatment

	Present study	Colombo et al.[7]	Bittner et al.[8]
Type of study	Open	Open	Placebo-controlled
Age (years)	18 ± 5	11 ± 2	17 ± 2
Dose (mg/kg per day)	20	10–15	10
ALT	-60%	-41%	-38%
Alkaline phosphatase	-44%	-19%	-28%
Nutritional state	Improved	No effect	No effect

similar to that found in primary biliary cirrhosis[5]. Colombo *et al.*[7] found a decrease of 41% with 10–15 mg/kg per day, and Bittner[8] a decrease of 38% with 10 mg/kg per day. For alkaline phosphatase a similar trend seemed to be apparent for the highest and lowest doses. Probably the lesser decrease in alkaline phosphatase in the Italian study was related to the patients' age due to the physiological spurt of alkaline phosphatase in the pre-pubertal period. Unfortunately, the age-dependent 5'-nucleotidase was not measured in these reports. The contention that high doses are required is reported in the reply to an editorial by Riely[18] in *Gastroenterology*, where Colombo *et al.*[19] claimed better results after increasing the dose to 20 mg/kg per day. This suggests that the maximal effect of UDCA therapy in cystic fibrosis patients requires higher doses than for other forms of cholestasis, and that the optimal dose is around 20 mg/kg per day. Whether still higher doses will be tolerated, and further improve cholestasis and nutrition in these patients, remains to be demonstrated, however. Furthermore, whether taurine adds any benefit remains to be formally proven.

Perhaps the highest clinical significance was the finding that the usage of higher doses of UDCA resulted in a sustained improvement of several nutritional parameters, including both body weight and body mass index even when excluding pre-pubertal patients from analysis. The mechanism of this nutritional improvement is still not clear; a higher duodenal pH due to the bicarbonate-rich choleresis could improve the activity of pancreas enzyme substitution, as demonstrated by adding bicarbonate to the pancreatic enzymes[20]. Indeed, an increase in duodenal pH in ursodeoxycholate-treated patients has been described[7]. However, other mechanisms such as an increase in the caloric intake, or a decrease in the caloric need, have to be considered. The decrease in liver inflammation could affect both these factors. Finally it is possible that body weight is affected by liver involvement only in the late stages of hepatobiliary disease; before this point is reached, body weight could mainly depend on malabsorption and chronic lung disease.

Nutritional state was apparently not influenced in the two other studies compared in Table 2. This could be related to dose (see above), to the mode of administration and/or to the differences in the patients studied. Both the Italian[7] and the German[8] groups studied younger patients and used lower doses. We chose to administer ursodeoxycholate in four divided doses since we wanted to avoid UDCA-induced diarrhoea at such high dosage. Moreover, the absorption of UDCA seems to be dose-dependent in normal humans (A. Stiehl, discussion contribution during this meeting). Which of these factors is responsible for these different findings remains to be determined.

The serum bile acid composition before treatment in the current report is comparable to previous studies in a patient with cystic fibrosis[21], and confirms the increased concentration of chenodeoxycholic acid. After high-dose UDCA treatment, plasma enrichment of this bile acid increased from about 2% before treatment to 60% during treatment, a similar enrichment as that found in other cholestatic diseases[22,23]. Plasma enrichment and bile enrichment of UDCA are lower in younger patients receiving a lower dose[7]. Whether this is due only to the lower dose used, or a unique factor in cystic fibrosis patients, remains to be determined. Faecal loss of bile salts is well known to be increased in cystic fibrosis[20,24] and is related to steathorrhoea[20], since both ileal transport of bile acids[25] and biliary secretion rates[26] are maintained at normal levels. Morever, faecal loss of UDCA in the Italian study ranged from 0.8 to 16 mg/kg per day with a mean of 5 mg/kg per day, representing at least a third of the administered doses[7]. This could also explain the fact that cystic fibrosis patients require higher doses of UDCA.

Of the total of 48 published[6-8] patients with cystic fibrosis treated with UDCA, all but one tolerated the drug very well. One patient in the study by Bittner *et al.*[8] complained of diarrhoea and vomiting. Thus the use of high-dose UDCA therapy appears quite safe.

Finally, should we now advocate bile acid therapy with UDCA in all patients with cystic fibrosis? From our point of view such a recommendation is premature. However, with the results accumulated during the past 5 years in different chronic liver diseases, we do not think that a placebo-controlled study could be ethically justified for patients with cystic fibrosis and advanced liver disease. In this group of patients both optimization of the dose and mode of administration have to be confirmed, and combination treatment with bicarbonate and/or taurine should be evaluated. Ethical considerations make it imperative to study prevention of cholestatic disease by UDCA in placebo-controlled studies. Such a study is under way in our departments.

Acknowledgements

This work was supported in part by a grant from Swiss National Foundation for Scientific Research to J.R. (Nos 32.9365 and 32.30168). J.C. was supported by a grant from the Berne Liver Foundation. The artwork by Ms M. Kappeler is gratefully acknowledged. We thank the nurses of our outpatient department, Ms E. Bühlmann, Ms A. Leu and Ms B. Ritschard, for the excellent care they provided to our patients, and for their accurate work in performing the quantitative liver function testing.

References

1. Duncan FR, Hodson ME, Batten JC. Cystic fibrosis – survival into adult life. Eur J Pediatr. 1981;137:125–31.
2. Matthews LW, Drotar D. Cystic fibrosis – a challenging long-term chronic disease. Pediatr Clin N Am. 1984;31:133–52.

3. Scott JP, Higenbottam TW, Penketh ARL, Hodson M, Steward S, Wallwork J. Heart-lung transplantation for cystic fibrosis. Lancet. 1988;2:192–4.

4. Psacharopoulos HT, Mowat AP. The liver and biliary system. In: Hodson ME, Normann AP, Batten JC, eds. Cystic fibrosis. London: Baillière & Tindall; 1983:164.

5. Poupon R, Chrétien Y, Poupon RE, Ballet F, Calmus Y, Darnis F. Is ursodeoxycholic acid an effective treatment for primary biliary cirrhosis? Lancet. 1987;2:834–6.

6. Cotting J, Lenze MJ, Reichen J. Effects of ursodeoxycholic acid therapy on nutrition and liver function in patients with cystic fibrosis and long-standing cholestasis. Gut. 1990;31:918–21.

7. Colombo C, Setchell KDR, Podda M, Crosignani A, Roda A, Curcio L, Ronchi M, Giunta A. Effect of ursodeoxycholic acid therapy for liver disease associated with cystic fibrosis. J Pediatr. 1990;117:482–9.

8. Bittner P, Posselt HG, Sailer T, Ott H, Magdorf K, Wahn U, Arleth S, Bertele-Harms RM, Wolf A, Krawinkel M, Lindemann H. The effect of treatment with ursodeoxycholic acid in cystic fibrosis and hepatopathy: results of a placebo-controlled study. In: Paumgartner G, Stiehl A, Gerok W, eds. Bile acids as therapeutic agents: from basic science to clinical practice. Lancaster: Kluwer Academic Publishers; 1991:345–8.

9. Stellaard F, Sackmann M, Sauerbruch T, Paumgartner G. Simultaneous determination of cholic acid and chenodeoxycholic acid pool sizes and fractional turn-over rates in human serum using ^{13}C-labelled bile acids. J Lipid Res. 1984;25:1313–19.

10. Snedecor GW, Cochran WG. Statistical methods. Ames, IA: Iowa State University Press; 1967.

11. Oppenheimer EH, Esterly JR. Pathology of cystic fibrosis: a review of the literature and comparison with 146 autopsied cases. Perspect Pediatr Pathol. 1975;2:241–78.

12. Farber S. Pancreatic function and disease in early life; V: pathologic changes associated with pancreatic deficiency. Arch Pathol. 1944;37:238–50.

13. Roy CC, Weber AM, Morin CL, Lepage G, Brisson G, Yousef I, Laselle R. Hepatobiliary disease in cystic fibrosis: a survey of current issues and concepts. J Pediatr Gastroenterol Nutr. 1982;1:489–98.

14. Strandvik B, Samuelson K. Fasting serum bile acid levels in relation to liver histopathology in cystic fibrosis. Scand J Gastroenterol. 1985;20:381–4.

15. Dumont M, Erlinger S, Uchman S. Hypercholeresis induced by ursodeoxycholic acid and 7-ketolithocholic acid in the rat: possible role of bicarbonate transport. Gastroenterology. 1980;79:82–9.

16. Stiehl A, Raedsch R, Rudolph G. Acute effects of ursodeoxycholic and chenodeoxycholic acid on the small intestinal absorption of bile acids. Gastroenterology. 1990;98:424–8.

17. Marteau P, Chazouilleres O, Myara A, Rian R, Rambaud JC, Poupon R. Effect of chronic administration of ursodeoxycholic acid on the ileal absorption of endogenous bile acids in man. Hepatology. 1990;12:1206–8.

18. Riely CA. Cystic fibrosis: another use of Urso? Gastroenterology. 1991;100:1476–7.

19. Colombo C, Crosignani A, Podda M, Setchell KDR, Giunta A. Gastroenterology. 1991;100:1477.

20. Weber AM, Roy CC, Morin CL, Lasalle R. Malabsorption of bile acids in children with cystic fibrosis. N Engl J Med. 1973;289:1001–5.

21. Nakagawa M, Colombo C, Setchell KDR. Comprehensive study of the biliary bile acid composition of patient with cystic fibrosis and associated liver disease before and after UDCA administration. Hepatology. 1990;12:322–34.

22. Makino I, Nagakawa S. Changes in biliary lipid and biliary bile acid composition in patients after administration of ursodeoxycholic acid. J Lipid Res. 1978;19:723–8.

23. Chretien Y, Poupon R, Gherardt MF, Chazouilleres O, Labbe D, Myara A, Trivin F. Bile acid glycine and taurine conjugates in serum of patients with primary biliary cirrhosis: effect of ursodeoxycholic treatment. Gut. 1989;30:1110–15.

24. Watkins JB, Tercyak AM, Szczepanic P, Klein PD. Bile salt kinetics in cystic fibrosis: influence of pancreatic enzyme replacement. Gastroenterology. 1977;73:1023–8.

25. Thomson GN, Davidson GP. In vivo bile acid uptake from terminal ileum in cystic fibrosis. Pediatr Res. 1988;23:323–8.

26. Robb TA, Davidson GP, Kirubakaran C. Conjugated bile acids in serum and secretions in response to cholecystokin/secretin stimulation in children with cystic fibrosis. Gut. 1985;26:1246–56.

38
Ursodeoxycholic acid prevents the hepatobiliary dysfunction associated with total parenteral nutrition

J. B. DAS, C. M. COSENTINO, G. G. ANSARI and
J. G. RAFFENSPERGER

INTRODUCTION

Since the introduction of parenteral feeding for total nutritional support in the critically ill infant, an iatrogenic syndrome, 'parenteral nutrition-associated cholestasis' (PN-AC), has been seen with a disturbing frequency[1]. The hallmark of PN-AC is a diminished capacity for the biliary secretion of organic anions (bile pigments and bile acids in particular), accompanied by a decrease in canalicular bile flow. In the early stages of PN-AC these defects result from functional changes in hepatocytes. In a rabbit model of early PN-AC developed in our laboratory, total parenteral nutrition (TPN) over 5 days produced a significant reduction of basal bile flow and bile acid secretion rate. Compartmental analysis of the hepatic transport kinetics of the exogenous organic anion, sulphobromphthalein (BSP), showed the fractional transfer rates for hepatic uptake and biliary secretion of the dye to be significantly depressed, with canalicular secretion being the rate-limiting step[2]. We also concluded that this is a reproducible animal model for the hepatobiliary dysfunction associated with TPN in infants.

In this study we examined the efficacy of ursodeoxycholic acid (UDCA) in the prevention or alleviation of the hepatobiliary dysfunction (PN-AC) induced by intravenous feeding in the young rabbit.

That UDCA can be of therapeutic advantage in cholestatic disease has gained credence since the report of the amelioration of symptoms with marked improvements in liver function in adults in the early stages of primary biliary cirrhosis[3]. Whereas the elevated levels of total serum bile acids did not change, the UDCA content as a percentage of total bile acids increased from 0 to 58 after 2 years of treatment, protecting the hepatocyte from the toxic effects of endogenous bile acids.

MATERIALS AND METHODS

Female, prepubescent NZW rabbits (1.8–2.5 kg body weight) were housed in individual cages with grid floors, under controlled conditions of 12 h light/dark cycles and room temperature of 21–22°C.

The control animals (LCF) consumed standard laboratory rabbit chow *ad lib*. The experimental groups were nourished by total intravenous feeding via a jugular vein for 5 days: one subset was maintained on TPN alone (PN5-O), and a second subset had concurrent jejunal infusions of UDCA (200 μmol/kg over 8 h daily), during the 5 days of TPN (PN5-U). The UDCA solution was delivered by a Silastic tube placed in the duodenum surgically. The venous and jejunal lines were tunnelled under the skin to the back of the neck and attached to a swivel-infusion assembly[2]. This afforded full mobility to the rabbit within its cage. All animals were allowed water *ad lib*.

The TPN solution provided amino acids (protein) 3.6 g, dextrose 14.4 g and lipids (soybean/egg phospholipid emulsion) 4 g per kg per day, and the daily requirements of electrolytes, trace elements and vitamins. It provided 110 kcal/kg per day.

The UDCA was dissolved in 0.1 mol/l Na_2CO_3 and 0.15 mol/l NaCl (1 : 1 v/v), with pH adjusted to 8.4[4]. All solutions were delivered by metered pumps.

The morning after termination of the diet regimen, at laparotomy under ketamine–xylazine anaesthesia and mechanical ventilation, the cystic duct was clipped off. The common bile duct was cannulated for timed ($\times$ 10 min) collections of hepatic bile for the measurements of bile flow and the biliary secretion of bile acids, cholesterol and BSP. Gallbladder bile was aspirated for the determination of bile volume and composition. Core temperature was maintained at 38.5–39.5°C.

An initial baseline period of 40 min (4 $\times$ 10 min) allowed stabilization of bile flow. Basal bile flow was calculated as the average of the third and fourth aliquots.

After a bolus injection of BSP (5 mg/kg i.v.), plasma clearance and biliary secretion of the dye were determined over the following 60 min (6 $\times$ 10 min periods). Computer-assisted compartmental analysis of the biexponential plasma BSP-decay curve (assuming two pools, for plasma and liver, with an open-ended biliary run-off) yielded the 'plasma-to-liver' and 'liver-to-bile' fractional transfer rates[5]. The volume of dye distribution (plasma volume), the plasma clearance coefficient (K_e) for BSP, the liver uptake maximum (LU_{max}) and the time to reach LU_{max} (T_{ss}) were also calculated[6].

Total bile acids and cholesterol were measured in bile and plasma by standard enzymatic techniques[2], and the bile acid profiles in bile by HPLC[7]. BSP, in plasma and bile, was determined colorimetrically after alkalinization[8].

The results were expressed as means and SD. The significance of difference values between multi-group means were tested by one-way ANOVA and the Bonferroni method[9].

RESULTS

All the animals on intravenous feeding tolerated the TPN regimen. The incidence of hepatobiliary dysfunction with TPN alone, and its reversal with

Table 1 Hepatobiliary dysfunction during TPN: its prevention with UDCA. Mean (SD)

	Basal bile flow (μl/kg per min)	Basal biliary bile acid secretion (μmol/kg per min)	Serum total bile acids (μmol/l)	Serum total cholesterol (mmol/l)
LCF ($n = 6$)	65.6 (14.9)	0.832 (0.033)	7.04 (1.43)	1.37 (0.12)
PN5-O ($n = 6$)	27.2 (8.7)	0.456 (0.205)	7.20 (2.60)	5.06 (0.57)
PN5-U ($n = 6$)	78.4 (20.5)	1.477 (0.395)	9.40 (3.60)	3.57[a] (0.81)
ANOVA; p	= 0.0001	< 0.0001	n.s.	< 0.0001
LCF:PNF-O	< 0.01	= 0.03		< 0.001
LCF:PN5-U	n.s.	< 0.01		< 0.001
PN5-O:PN5-U	< 0.001	< 0.001		< 0.01

LCF = Labchow-fed; PNF-O = on TPN only × 5 days; PN5-U = on TPN × 5 days with concurrent UDCA daily. [a]The decrease in serum cholesterol with UDCA therapy is particularly significant because during TPN with intralipid it tends to increase, as seen in the PN5-O group.

Table 2 Plasma clearance of BSP during TPN without and with UDCA. Mean (SD)

	Plasma volume (ml/kg)	Steady-state plasma–BSP clearance (ml/kg per min)	T_{ss}[a] (min)	LU_{max}[b] (fraction of dose)
LCF ($n = 6$)	39.0 (7.8)	7.5 (2.6)	9.3 (2.0)	0.70 (0.11)
PN5-O ($n = 6$)	45.2 (5.1)	4.5 (1.3)	15.5 (3.8)	0.67 (0.08)
PN5-U ($n = 6$)	49.2 (9.3)	8.7 (0.8)	8.2 (1.4)	0.68 (0.06)
ANOVA p	= 0.0966	= 0.0024	= 0.0004	n.s.
LCF:PN5		< 0.05	< 0.01	
LCF:PN5-U	n.s.	n.s.		
PN5-O:PN5-U		< 0.01	< 0.01	

[a]T_{ss} = time to reach maximum uptake of BSP by liver. [b]LU_{max} = highest fraction of dose in liver, at T_{ss}. LU_{max} remained unchanged, implying no damage to hepatocytes. The changes in plasma volume with TPN were not statistically significant ($p = 0.0966$).

a concurrent infusion of UDCA, are shown in Table 1. Bile flow and basal biliary bile acid secretion rates decreased, and serum cholesterol concentrations increased with TPN alone. When UDCA was added to the TPN regimen, serum cholesterol levels decreased, while the other three variables (bile flow, biliary bile acids, and serum bile acids) showed UDCA-induced increases.

Plasma disappearance of BSP was slow in the PN5-O group. Steady-state plasma-BSP clearance, plasma clearance coefficient for BSP and the plasma → liver and liver → bile transfer rates were low in PN5-O while the time to reach maximum uptake of BSP was prolonged in comparison to the labchow-fed animals; all these variables were normalized when UDCA was given concurrently with the TPN (Table 2, Figs 1 and 2).

The cumulative secretion of BSP over the 60 min following the i.v. bolus of dye was 48 (SD 8)% of the injected dose in PN5-O, and significantly different from the 75 (SD 7)% seen in LCF. In contrast to LCF, where most of the dye secretion occurred in the first $\frac{1}{2}$ h, in PN5-O most of the dye was

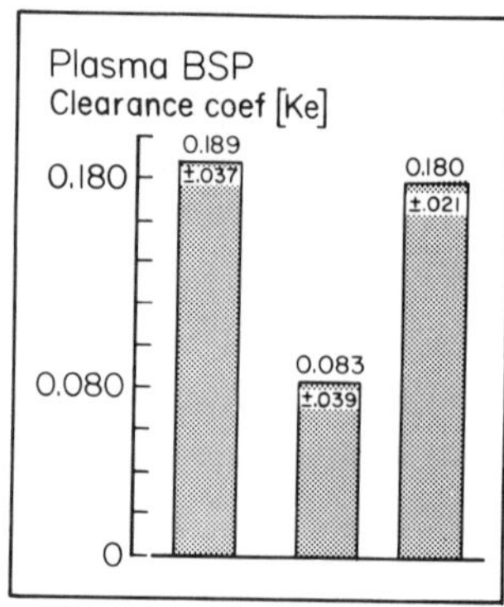

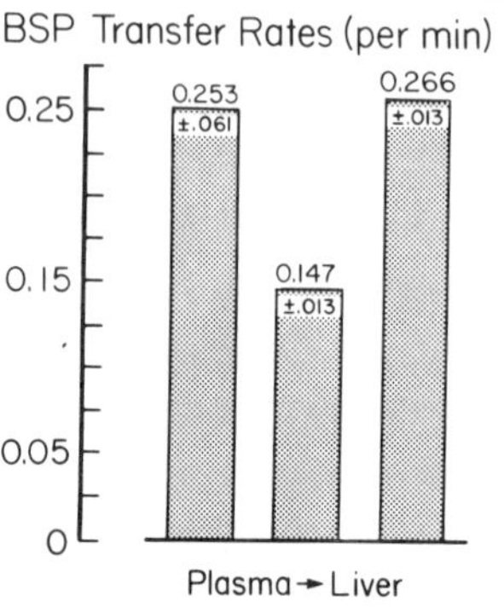

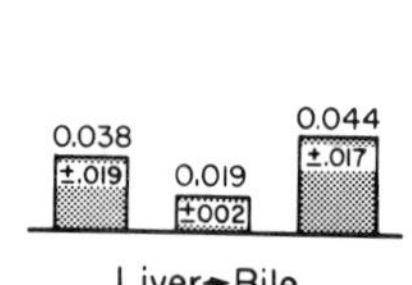

Fig. 1 Plasma BSP clearance coefficient and transfer rates. Hepatic uptake and canalicular secretion of BSP diminished after 5 days of TPN alone. When UDCA was given jejunally along with the TPN, both these variables remained normal. The changes in hepatic uptake reflected the changes in plasma clearance of dye. In each bar chart the left column is LCF, the middle column PN5-O and the right column PN5-U

secreted in the second $\frac{1}{2}$ h (Fig. 3). In the PNF5-U group, both the percentage and the pattern of dye secretion were similar to those in LCF.

The percentage of glyco-conjugated UDCA in hepatic and gallbladder biles increased markedly, with a reciprocal decrease disease in glyco-DCA, the dominant bile acid in the rabbit (Tables 3 and 4). The volume of bile sequestered in the gallbladder was increased in the TPN groups, especially in the PN5-U animals.

DISCUSSION

In the young rabbit, basal bile flow and bile acid secretion rates were significantly reduced over the 5 days of TPN. The fractional rates for hepatic uptake and canalicular secretion of BSP were depressed. UDCA increased the basal bile acid secretion rate, and normalized the plasma clearance of BSP and the biliary secretion of the dye to the control values seen in labchow-fed rabbits (Fig. 2). Compartmental analysis further showed that with UDCA administration during the 5 days of TPN, the biliary organic anion-transport kinetics equalled that in the LCF group.

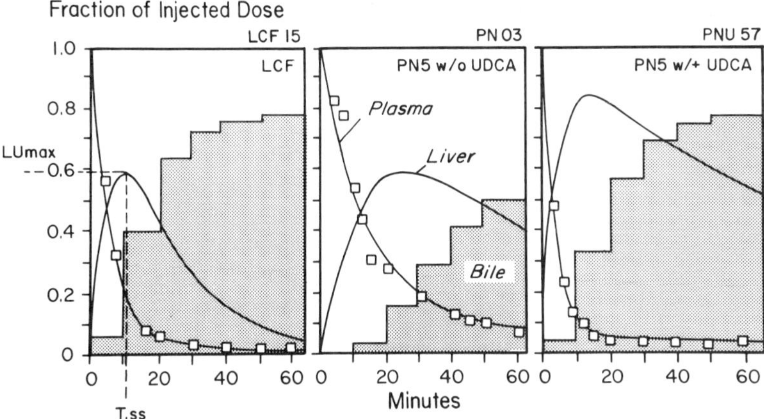

Fig. 2 Computer-generated curves for fraction of BSP dose in the plasma and liver compartments, and the cumulative secretion of BSP in bile, following injection of dye at $t = 0$. Data are shown for one animal from each of the three groups studied

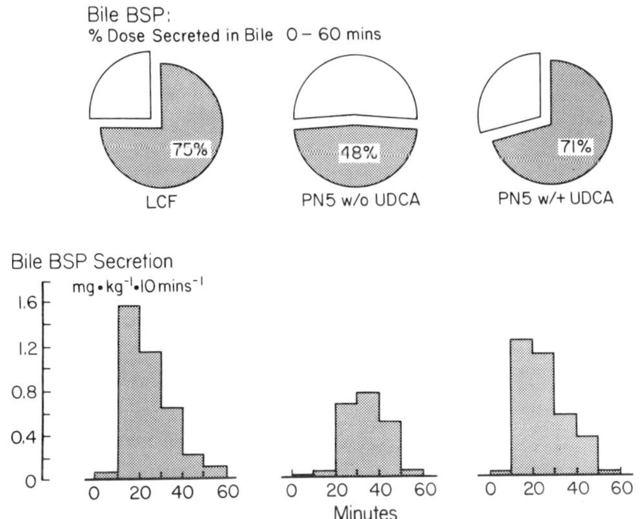

Fig. 3 BSP secretion in bile following a bolus injection of 5 mg/kg i.v. Percentage of dose secreted in the first hour (upper panel); pattern of bile-BSP secretion (lower panel)

Organic anion secretion is enhanced by bile acids through an effect on the BSP transport system[10]. It has been postulated that UDCA, in contrast to taurocholate, may be transported into and out of the hepatocyte along the bilirubin–BSP transport system[11]. An interaction of UDCA with the BSP carrier can account for the enhanced biliary secretion of BSP ('facilitated transport') when the transhepatic flux of the bile acid was augmented by the jejunal perfusion of UDCA.

Table 3 Substitution of glyco-DCA by glyco-UDCA in hepatic bile. Mean (SD)

	Total conjugated bile acids (TCBA) (mmol/l)	Glyco-DCA		Glyco-UDCA	
		mmol/l	Percentage of TCBA	mmol/l	Percentage of TCBA
LCF ($n = 6$)	5.53 (1.73)	4.56 (1.85)	80 (12)	0.31 (0.25)	3 (1)
PN5-O ($n = 6$)	6.33 (2.56)	4.58 (1.96)	72 (7)	0.75 (0.63)	4 (3)
PN5-U ($n = 6$)	7.02 (2.06)	1.77 (0.36)	25 (3)	4.68 (1.66)	66 (4)

As glyco-DCA decreased with the UDCA therapy, glyco-UDCA increased reciprocally.

Table 4 Substitution of glyco-DCA by glyco-UDCA in gallbladder bile. Mean (SD)

	Gallbladder volume (ml)	Total conjugated bile acids (TCBA) (mmol/l)	Glyco-DCA as percentage of TCBA	Glyco-UDCA as percentage of TCBA	GB-TBA[a] (μmol/kg)
LCF ($n = 6$)	0.493 (0.126)	203 (42)	80 (3)	< 1	34 (9)
PN5-O ($n = 6$)	0.895 (0.491)	406 (100)	84 (5)	< 1	101(36)
PN5-U ($n = 6$)	1.323 (0.433)	313 (73)	50 (11)	39 (6)	261(86)

[a]GB-TBA = total bile acids sequestered in gallbladder, expressed as μmol/kg body weight.

UDCA maximized the basal biliary secretion of bile acids, and accounted for 66% of the total conjugated bile acids secreted in the resting state (Table 3). The dilution of the endogenous bile acid pool of glyco-DCA by glyco-UDCA protected the hepatocytes against the putative, toxic effects of the TPN infusate. The increase in biliary bile acid secretion with UDCA maintained the dynamics of the enterohepatic circulation, which is impaired during the enteral fast of TPN. Bile flow was normalized by the unique choleretic potential of UDCA to increase both the bile acid-induced and the electrolyte (bicarbonate)-stimulated components of bile secretion[12,13] by cholehepatic cycling[14]. Prior alkalinization of the UDCA solution (to pH 8.4) increased the bioavailability of the duodenally administered bile acid.

Another observation in the TPN animals, with and without concurrent UDCA, was the increase in gallbladder volume with an associated sequestration of bile acids (Table 4). The increase in the amount of bile acids sequestered was due to an increase in gallbladder bile volume, and not due to any significant increase in total bile acid concentration. In the PN5-O group, suppression of the release of endogenous cholecystokinin (CCK), mediated by the enteral fast, could have caused the 'atony' of the gallbladder, a condition seen during TPN in humans[15]. It was surprising, however, to observe further increases in the volume of the gallbladder bile with bile acid sequestration in the PN5-U group, where the enterohepatic circulation had been re-established. In humans and dogs an increase in the duodenal content of bile acids interferes with the release of gut hormones including CCK, and decreases gallbladder motility[16]. Similarly, during the treatment of gallstones with UDCA, increased gallbladder fasting volumes and delayed gallbladder emptying have been reported[17]. Therefore, although the enrichment of the UDCA pool improves the choleretic potential of the hepatocyte, UDCA may down-regulate gallbladder motility at the same time.

In conclusion, UDCA prevented the depression in the hepatic transport of the cholephilic dye, BSP, induced by TPN, and maintained normal bile flow. By inference, UDCA should improve the biliary secretion of the related, endogenous organic anion, bilirubin, the plasma accumulation of which results in cholestatic jaundice during TPN. As gallbladder dyskinesia appears to be a side-effect of UDCA therapy, however, CCK or one of its analogues should form a therapeutic adjunct to ursodeoxycholic acid in the treatment of cholestasis.

Acknowledgements

This work was supported by the Children's Surgical Foundation Inc, Chicago, IL. We thank Santibrata Ghosh, PhD, of the Department of Cell, Molecular and Structural Biology, Northwestern University Medical School, Chicago, for the computer analysis of the plasma BSP clearance data.

References

1. Bell RL, Ferry GD, Smith EO, Shulman RJ, Christensen BL, Labarthe DR, Wills CA. Total parenteral nutrition-related cholestasis in infants. J Parent Ent Nutr. 1986;10:356–9.
2. Das JB, Ghosh S, Cosentino CM, Ansari GG. Hepatic organic anion transport kinetics and bile flow during short-term total parenteral nutrition in the rabbit. Proc Soc Exp Biol Med. 1990;195:274–8.
3. Poupon R, Chretien Y, Poupon RE, Ballet F, Calmus Y, Darnis F. Is ursodeoxycholic acid an effective treatment for primary biliary cirrhosis? Lancet. 1987;1:834–6.
4. Gurantz D, Hofmann AF. Influence of bile acid structure on bile flow and biliary lipid secretion in the hamster. Gastroenterology. 1984,247:G736–48.
5. Barber-Riley G, Goetzee AE, Richards TG, Thomson JY. The transfer of bromsulphthalein from the plasma to the bile in man. Clin Sci. 1961;20:149–59.
6. Clarkson MJ, Richards TG. Steady-state plasma clearance of bromsulphthalein and indocyanine green measured by single injection. Res Vet Sci. 1967;8:454–62.
7. Rossi SS, Converse JL, Hofmann AF. High pressure liquid chromatographic analysis of conjugated bile acids in human bile: simultaneous resolution of sulfated and unsulfated lithocholyl amidates and the common conjugated bile acids. J Lipid Res. 1987;28:589–95.
8. Gaebler OH. Determination of bromsulphthalein in normal, turbid, hemolyzed or icteric serums. Am J Clin Pathol. 1945;15:452–5.
9. Godfrey K. Comparing the means of several groups. N Engl J Med. 1985;313:1450–6.
10. Binet S, Delage Y, Erlinger S. Influence of taurocholate, taurochenodeoxycholate, and taurodehydrocholate on sulfobromophthalein transport into bile. Am J Physiol. 1979;236:E10–14.
11. Berk PD, Isola LM, Jones EA. Specific defects in hepatic storage and clearance of bilirubin. In: Ostrow JD, editor. Bile pigments and jaundice: molecular, metabolic and medical aspects. New York: Marcel Dekker, 1986:279–316.
12. Dumont M, Erlinger S, Uchman S. Hypercholeresis induced by ursodeoxycholic acid and 7-ketolithocholic acid in the rat: possible role of bicarbonate transport. Gastroenterology. 1980;79:82–9.
13. Renner EL, Lake JR, Cragoe EJ Jr, van Dyke RW, Scharschmidt BF. Ursodeoxycholic acid choleresis: relationship to biliary HCO3 and effects of Na+/H+ exchange inhibitors. Am J Physiol. 1988;254:G232–41.
14. Yoon YB, Hagey LR, Hofmann AF, Gurantz D, Michelotti FL, Steinbach JH. Effect of side-chain shortening on the physiologic properties of bile acids: hepatic transport and

effect on biliary secretion of 23-Nor-ursodeoxycholate in rodents. Gastroenterology. 1986;90:837–52.

15. Messing B, Bories C, Kunstlinger F, Bernier J-J. Does total parenteral nutrition induce gallbladder sludge formation and lithiasis? Gastroenterology. 1983;84:1012–19.

16. Gomez G, Upp JR, Lluis F, Alexander RW, Poston GJ, Greeley GH, Thompson J. Regulation of the release of cholecystokinin by bile salts in dogs and humans. Gastroenterology. 1988;94:1036–46.

17. Festi D, Frabboni R, Bazzoli F, Sangermano A, Ronchi M, Rossi L, Parini P, Orsini M, Primerano AMM, Mazzella G, Aldini R, Roda E. Gallbladder motility in cholesterol gallstone disease. Gastroenterology. 1990;99:1779–85.

Index